STRABISMUS AND PEDIATRIC OPHTHALMOLOGY

STRABISMUS AND PEDIATRIC OPHTHALMOLOGY

GARY R. DIAMOND, MD, FACS
Associate Professor of Ophthalmology and Pediatrics
Hahnemann University
Philadelphia, PA

HOWARD M. EGGERS, MD
Associate Professor of Clinical Ophthalmology
Columbia University
New York, NY

VOLUME

5

TEXTBOOK OF OPHTHALMOLOGY
EDITED BY

STEVEN M. PODOS, MD, FACS
Professor and Chairman
Department of Ophthalmology
Mt. Sinai School of Medicine
New York, NY

MYRON YANOFF, MD, FACS
Professor and Chairman
Department of Ophthalmology
Hahnemann University
Philadelphia, PA

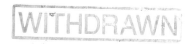 MOSBY

London St. Louis Baltimore Boston Chicago Philadelphia Sydney Toronto

IV

For full details of all Mosby-Year Book Europe, Limited titles please write to:
Mosby-Year Book Europe, Limited, Brook House, 2-16 Torrington Place, London WC1E7LT, England.

LIBRARY OF CONGRESS CATALOGING-IN-PUBLICATION DATA
(Revised for vol. 5)

Textbook of ophthalmology.

    Includes bibliographical references and indexes.
    Contents: v. 1. Optics and refraction / David Miller
—v. 5. Strabismus and pediatric ophthalmology /
[edited by] Gary R. Diamond, Howard M. Eggers.
    1. Ophthalmology. 2. Ophthalmology. I. Podos, Steven M. II. Yanoff, Myron
[DNLM: 1. Ophthalmology WW 100 T355]
RE46.T26   1991   617.7   91-34425
ISBN 1-56375-011-2 (v.1)
ISBN 1-56375-097-X (v.5)

BRITISH LIBRARY CATALOGUING-IN-PUBLICATION DATA
A catalogue record for this book is available from the British Library.

ISBN Volume 5: 1-56375-097-X
ISBN Set: 0-397-44692-6

Project Manager: DIMITRY POPOW
Editor: SHARON RULE
Art Director and Cover Design: KATHRYN GREENSLADE
Interior Design and Layout: NANCY BERLINER, JEFFREY S. BROWN
Illustration Director: CAROL KALAFATIC
Illustrator: WENDY JACKELOW

Originated in Hong Kong by Bright Arts
Printed and bound in Singapore
Produced by Imago Productions, Pte., Ltd.

EDITORS' PREFACE

As we approach the twenty-first century it is apparent that the half-life of medical knowledge is continuing to shrink and the amount of current dogma is continuing to expand. Packaging today's relevant ophthalmic knowledge is a difficult chore, yet one that periodically demands doing. Every editor or author desires to accomplish this task in a new and unique fashion. This ten-volume series represents our vision of a *Textbook of Ophthalmology* for the 1990s: one that integrates the basic visual science and clinical information of each subspecialty in a separate volume that is edited or written by noted basic scientists and clinicians; one that is manageable, readable, and affordable for the ophthalmic expert as well as the neophyte; and one that contains original diagrams, figures, and photographs—all in full color—designed to depict the necessary knowledge we hope to impart.

We are grateful to our associate editors and authors for sharing their superb expertise in the compilation of this unique ophthalmic resourse, to our assistants Barbara Zoldessy and Roe Brennan for their unstinting efforts in organizing and coordinating this project, and to our wives Wendy Donn Podos and Karin L. Yanoff for their continued patience and encouragement throughout the many phases of this endeavor.

STEVEN M. PODOS, MD, FACS
DEPARTMENT OF
OPHTHALMOLOGY
MT. SINAI SCHOOL OF MEDICINE
NEW YORK, NY

MYRON YANOFF, MD, FACS
DEPARTMENT OF
OPHTHALMOLOGY
HAHNEMANN UNIVERSITY
PHILADELPHIA, PA

AUTHORS' PREFACE

GARY R. DIAMOND, MD, FACS

ASSOCIATE PROFESSOR
OF OPHTHALMOLOGY
AND PEDIATRICS
HAHNEMANN UNIVERSITY
PHILADELPHIA, PA

HOWARD M. EGGERS, MD

ASSOCIATE PROFESSOR
OF CLINICAL OPHTHALMOLOGY
COLUMBIA UNIVERSITY
NEW YORK, NY

This volume represents a labor of love and the realization of a privilege given to very few: the recording of their experiences and opinions for others to consider. *Strabismus and Pediatric Ophthalmology* is not intended to be encyclopedic. Instead, the authors hope to have created an up-to-date book that will be welcomed by the initiate and experienced ophthalmologist alike. The topic choices are somewhat arbitrary, but topics not found in this volume do appear elsewhere in the *Textbook of Ophthalmology* series.

The authors are grateful for Dr. Robert W. Lingua's gracious willingness to permit our use of his excellent text and photographs of representative strabismus surgical procedures. Equally grateful are they to Drs. James J. Augsburger and Myron Yanoff for their excellent chapters on retinoblastoma.

Dr. Diamond would like to thank the teachers who had the most impact on his professional life: Dr. Irene Maumenee, who lives her dictum that every child counts; Dr. Marshall Parks, who helped it all make sense to him and generations of ophthalmologists; and Dr. A. Edward Maumenee, last of the Renaissance ophthalmologists, for whom no corner of the specialty is left unexplored or unenlightened. Appreciation is due to his colleagues in the Department of Ophthalmology, Hahnemann University, for the time and resources they invested to complete this work. Finally, he would like to thank his wife, Sherry, and his children, Jennie Beth and Scott, for understanding his unavailability for much of the past nine months.

Dr. Eggers would like to recall the teachers who influenced him towards research: Dr. Sara Luse, who demonstrated the demands one can place on oneself; and Dr. Harry Grundfest, who demonstrated the rigor one needs to reach complete understanding. Special thanks are due to Dr. Philip Knapp, for making strabismus attractive by showing that there is an underlying rationality in its motor and sensory aspects.

CONTRIBUTORS

James J. Augsburger, MD
Associate Clinical Professor of Ophthalmology
Wills Eye Hospital
Thomas Jefferson University
Philadelphia, Pennsylvania

Robert W. Lingua, MD
Associate Clinical Professor of Ophthalmology
Loma Linda University
Loma Linda, California
Pediatric Ophthalmology Consultants, Inc.
Santa Ana, California

Myron Yanoff, MD, FACS
Professor and Chairman
Department of Ophthalmology
Hahnemann University
Philadelphia, Pennsylvania

CONTENTS

1 | OCULAR EMBRYOLOGY

Gary R. Diamond

Ocular embryology can be divided into four periods of development: pre-embryonic, encompassing the first 3 weeks after fertilization; embryonic, from 4 to 8 weeks; fetal, from 9 weeks until birth; and postnatal, from birth until 4 to 6 months of life, during which time final structural differentiation occurs.

During the first 3 weeks after fertilization, mitotic activity and cell differentiation form an embryonic plate, yolk sac, and amniotic cavity, all resting on a bed of endoderm. The growing plate develops a primitive streak encompassed laterally by ectoderm, which thickens to form the neural plate. The neuroectoderm lying anterior to the primitive streak forms the brain and the eyes in response to appropriate biochemical and mechanical stimulation by underlying mesoderm ("induction"). Folds develop in the lateral neural plate, grow over the plate, and fuse during the third week, thus leaving surface ectoderm externally, neural ectoderm within, and neural crest cells at the summit of the fold (Fig. 1.1). As

1.1 | Day 25. As the neural tube closes superiorly, neural crest cells begin migrating into the optic pits or vesicles. The central space is the developing neural tube.

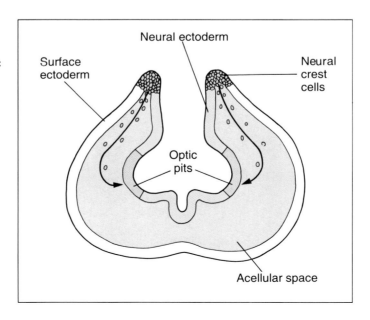

the neural tube closes superiorly, optic vesicles develop in the cephalic portions (25 days after fertilization), and neural crest cells begin migration into the optic vesicles, losing continuity with surface cells.

The optic vesicles are cylindrical outpouchings containing a single layer of neuroectoderm in the anterior aspects of the neural folds. As the neural tube closes, the vesicles move laterally.[1] Expansion does not occur in the stalk connecting these vesicles to the developing neural tube. Further invagination of the optic vesicle during the fifth week forms the optic cup. Neuroectodermal tissue induces a focal thickening of the overlying cells of the surface ectoderm, the lens placode (26 to 28 days). The lens placode moves inward but remains attached to surface ectoderm as the lens vesicle (fifth week)[2] (Fig. 1.2) .

The outer layer of the optic cup (neuroectoderm) will form the retinal pigment epithelium and the inner layer the neurosensory retina. An inferior fissure in the developing optic cup permits the hyaloid vascular system to be enveloped by the globe. Fusion of the lips of the fissure begins at the equator of the primitive globe and proceeds anteriorly and posteriorly. Incomplete closure leads to coloboma of the disc, choroid, ciliary body, or iris, depending on the location (Fig. 1.3).

Neural crest cells contribute most connective tissue components of the eye and orbit, including sclera, uveal melanocytes, ciliary body muscle, iris stroma, corneal endothelium and stroma, optic nerve sheath, orbital fat, extraocular muscle sheaths, and the Tenon capsule.[3] Exceptions are neuroectodermal components (neurosensory retina, retinal pigment epithelium, iris pigment epithelium), surface ectodermal components (corneal epithelium, lens, lacrimal gland and drainage system, glands of the conjunctiva and lids), and mesodermal components (extraocular striated muscle fibers, endothelial vascular cells).

1.2 | Days 26–28. Neuroectodermal tissue induces the lens placode from surface ectoderm.

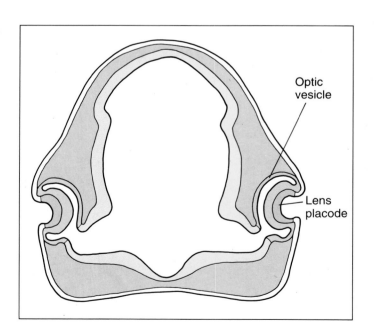

Optic vesicle

Lens placode

First appearing as a placode of surface ectoderm on the optic vesicle (at 26 to 28 weeks), the epithelial cells contained within a basement membrane elongate and grow inward. In the sixth week the lens vesicle, consisting of a single layer of cells covered by capsule, separates from the surface ectoderm. By the seventh week, the cells lengthen to fill the cavity of the vesicle and are termed primary lens fibers. The outer cells migrate to the equator, where they produce the secondary lens fibers. These dissect between the lens capsule and primary lens fibers and meet in the upright anterior Y suture and the inverted posterior Y suture by the ninth week. The lens contained within these sutures is the embryonic nucleus.[4]

As secondary fibers are added, the Y sutures become more complex and the lens more ellipsoid. In the third month, the nuclei of the deep lens cells are lost. Growth and maturation of lens fibers continues throughout life.

LENS

After lens induction and descent into the optic vesicle, the overlying corneal anlage remains as a layer of epithelial cells and their basement membrane. Neural crest cells migrate beneath the epithelium (sixth week) and form the endothelium. Further waves of neural crest cells separate these two layers to form stroma.[5] The original acellular fibrillar layer remains as the Bowman layer; Descemet's membrane develops as the basement membrane of the endothelium during the sixth month.

Neural crest cells condensing posteriorly form sclera (seventh week), lamina cribrosa (fifth month) and extraocular muscle capsules near the equator of the globe. By the end of the first year of postnatal life, uveal pigment appears in the scleral canals.

CORNEA AND SCLERA

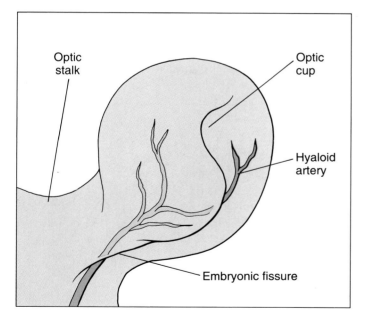

1.3 | The embryonic fissure permits the hyaloid vascular system to be incorporated into the globe.

Optic stalk

Optic cup

Hyaloid artery

Embryonic fissure

NEUROSENSORY RETINA

The retina initially consists of two zones, primitive and marginal, both arising from the invaginated layer of neuroepithelial cells in the fifth week. The primitive layer lies near the cavity of the optic vesicle and consists of tightly packed nuclei eight to ten layers deep, separated from the vitreous cavity by a fibrillar marginal layer. In the deeper primitive layer, nuclei migrate towards the central cavity of the globe and develop two neuroblastic layers, reaching the future region of the ora serrata by the twelfth week.[6] These two layers are separated by a transient fibrillar nerve fiber layer (Chievitz) that disappears by the tenth week except in the fovea where it persists until birth (Fig. 1.4).[7] Immature bipolar cells from the inner neuroblastic layer migrate centrally; thus three nuclear layers and intervening nerve fiber layers exist by the twelfth week. The outer neuroblastic layer forms the photoreceptors and the cilia that develop on their outer portion. Cones begin differentiation in the third month and rods in the seventh. By the sixth week, ganglion cell processes begin to grow toward the optic nerve.

The development of the macular retina begins in the fifth month, displacing peripheral ganglion cells; by the time of birth, only the outer plexiform layer and a few nuclear cells overlie the macular photoreceptors. By the fourth postnatal month, the layer of Chievitz is gone from the foveal pit and the retinal internal limiting membrane is apposed to the axons (outer plexiform layer) of the macular photoreceptors.

VASCULAR SYSTEM

The hyaloid artery, a branch of the primitive dorsal ophthalmic artery, arises at the junction of the optic stalk and cup at the time of closure of the embryonic fissure. It forms the anterior annular vascular system and several branches surrounding the lens (tunica vasculosa lentis)[8] (Fig. 1.5). The primitive dorsal ophthalmic artery becomes the ophthalmic artery during the sixth week, providing the short posterior ciliary arteries, central retinal artery, and temporal long posterior ciliary artery; the primitive ventral ophthalmic artery survives only as the nasal long posterior artery. The major anterior circle of the iris develops near the annular artery, sending branches

1.4 | The transient nerve fiber layer of Chievitz lies within the two neuroblastic layers of the primitive retinal layer.

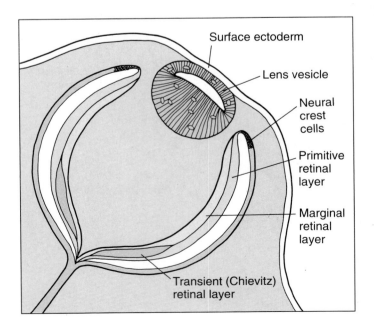

Surface ectoderm

Lens vesicle

Neural crest cells

Primitive retinal layer

Marginal retinal layer

Transient (Chievitz) retinal layer

to form the pupillary membrane of radial vascular loops on the iris and lens surface; these vessels disappear centrally, but persist peripherally as the minor vascular iris circle.

The disc vascular channels penetrate into inner retina by the fourth month and form the retinal arterial system; growth and remodeling continue into the ninth month. Nasal retinal vasculature is completed by the beginning of the 36th week as the optic nerve is closer to the nasal ora serrata; temporal vasculature is not complete until 42 to 46 weeks of gestational age.[9] By the seventh month the hyaloid vascular system and tunica vasculosa lentis begin to atrophy. In the absence of intraocular inflammation, the degree of persistence of the tunica is an indication of fetal age.

By the sixth week, the cavity of the optic cup is filled with primitive mesenchyme and hyaloid vessels. The primary vitreous fibrils have been attributed to lenticular (surface ectodermal) and retinal (neuroectodermal) origin, but probably contain a few cells of both neural crest and mesodermal origin. Secondary vitreous is added by the second and third month, consisting of a paucicellular, avascular fibrillar gel arising from vascular adventitial fibroblasts, hyalocytes, and occasional monocytes.[10]

By the fifth month, ciliary body nonpigmented epithelium produces collagen at the optic cup rim which grows centrad to join the lens as zonular fibers (tertiary vitreous).[11] At this time, the primary vitreous is compressed by a growing secondary vitreous into a small central zone (Cloquet's canal); therefore, in the term eye most of the vitreous body is secondary vitreous.

VITREOUS BODY

1.5 | The hyaloid artery provides branches to the vitreous cavity and the lens (tunica vasculosa lentis).

RETINAL PIGMENT EPITHELIUM

The outer layer of neuroectoderm (the future retinal pigment epithelium) develops melanin by the sixth week of gestation, the first cells in the body to do so.[12] The basement membrane of the retinal pigment epithelium becomes the inner portion of Bruch's membrane; the outer basement membrane portion of Bruch's membrane is formed by the endothelium of the choriocapillaris.[13] The retinal pigment epithelium induces normal development of the choroid, sclera, and neurosensory retina (absence of pigment epithelium in colobomas is the most important factor in defining the extent of defects in the above structures).

OPTIC NERVE

By the sixth week 6, ganglion cell axons have reached the optic nerve, and one week later they reach the chiasm. Glial cells develop from disc surface neuroectoderm and extend back into the nerve and forward into the vitreous to form a scaffold for the hyaloid arterial system. By the sixth month, disc glial development is at its most prominent and begins to recede; persistent glial disc remnants are termed the Bergmeister papilla. Neural crest cells form the optic nerve sheath beginning in the seventh week. Medullation begins at the chiasm in the seventh month and is complete to the lamina cribrosa by one month after term.[14]If medullation continues into the retinal nerve fiber layer, such persistent medullation will be noted as a white retinal lesion with feathered edges, which causes visual field defects by shielding light from the underlying photoreceptors.

FILTRATION ANGLE STRUCTURES

At about the seventh week a capillary layer forms between cornea and lens.[15] Shortly before, neural crest cells begin to differentiate into trabecular meshwork, the Schlemm's canal, anterior chamber angle, iris stroma, ciliary body stroma, and ciliary musculature. The sphincter differentiates from the tip of the optic cup neuroectoderm in the fourth month. The iris pigment epithelium develops pigment granules in the tenth week. Iris stromal melanocytes begin pigment formation just before birth and continue for several months thereafter.

LIDS

Neural crest cells from the frontonasal and maxillary processes form folds over the globe in the seventh week, fusing in the eighth week. Separation begins in the fifth month at the same time that the sebaceous glands of the lids begin mucus formation.[16]

2 | EVALUATING VISION IN PREVERBAL AND PRELITERATE INFANTS AND CHILDREN

Gary R. Diamond

HISTORICAL AND OBSERVATIONAL TECHNIQUES

Much can be learned from historical descriptions of a young child's visual behavior towards family members and at playtime. Parents or caretakers should be asked if the child responds to a silent smile, enjoys silent mobiles, and follows objects around the environment. Pertinent observations include strabismus, nystagmus, persistent staring, and inattention to objects. A younger sibling's visual behavior can be compared with that of an older child.

The pupillary light response is not equivalent to visual ability, but its presence indicates intact afferent visual neurological pathways to the level of the brachium of the superior colliculus, and efferent pathways to the iris sphincter. This reflex is present in premature infants over 29 to 31 weeks of gestational age.[1] Visualization sometimes requires a magnifying glass in very young children, as their pupils are smaller than those of older children (because of decreased sympathetic tone) and the light responses are of small amplitude. Dilatation to direct illumination has been described in Leber congenital amaurosis, optic nerve hypoplasia, congenital cone dystrophy, and congenital stationary night blindness.[2] Nystagmus is absent in cortical blindness[3] and often with unilateral visual defects.

The blink to a bright light is a reflex learned by 30 weeks of gestational age and is occasionally present in decorticate infants. The blink to a threatening gesture is another learned reflex, usually present by 5 months; care must be taken not to brush air against the child's corneas and elicit a blink by that mechanism.

FIXATION TARGETS

Visual fixation abilities can be demonstrated in term newborns if the appropriate target, such as a human face, is utilized. A flashlight is a poor target, as it has no edges; stripes, dots, checkerboards, or human faces are superior. Term infants under 3 months of age follow by means of hypometric saccades when the target is small; they can generate smooth pursuit movements to a large target, such as an opticokinetic drum. Because saccadic palsies are common in young children with central nervous system damage, spinning an upright child will demonstrate presence of saccades as the rapid recovery phase of the spin-induced nystagmus. If no rapid phase can be stimulated, the child's vision cannot be evaluated by its ability to "follow" a small target, as it has neither a saccadic nor a smooth pursuit system available. In addition, a child with normal fixational behavior should dampen spin-induced nystagmus in 3 to 5 seconds; a blind or poorly sighted child cannot use fixational dampening and will beat for 15 to 30 seconds until mechanical dampening occurs.

In somewhat older children, small, colorful, nonthreatening familiar toys generate the best, albeit often momentary, interest. Small coins and breakfast cereals have often been used to roughly quantitate visual acuity with success, but the rule remains: "One toy earns one look" (Fig. 2.1).

OPTICOKINETIC NYSTAGMUS

Evaluation of the presence or absence of opticokinetic nystagmus represented the first "technological" approach to acuity measurement in preverbal children; sinusoidal gratings placed on arcs were moved across an infant's visual field.[5] Standardized drums containing stripes that subtend small fractions of the infant's visual field are available but often do not hold interest, frequently are spun at varying and noncalibrated rates, and are bathed in varying illumination (Fig. 2.2). More disturbing is the realization that occasional decorticate infants can generate normal responses,[6] indicating that subcortical areas of the occipital cortex can generate opticokinetic responses. When determination is performed binocularly, term infants have approximately 20/400 acuity at birth and reach 20/20 by 26 to 30 months. This method measures acuity by means of a motor response technique (eye movement), and can underestimate the acuity in some children who have disturbed oculomotor systems. Whereas the horizontal saccadic system is present at term birth, the vertical saccadic system does not develop until 4 to 6 weeks later; therefore, vertical responses are not present until that time.

Because the testing drums are reasonably priced, portable, and rarely break, this technique remains a quick and easy method to evaluate infant acuity.

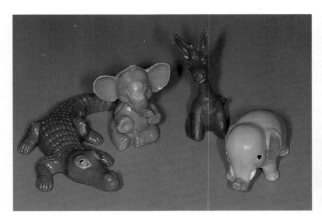

2.1 | A selection of colorful toys for attracting infant fixation.

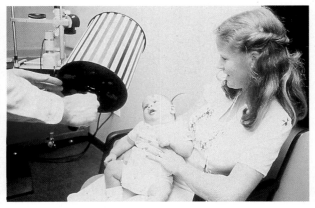

2.2 | Infant responding to OKN drum.

On the basis of the observation that visual stimuli yield a measurable electroencephalographic pattern received by occipital scalp electrodes, various methods, including bright-flash stimuli, square-wave gratings, and phase-alternating checkerboards, have been used to evaluate acuity. Only the two latter targets can be calibrated, and many investigators have found 20/200 acuity in term newborns.[7] Acuity of 20/20 can be demonstrated by 6 to 12 months, considerably earlier than the age indicated by opticokinetic nystagmus testing, perhaps reflecting the fact that this electrophysiological test evaluates acuity by direct recording of sensory afferents, the only test to do so.

Visual evoked potential testing has been used to evaluate acuity in aphakic,[8] amblyopic,[9] and strabismic children, and in those who have large refractive errors. Although the test directly evaluates vision by means of a sensory process, a normal-appearing waveform has been recorded occasionally in decorticate infants who later behaved as if blind, implying a subcortical contribution; the exact origin of the response remains unknown.[10] As the response waveform changes markedly between 1 and 6 months, care must be taken to compare waveforms with age-matched controls.

Difficulties with this test include reliance on expensive, delicate equipment and the subsequent need for technical assistance, and lack of standardization of equipment. Intense interest in this technique still continues, as do technological improvement and miniaturization (Figs. 2.3–2.5)

VISUAL EVOKED POTENTIALS

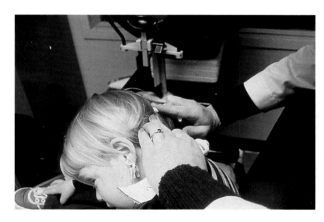

2.3 | Occipital electrodes being placed for evoked potential test.

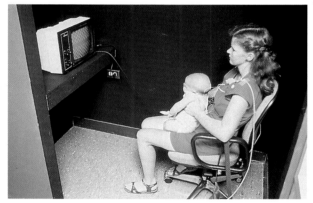

2.4 | Infant responding to checkerboard pattern for evoked potential test.

2.5 | Waveform of typical visual evoked potential. The amplitude of the major positive wave, and elapsed time from stimulus onset to this wave, are the most important features of the visual evoked potential.

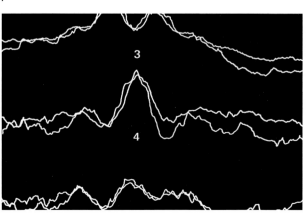

FORCED-CHOICE PREFERENTIAL LOOKING

This behavioral technique is based on the observation that infants prefer to view a pattern stimulus rather than a homogeneous field.[11] By creating flat, calibrated, sine-wave gratings, this tendency can be observed by a trained individual.[12] Similar to the opticokinetic nystagmus test results, a term newborn will differentially respond to 20/400 gratings and to 20/20 gratings at 18 to 24 months.[13] By unmasking the target presenter, a smaller and simpler apparatus was devised which is more suitable for clinical applications[14] (Figs. 2.6 and 2.7).

The child must be alert and able to generate neck and eye movements, disqualifying many whose hypotonia and inattention prevents this type of purposeful movement; this is a significant limitation in the evaluation of developmentally delayed infants. Thus, as with the opticokinetic nystagmus technique, vision is evaluated by means of a motor response. In addition, this test presents a resolution acuity task, not a recognition acuity task, and therefore may be less than ideal for the detection of amblyopia than the visual evoked response test. However, the testing cards are simple, portable, and cannot lose calibration; the testing of both eyes in a typical child often takes less than 20 minutes. Evidence exists of experiential effects, and because the cards can only be presented with the stripes in one orientation (vertical), some optically uncorrected astigmatic children may have erroneous estimates of acuity by this technique.

GRADED OPTOTYPES

Although rare children as young as 18 months have responded to Snellen optotypes, it is uncommon for children under 4.5 years to read dependably a standardized Snellen acuity chart. Tests useful in the 2.5- to 4.5-year range include Allen picture cards, Landolt rings, the HOTV test, and the Tumbling E test.

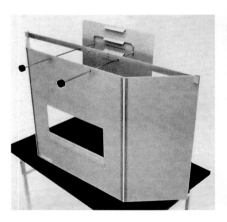

2.6 | Forced choice preferential looking device (Teller Acuity Cards) available from Visitech Consultants, Inc., 1372 North Fairfield Road, Dayton, OH 45432-2644.

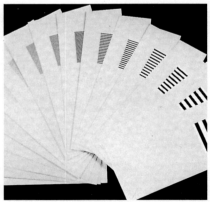

2.7 | Teller Acuity Cards.

Allen picture cards are quite useful (the near test card is a bit easier for the younger child) but have certain disadvantages: the pictures are not constructed according to the Snellen formula (each element in the target's subtending 1 minute of visual angle); some (the telephone) may not be as familiar to modern children owing to their antiquated form; the targets are variably larger than the corresponding Snellen letter target; and the smallest target size is labeled 20/30. Despite these difficulties, many children respond readily to this familiar and easily obtainable test (Fig. 2.8).

The HOTV test requires pattern recognition and matching of progressively smaller optotypes with ones on a hand-held card. These letters were chosen to be of average recognition difficulty and have a vertical axis of symmetry, obviating the issue of right–left confusion so common in this age group. An advantage is the exact correspondence of the target to the graded Snellen optotypes (Fig. 2.9).

Landolt rings are discontinuous circles; the child points to a similar ring on a hand-held card. The test is often confusing to the younger child and is perhaps more useful for illiterate adults, but it does have the advantage of corresponding directly to the Snellen chart.

The familiar Tumbling E test requires matching orientation of the letter E with a figure or the child's fingers; unfortunately, right–left disorientation is common in this age range and limits the usefulness of the test. Its major advantage is the direct correspondence to graded Snellen optotypes (Fig. 2.10).

Some children respond to isolated Snellen optotypes, or to graded numerical optotypes, before linear Snellen presentations.

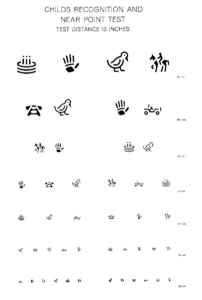

2.8 | Allen picture cards.

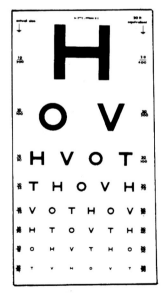

2.9 | HOTV test.

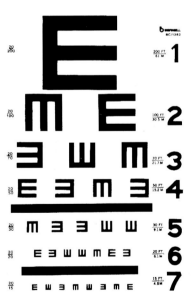

2.10 | Tumbling E test.

MATURATION OF VISUAL ACUITY

Although the central cones are functioning at term birth, acuity as measured by the above techniques does not approach 20/20 until between 6 and 30 months (depending on the examination technique used) (Fig 2.11). Reasons for this delay include continuing photoreceptor development and specialization, synaptic maturation in the inner retinal layers, and continuing myelination of the upper visual pathways. Foveal cones do not attain adult appearance until 4 months after term birth,[15] and visual pathway myelination continues until 2 years of age.[16] Interestingly, ambient illumination increases the rate of visual system myelination.[17]

Occasionally, infants fail to develop visual fixational abilities for up to 6 to 12 months, but at that later age develop normal visual behavior. These challenging children, often small for gestational age or developmentally delayed, have a normal or sluggish pupillary response, no nystagmus, and normal globe structure. The electroretinogram is completely normal; the visual evoked response has been variably reported as normal,[18] reduced in amplitude, or absent.[17] These children are postulated to have a cortical synaptic developmental delay. No clear explanation exists for those children who have normal visual evoked response tests who present with visual inattention and this syndrome. The parents should be reassured and the child examined frequently during this time period until visual attention becomes as expected.

Interest among researchers concerning potential precocity of visual development in premature infants has led to the following findings: no precocity in expected acuity as measured by the opticokinetic nystagmus and forced choice preferential looking techniques has been found, but initial precocity of attained acuity, as measured by visually evoked potentials, has been demonstrated. Premature infants tested by the latter lead similarly aged term infants for approximately 6 months, but then acuity development slows to match acuity of the term infants.

Figure 2.11. Visual Acuity of Infant Eyes

	BIRTH	2 MONTHS	4 MONTHS	6 MONTHS	1 YEAR	AGE OF 20/20 ACUITY ATTAINMENT
OKN	20/400	20/400	20/200	20/80		24 to 30 months
FCPL	20/400	20/200	20/200	20/50		18 to 24 months
VER	20/200	20/80	20/60–20/20	20/40–20/20		6 to 12 months

OKN = opticokinetic nystagmus test; FCPL = forced choice preferential looking test; VER = visual evoked response test.

3 | ANATOMY AND PHYSIOLOGY

Howard M. Eggers

EMBRYOLOGY

The extraocular muscles arise from three distinct masses of primordial cells.[1,2] In the presomite human embryo, cells proliferate laterally from a central mass located at the anterior end of the notochord (the prechordal plate). In the 25-day-old human embryo (14 somites) a pair of premandibular condensations can be seen, which give rise to the eye muscles later innervated by the oculomotor nerve (superior, medial, and inferior recti and the inferior oblique). The lateral rectus and superior oblique each arises from its own adjacent tissue mass in the maxillo-mandibular mesoderm.

At 1 month the three ocular motor nerves reach their respective muscles. Muscle striations appear early in the second month. The trochlea begins to form at 6 weeks of gestational age.

At about 3 months the muscles have become enveloped by collagen fibers, representing the earliest fascia. The levator palpebrae develops as a separate lamination from the superior rectus during the third and fourth months. Connective tissue septa are formed by the end of the fourth month and continue to enlarge through the second trimester, along with the muscle fascia.

The orbital mesenchyma differentiates last.[3] In the fifth month adipose cells arise about capillary beds in areas of loose mesenchyma between the connective tissue septums. By 6 months the muscles are in their final positions, and thereafter all the existing tissues and structures simply enlarge further.

GROSS ANATOMY

The orbits are symmetrically arranged about the midline. The orbital axes diverge, and the medial walls are approximately parallel to each other. To be parallel to each other, the visual axes must each be adducted by 22.5° relative to the orbital axes[4] (Fig. 3.1).

The six extraocular muscles, four rectus and two oblique, attach to and rotate the eye. Anatomically and functionally the muscles are organized into three pairs: medial and lateral rectus, superior and inferior rectus, and superior and inferior oblique.[5-7]

The rectus muscles (medial, lateral, superior, and inferior) are flat strips, having a width six times their thickness, that take origin at an oval, fibrous ring at the orbital apex, the annulus of Zinn, which overlies the optic foramen and the medial portion of the superior orbital fissure (Fig. 3.2). Through the annulus of Zinn pass the abducens nerve, the upper and lower divisions of the oculomotor nerve, the optic nerve and ophthalmic artery, and the nasociliary branch of the ophthalmic nerve.

The rectus muscles course forward in a cone-like configuration and insert in the sclera a few millimeters posterior to the corneal limbus, through tendons a few millimeters long[8-11] (Fig. 3.3). The distance of the insertions from the lim-

3.1 | Orbital geometry. The medial walls of the orbit are approximately parallel to each other and are symmetrically arranged with respect to the midsagittal plane. The lateral walls form an approximate 45° angle to the medial walls and, therefore, 90° with each other. The central axis of each orbit therefore diverges from the midline by about 22.5° and from the axis of the other orbit by about 45°.

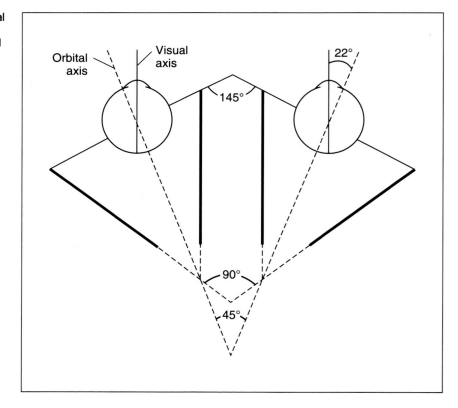

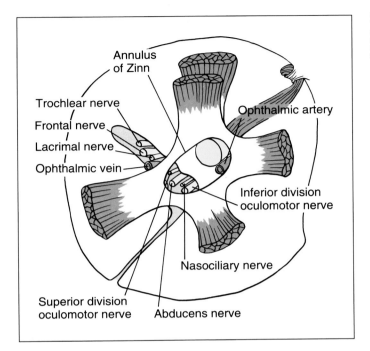

3.2 | Annulus of Zinn and the orbital apex. The extraocular muscles insert into the annulus of Zinn at the orbital apex. The locations of various vessels and nerves are shown.

Figure 3.3. Anatomy and Function of Extraocular Muscles[8–11]

Muscle	Origin	Insertion	Muscle Length (mm)	Tendon Length (mm)	Width of Insertion (mm)	Direction of Pull to Sagittal Plane (deg)	Action: Primary Secondary Tertiary	Innervation (Cranial Nerve)
Medial rectus	Annulus of Zinn	5.5 mm behind nasal limbus	41	3.5	10.3	90	Adduction	Lower III
Inferior rectus	Annulus of Zinn	6.5 mm behind inferior limbus	40	4.5	9.8	23	Depression Extorsion Adduction	Lower III
Lateral rectus	Annulus of Zinn	6.9 mm behind lateral limbus	41	8	9.2	90	Abduction	VI
Superior rectus	Annulus of Zinn	7.7 mm behind superior limbus	42	5	10.6	23	Elevation Intorsion Adduction	Upper III
Superior oblique	Fronto-ethmoidal suture above annulus of Zinn	Posterior, lateral, superior octant	32	26	10.8	54	Intorsion Depression Abduction	IV
Inferior oblique	Posterior to lacrimal fossa	Posterior, lateral, inferior octant	35	1	9.6	51	Extorsion Elevation Abduction	Lower III

bus increases in sequence from the medial to the inferior, to the lateral, and to the superior rectus, a progression known as the spiral of Tillaux[12] (Fig. 3.4).

The insertions vary somewhat in shape and location (Fig. 3.5). The exact muscle length depends on eye position, but at rest, as under anesthesia or in deep sleep, the rectus muscles are approximately 40 mm in length, the superior oblique is 32 mm, and the inferior oblique is 35 mm.

The two oblique muscles approach the eye from the front.[13] The superior oblique muscle is fusiform in shape and arises near the annulus of Zinn over the fronto–ethmoidal suture, superomedial to the origin of the medial rectus. It courses forward along the junction of the orbital roof and medial wall. Its tendon passes through a pulley, or trochlea, and is redirected posteriorly, passing inferior to the superior rectus muscle and inserting on the posterior, superior, and lateral octant of the globe (Fig. 3.6). The trochlea is the functional origin of the superior oblique.

3.4 | The Spiral of Tillaux. The insertions of the rectus muscles increase in distance from the limbus in the sequence medial, inferior, lateral, and superior. The vertical recti have the centers of their insertions slightly lateral to the vertical corneal meridian. The lateral portions of the vertical rectus tendons also are slightly more posterior than the nasal sides.

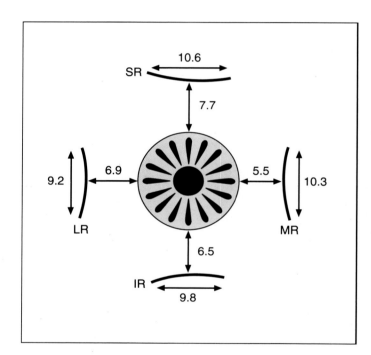

3.5 | Variations in muscle insertions. This schematic diagram of the area over which each muscle has been found to insert is based on a dozen dissections. The obliques are the least consistent, followed by the vertical recti. The medial rectus is the most consistent.[5]

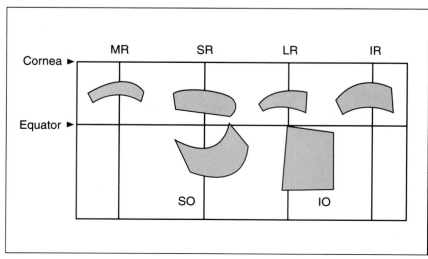

The inferior oblique arises behind the lacrimal fossa from the orbital plate of the maxilla and proceeds backwards laterally in a direct path to its insertion in the posterior, inferior, and lateral octant of the globe. It passes inferior to the inferior rectus.

In childhood the eye muscles grow along with the orbit and the eye[15] (Fig. 3.7). The muscle lengths increase by about 40%–50%, but, while the dimensions

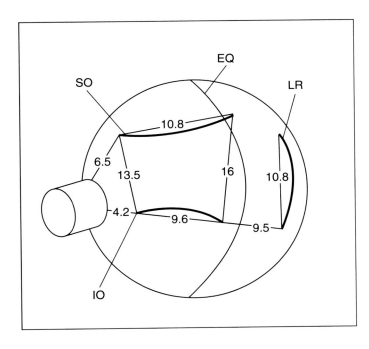

3.6 | Posterior surface of the eye. The posterior surface of a right eye showing the average insertions of the oblique muscles. Dimensions are given in mm.[14]

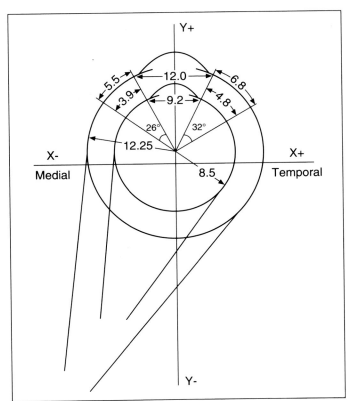

3.7 | Growth of the eye and extraocular muscles. Dimensions are in mm. With aging, the angular relationships are preserved even though the lengths change. (Adapted from Muhlendyck H: Wachstum und Lange der ausseren Augemuskeln. *Berl Dtsch Ophthalmol Ges 1978;75:449-452.*)

change, the angular relationships stay the same. This growth pattern ensures that the percent contraction of each muscle stays the same for a given size of eye movement. The central innervation patterns are thus independent of growth.

BLOOD SUPPLY

Two branches of the ophthalmic artery supply the extraocular muscles. One branch supplies the lateral and superior recti and the superior oblique, and the other supplies the medial and inferior recti and the inferior oblique. The lacrimal artery may partially supply the lateral rectus and the infraorbital artery may partially supply the inferior rectus and oblique. The anterior ciliary arteries, which supply blood to the anterior segment of the eye, arise from the rectus muscles and penetrate the sclera at the muscle insertions. The lateral rectus contains one anterior ciliary artery and the other recti two each. A clinical rule of thumb is to avoid surgery on more than two rectus muscles at a time to avoid the risk of anterior segment ischemia from interruption of the anterior ciliary arteries. With time, collateral circulation may develop through the long posterior ciliary arteries. The venous drainage of the extraocular muscles is into the superior and inferior orbital veins.

INNERVATION

The third cranial nerve (oculomotor) divides within the orbit into superior and inferior branches (Fig. 3.8). The superior division innervates the superior rectus and levator palpebrae and the inferior division innervates the inferior and

3.8 | The III cranial nerve gives off a superior division and an inferior division. The muscles are innervated at the junction of the middle and posterior thirds, except for the inferior oblique, which is innervated at the middle.

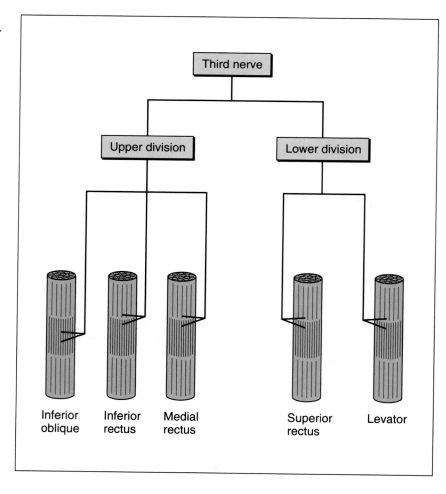

Third nerve

Upper division

Lower division

Inferior oblique   Inferior rectus   Medial rectus

Superior rectus   Levator

medial recti and inferior oblique. The nerves enter these three rectus muscles from within the muscle cone at approximately the junction of the middle and posterior thirds of the muscle. The VI cranial nerve (abducens) innervates the lateral rectus and enters that muscle from within the muscle cone just posterior to the middle of the muscle. The trochlear nerve innervates the superior oblique and enters that muscle from its orbital surface, in several branches in the anterior half of the posterior third of the muscle. The nerve to the inferior oblique enters the muscle at about the middle of the posterior border.

ORBITAL TISSUES

The globe and extraocular muscles are enveloped by a connective tissue layer called Tenon's capsule.[16] This capsule forms a potential space next to the sclera that is free of any tissue attachments that might restrict globe rotation. Beyond small rotations Tenon's capsule rotates with the eye. The orbital fat is prevented from attaching to the globe by Tenon's capsule. Sometimes Tenon's capsule is perforated during surgery and the orbital fat is sufficiently traumatized that adhesions can form between the fat and the globe. Such an adhesive syndrome significantly impairs eye rotations. Penetration of Tenon's capsule can release fat as far forward as 10 mm behind the limbus.

The anterior portion of Tenon's capsule lies anterior to the rectus muscle insertions. It is thin and adherent to the globe and extends almost to the corneoscleral limbus, where it links with conjunctiva. The posterior Tenon's capsule is attached to the orbital fat and connective tissue network. It is penetrated by the extraocular muscles, the optic nerve, and the blood vessels and nerves serving the globe. The rectus muscles pass through Tenon's capsule anterior to the equator of the globe and pick up sleeve-like extensions of the capsule. The intracapsular portion of the rectus muscles is 7–10 mm in length. After passing through the capsule each muscle gives off falciform, fascial expansions from its edges which attach to the overlying Tenon's capsule and insert into the sclera (Fig. 3.9). Small attachments between the undersurface of the muscle and the sclera just behind the muscle insertion are called

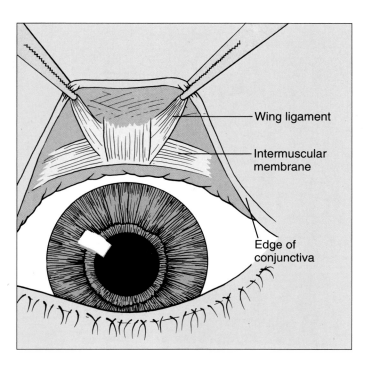

Wing ligament

Intermuscular membrane

Edge of conjunctiva

3.9 | The muscles are surrounded by Tenon's capsule. During muscle surgery the conjuctiva is elevated and Tenon's capsule is dissected free from the muscle. Under traction, Tenon's capsule drapes in folds radiating from the muscle edge, known as wing ligaments.

footplates. Posterior to the capsular passage, for a distance of some 10–12 mm, the muscle sheaths give off lateral expansions that join to the adjacent muscles, forming an intermuscular membrane.

Thin connective tissue bands from the medial and lateral rectus muscle sheaths are known as check ligaments. Strands from the lateral rectus attach on the zygomatic tubercle and strands from the medial rectus attach on the lacrimal bone behind the lacrimal crest. Unless scarred, these bands do not limit eye rotations but help to anchor the whole fascial apparatus in position.

The sheath of the superior rectus blends with that of the levator palpebrae superioris and through this mechanical coupling helps to produce synergic movement between the two muscles. It explains the apparent or pseudoptosis that accompanies a hypotropia. A forward expansion of the inferior rectus sheath passes from the inferior surface of the muscle and inserts between the tarsus and orbicularis oculi muscle. This mechanical linkage helps to lower the lower lid on downgaze. It explains the change in lid fissure width after inferior rectus surgery. Resections of this muscle tend to raise the lower lid and narrow the lid fissure, whereas recessions tend to widen the lid fissure by lowering the lid. Each rectus muscle sends connective tissue expansions that move the conjunctival cul-de-sac in the direction of eye movement.

The periocular and retroocular orbital spaces are filled with fat pads organized as adipose tissue spaces, surrounded by collagenous strands and septa.[17] The septa are 0.3 mm or more in thickness and subdivide the orbital volume. Around the globe the septa are radial to the eye and attach to Tenon's capsule and the intermuscular membrane (Figs. 3.10 and 3.11). A system of connective tissue septa exists for each muscle, which serves to anchor the muscle and support the blood vessels. The suspensory ligament of Lockwood is an expansion of the inferior rectus sheath to the surrounding septa to form a part of this system.

3.10 | Connective tissue septa of the anterior orbit. *1* = periorbita; *2* = connective tissue strands; *3* = intermuscular membrane; *4* = Tenon's capsule. Asterisks indicate where smooth muscle cells were found. (Adapted from Koorneef L: Details of the orbital connective tissue system in the adult *Acta Morphol Neerl Scand 1977;15:1-34.*)

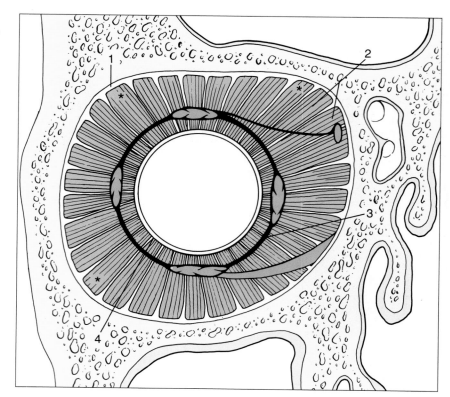

The anatomy of eye muscles has always been a complex and difficult subject owing to the differences among species. The eye muscles also are anatomically different from skeletal muscle.[18,19] The unique anatomic features of eye muscle derive from its unique functional properties: constancy of activity (orbital layer of small, constantly active fibers, great orbital surface vascularity), rapidity of contraction (parallel arrangement of muscle fibers, large twitch fibers using anaerobic metabolism), and fine gradation of contraction (low ratio of muscle cells to nerve terminals, rich nerve supply).

The eye muscles have a histologic structure different from that of skeletal muscle.[18] Each muscle fiber (cell) is surrounded by connective tissue. Adjacent to the cell surface is a 50-nm layer of mucopolysaccharide. This is surrounded in turn by delicate argyrophilic (collagen) and elastin fibers (Fig. 3.12). The connective tissue surrounding the muscle fibers contains many

MICROSCOPIC ANATOMY

CONNECTIVE TISSUE

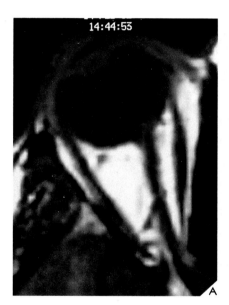
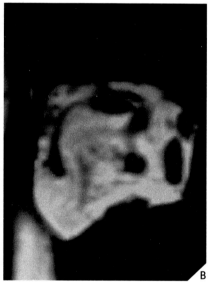

3.11 | Nuclear magnetic resonance images of a normal orbit. *A:* Horizontal section. *B:* Transverse section of right orbit seen from the front. The muscles are generally strap-like in shape but the thickest portion can be seen to be posterior to the globe. The orbital septa can be seen stretching between several of the muscles. (Courtesy of Dr. M. Kazim.)

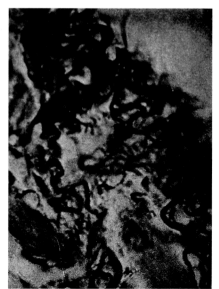

3.12 | Longitudinal section of human extraocular muscle shows elastin fibers.[18]

small nerves and blood vessels. At the surface of the muscle this tissue blends with the muscle sheath. The muscle sheath is thin for 2 cm from the muscle origin, and becomes thicker and more opaque towards the back of the globe. The inner layer has longitudinal fibers and the outer layer circumferential fibers, which fuse with Tenon's capsule. Capillary blood vessels are most numerous on the orbital surface of the muscle, which contains more small muscle cells that are constantly active.

MUSCLE FIBERS

The muscle fibers or cells are roughly cylindrical, each cell running most of the length of the muscle and inserting into the muscle tendon. This pattern stacks the sarcomeres end to end for the entire length of the muscle and sums the contraction of each, producing maximal velocity of contraction and maximal distance of shortening, and, therefore, of eye rotation.

Two broad classes of muscle cell exist in extraocular muscle, each having different fuctional characteristics: singly innervated cells, which respond with an all-or-none twitch to a conducted action potential; and multiply innervated cells, which have a graded, tonic contraction proportional to the nerve impulse rate, without a conducted action potential.[20-24] Light microscopy shows two anatomic patterns of contractile fibrils within the muscle fibers that correspond to these two innervation patterns. The singly innervated twitch fibers have myofibrils in discrete bundles, separated by sarcoplasmic reticulum and lying in register to produce a striated appearance (*fibrillenstruktur*). The multiply innervated tonic fibers have irregular, larger myofibrils that are partially fused producing a more homogeneous appearance (*felderstruktur*).

These two types of cell can be subclassified by electron microscopy into five or six different groups on the basis of features such as development of endoplasmic reticulum, number of mitochondria, size and arrangement of transverse tubules, and fine structure of fibrils.[23-27] These subcellular anatomical differences relate directly to the functional capacities of each cell type (Fig. 3.13).

In cross-section, extraocular muscle shows a layered organization, in which the smaller diameter cells tend to lie on the orbital surface and the larger cells adjacent to the globe. The orbital surface layer of the muscle contains smaller-diameter fibers, both twitch and tonic, containing many mitochondria, implying the capability of prolonged contractile activity. The global layer contains twitch fibers of three types: "red," "intermediate," and

3.13 | Electron micrograph of a "red" twitch fiber in human extraocular muscle. The diagram shows how the filaments produce the banding pattern. The A-bands are optically anisotropic and contain myosin. The I-bands are optically isotropic and contain actin, troponin, and tropomyosin. The sarcomere extends from Z-line to Z-line and varies in length from 1.5–3.5 μm depending on the amount of shortening of the muscle. The H zone is free of thin filaments.

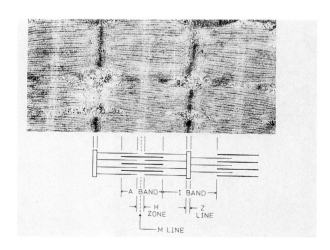

"white," according to mitochondrial content, development of sarcoplasmic reticulum, and diameter. In addition, a "white," multiply innervated tonic fiber occurs in the global layer. If the red twitch fibers in the orbital and global layers are considered to be the same type, altogether only five types of muscle fiber occur (Fig. 3.14).

Fibrillenstruktur fibers are about 25–50 μm in diameter and show myofibrils that are distinctly separated from one another by agranular cytoplasm. Mitochondria lie in rows between fibrils or adjacent to the sarcolemma. The sarcoplasmic reticulum and transverse tubule system are well developed, and the motor endplates resemble the *en plaque* nerve terminals of skeletal muscle and are located in the middle third of the muscle (Fig. 3.15). The axons innervating these cells are myelinated and range from 9–13 μm in diameter.[28–30]

Felderstruktur fibers are about 9–15 μm in diameter and have less sarcoplasm and fewer mitochondria than the *fibrillenstruktur* fibers. The mitochondria lie in peripheral areas of sarcoplasm free of fibrils. The transverse tubule system is less evident but still present. The myofibrils are poorly demarcated. The nerve endings are multiple, *en grappe,* distributed along the length of the muscle, and number eight to ten per cell (see Fig. 3.15).

Histochemistry of extraocular muscles shows three types of cell: granular (global "intermediate" and "red" twitch, orbital tonic), fine (global tonic and "white" twitch), and coarse (orbital twitch, global "red" twitch).[31] Human skeletal muscle shows a reciprocal relationship between phosphorylase (anaerobic glycolysis) and oxidative enzyme content. The granular fibers are large, fast-

Figure 3.14. Muscle Fiber Types

ORBITAL LAYER
Small, singly-innervated twitch fiber, many mitochondria ("red")
Small, multiply-innervated tonic fiber, many mitochondria ("red")

GLOBAL LAYER
Small, singly-innervated twitch fiber, many mitochondria ("red")
Medium, singly-innervated twitch fiber, moderate mitochondria ("intermediate")
Large, singly-innervated twitch fiber, few mitochondria ("white")
Variable sized, multiply-innervated twitch fiber, few mitochondria ("white")

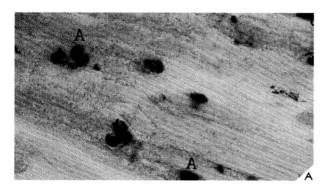
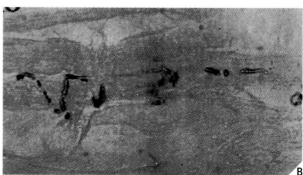

3.15 | Acetylcholinesterase stain of human extraocular neuromuscular junctions. *A: En plaque* nerve terminals occur on twitch fibers. *B: En grappe* nerve terminals occur on tonically contracting fibers.[28]

twitch fibers ("white"). They have few mitochondria and show high phosphorylase activity. They are thought to be recruited only when a large muscle force is required and rely on glycolysis to provide the needed ATP. These cells fatigue rapidly. During rest, the mitochondria replenish the cell's energy stores. The fine fibers are smaller, slower-twitch fibers ("red") that have more mitochondria. They are more fatigue resistant and capable of continuous activity. The coarse fibers correspond to the tonic fibers. They have a high level of oxidative enzymes, as required by constant contractile activity.

The laminated organization of the rectus muscles into orbital surface and global layers is well demonstrated by histochemistry. The orbital surface layer contains roughly 90% coarse fibers; the remainder are mostly granular. The global layer shows roughly 55% granular, 12% fine, and 33% coarse. The percentage representation of fiber types is the same in all six oculorotary muscles. Assuming that the small nerve fibers innervate the tonic muscle fibers and the large nerve fibers innervate the twitch fibers, there results a ratio of three or four muscle cells per nerve axon for the tonic fibers, and ten per nerve axon for the twitch fibers.

PROPRIOCEPTORS

Muscle spindles in the extraocular muscles occur in the proximal or distal third of the muscle[31,32] (Fig. 3.16). The spindle in extraocular muscle is smaller, more delicate, and simpler than that in skeletal muscle, containing only one type of intrafusal muscle fiber and motor nerve terminal. Human extraocular muscle contains spiral nerve endings that wrap around extrafusal muscle fibers (Fig. 3.17). Formerly thought to be sensory structures ("atypical spindles"), these have been identified as a special type of motor terminal.[33] Golgi tendon organs do occur.[34] Unlike their arrangement in skeletal muscles, in human extraocular muscle both ends of the tendon organ have tendinous attachments. Also present are a small number of sensory endings with various other morphologies.[35,36] An exact functional role for any of the muscle proprioceptors is not established. Eye position is best signaled through the retina. Many experiments have shown that there is a nonretinal eye position signal available to the brain. This could come from motor outflow to the eye muscles (efference copy or corollary discharge) or from muscle proprioception, or both. In addition, muscle proprioception may play a role in visual development or in the long-term maintenance of control of the proper level of efferent signals.

3.16 | Longitudinal (A) and cross-sections (B) of human extraocular muscle spindles. The fusiform spindle capsule encloses the intrafusal fibers. The point of entry of a nerve trunk is shown. The cross-section shows three intrafusal fibers with nerve fibers and capillaries.[31]

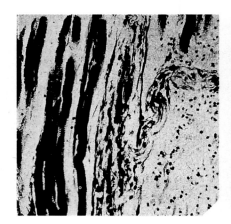
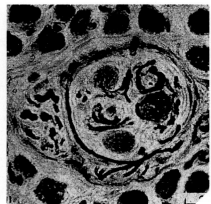

PHYSIOLOGY

The extraocular muscles have unusual contractile properties, determined by the various fiber types. The large twitch fibers are responsible for making the extraocular muscles the fastest contracting mammalian muscle.[37] Contraction times for the medial rectus range up to 10 msec and lead to a correspondingly high fusion frequency (350 Hz). At the fusion frequency the rate of stimulation is high enough that the cell does not have time to relax and successive twitches are overlapped (tetanus). On the other hand, when exposed to acetylcholine or depolarizing muscle relaxants, the extraocular muscles undergo a prolonged contracture owing to activation of the tonically contracting fibers.[38] The tonic fibers have a rise time of contraction of 25 msec and a contraction time of 25–50 msec. The contractions fuse at 200 pulses/sec or lower.[39–42]

The twitch fibers have a membrane and contractile physiology similar to that of skeletal muscles. A propagated action potential spreads down the muscle cell membrane. Depolarization of the sarcolemma leads to a release of calcium ions from the sarcoplasmic reticulum, which actively transports and stores calcium.

In tonic fibers the extent of contraction depends on the degree of depolarization. No propagation of an action potential occurs and the membrane between terminals is depolarized by passive electrotonic spread. The intensity of contraction is smoothly graded with the frequency of nerve impulses.

In normal function, the tonically contracting fibers provide a constant tonus which may play some role in reducing the elastic slack in series with the muscle, and thus speed up eye movements.

The load against which an eye muscle contracts—the inertia of the eye, the elasticity of the structures that attach to the eye, and the contractile force and viscous drag of the antagonist muscle—is approximately constant. The initial contraction of the agonist muscle is approximately isometric. As the eye moves, the muscle undergoes an isotonic contraction and the muscle then relaxes isometrically.

The contractile force produced by an eye muscle depends on the innervation (the number of action potentials per unit time) and the muscle length. These relationships can be summarized in a family of length–tension

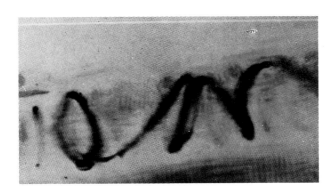

3.17 | Light micrograph of an atypical muscle spindle in human extraocular muscle. The terminal fiber wraps around the extrafusal muscle fiber and terminates in a small end bulb. These are now known to be a special type of motor end plate. (From Daniel P: Spiral nerve endings in the extrinsic eye muscles of man. *J Anat 1946;80:189–193.*)

curves[43] (Fig. 3.18). The interaction of the muscle length–tension curve with the three-dimensional geometry of the muscle and the innervation patterns of antagonistic muscles determines the actual direction in which the eye points. The muscle length at maximal developed tension is at the limit of the physiologic range of eye rotation and in primary position the length is about 85% of this. The force of muscle contraction decreases as the muscle shortens. This makes for a stable mechanical equilibrium because, when a muscle shifts to a new length–tension curve in response to a change in innervation, it pulls with more force against its antagonist at the given length. In response to the greater pull, the antagonist stretches but increases its force. The agonist shortens, reducing its force, and at some muscle length these opposing forces balance. The eye is then held in a new direction.

The muscle forces required to maintain fixation (Fig. 3.19) form a parabolic curve.[44,45] The agonist forces counteract both the orbital spring forces and antagonist stretch. Within 15° of primary position the muscle force changes very little. More than 15° out of its field of action, where the muscle is less innervated, muscle elongation increases the force in the muscle, even though it is less innervated. The developed force in the muscle is not directly related to the innervation but depends on the mechanical response of the muscle and eye. It is misleading to think of innervation as an increase in tension. The eye position is the result of an equilibrium of forces applied to the eye. Innervation changes move the eye by means of changes in the length–tension curves.

3.18 | Length–tension curves of a human lateral rectus muscle. The innervation is determined by the fixation effort of the fellow eye. The muscle was detached from the eye and the force required to stretch the muscle to various lengths was plotted for each innervation level. The dotted lines represent developed tension (total tension minus passive stretch, PM). N = nasal; T = temporal. (From Robinson DA, O'Meara DM, Scott AB, Collins CC: Mechanical components of human eye movements. *J Appl Physiol* 1969;26:548-553.)

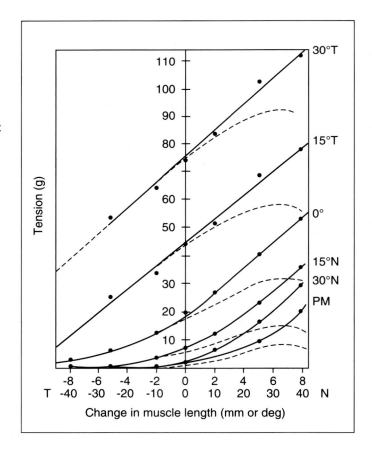

The predominant forces affecting globe rotation are an elasticity and a viscosity.[46] The elasticity (stiffness) is about 1.25 gram-force/degree of rotation, of which 0.5 is due to the passive tissues and 0.75 is due to the length–tension relationship of the horizontal rectus muscles. The viscosity is quite high, about 0.06 gram-force/degree/sec.[47]

The rotations of the eye are, to a close approximation, described by a ball-and-socket concept. For horizontal rotations, the instantaneous center of rotation moves with respect to both the orbit and the eye. Despite lateral and anteroposterior displacements relative to both the eye and orbit, the visual axis does pass through a point fixed in space, or nearly fixed. It is usually assumed for convenience that the eye rotates about a fixed point 13.5 mm behind the cornea on the visual axis.[48,49]

The specification of the orientation of the eye in space requires three coordinates, representing rotational positions about three axes. A coordinate system frequently used for this is Fick's (see Fig. 3.21), which is similar to longitude and latitude for horizontal and vertical positions, respectively. The third axis is orientation around the line of sight (torsion or cyclorotation). Primary position is gaze straight ahead. Secondary positions are gaze directly up, down, right, or left. Tertiary positions are in oblique directions away from primary position. Eye movement nomenclature is listed in Chapter 4. Rotations of one eye considered by itself are known as ductions. Rotations of both eyes in the same direction are known as conjugate movements or versions, and rotations in opposite directions are known as disjunctive movements or vergences.

KINEMATICS

3.19 | A family of human medial rectus length-tension curves, determined from indwelling strain-gauge measurements. The heavy line is the actual realized force. Note that minimum force is at 15° out of the field of action. The loop, showing force during a saccade, is approximated by an isometric contraction followed by an isotonic change in length, followed by an isometric relaxation. The rise in tension during the return saccade, when the muscle is inhibited, is due to viscosity. (Modified from Collins CC, Scott AB, O'Meara D: Muscle tension during unrestrained human eye movements. *J Physiol (Lond)* 1975;245:351-369.)

Donders discovered that the orientation of the eye about the fixation axis, measured in any coordinate system, is determined, in the absence of head tilt and for stationary fixation, solely by the horizontal and vertical coordinates.[50] This means that only two of the three rotational coordinates are independent. Preceding eye movements have no effect on the orientation. This law does not hold during a smooth pursuit movement.[51] If head tilt is allowed, countertorsion produces a torsional position at each direction of gaze which depends on the head tilt.

Listing's law goes on to specify exactly what the orientation is as a function of gaze direction.[52] Listing's plane is the frontal plane that passes through the center of rotation of the eye (Fig. 3.20). For a stationary erect head and fixation at infinity, the orientation is what it would be if the eye had rotated from primary position to its final position about a single axis lying in Listing's plane. Thus, in eccentric gaze, the end of the vertical corneal meridian that lies closest to primary position is tilted towards primary position.[53] No torsional disparity exists between the eyes. Listing's law does not apply in the presence of head tilt (which elicits countertorsion), optokinetic torsion, cyclofusional or cyclophoric torsion, or during convergence, which has its own associated extorsion. Projection of afterimage crosses, imprinted in primary position, on a spherical surface (to prevent distortion of the shape of the cross) shows almost 10° of tilt with respect to the objective vertical in gaze eccentric and 45° oblique.

3.20 | Listing's plane is the frontal plane that passes through the center of rotation of the eye. The torsional position of the eye in eccentric positions of gaze is what it would be if the eye had reached that position by a pure rotation (heavy arrow) around a perpendicular axis (dotted line) lying in Listing's plane.

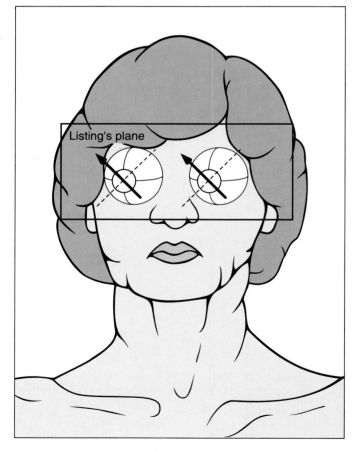

The vertical corneal meridian, in tertiary positions, will have an orientation to the vertical which is described differently in the various coordinate systems. This has caused endless confusion under the name of "false torsion." The eye, in moving from primary to tertiary positions, according to Listing's law clearly moves along the direction of one corneal meridian and in this sense undergoes no torsion. Although the Fick, Helmholtz, and Listing (or perimetric) coordinate systems agree as to the vertical in primary position, the verticals in tertiary positions are different (Fig. 3.21). Therefore, described in Fick or Helmholtz coordinates, tertiary positions show (false) torsion.[54]

The brainstem neuronal machinery that drives eye movements is organized into horizontal and vertical components. The nuclei serving horizontal movements are in the pons and those serving vertical movements are in the midbrain. A complex mapping is performed between commands for gaze in a particular direction and the exact stimulation required of each muscle to achieve it. The location of the mapping is unknown. Listing's law places a constraint on the mapping by specifying the orientation of the eye about its line of sight. That Listing's law does not hold during sleep implies that cortical activity is able to change the mapping, at least to some extent.[55] Although the brainstem machinery is separated into horizontal and vertical components, evidence from experiments with smooth pursuit tracking suggests that no preferential frame of reference occurs in cortical processing.[56]

Recordings from oculomotor neurons in the monkey show that the firing rate of individual neurons depends on both the eye position and the velocity of movement.[57,58]

$$\text{Firing rate} = k(E - E_t) + r \, \frac{dE}{dt},$$

where E is eye position and E_t is the threshold position at which the unit is recruited. From a large population of cells, mean k has been found to be about 4 (spikes/sec)/degree and r about 0.9 (spikes/sec)/(degrees/sec). The thresholds all are below 25° into the field of action, and some motor units (16%) are still active when the muscle is fully out of its field of action. The same firing rate rule holds for all oculomotor neurons during all types of eye movement: fixation, saccades, pursuit, vergence, and vestibularly induced movements. The firing rate rule is strong evidence against the idea that the various types of muscle fiber serve different kinds of eye movement. A fixed, definite angle of recruitment exists for every motor unit regardless of the kind of movement being made. A distinction between "tonic" and "phasic" units is of little value because it arises from the chance event of whether or

CENTRAL INNERVATION PATTERNS

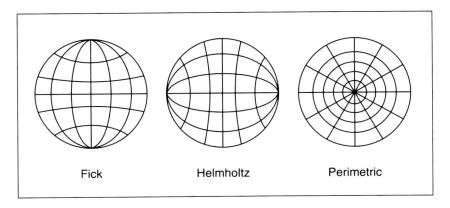

Fick   Helmholtz   Perimetric

3.21 | Commonly used coordinate systems for specifying eye position. In Fick's coordinates the horizontal gaze angle is specified first, in Helmholtz's the vertical. The perimetric system is simplest for Listing's law.

not a unit's recruitment threshold was crossed for a particular eye movement. All units follow the same rule, but with variation in the parameters of the equation. The same behavior of single oculomotor units has been found electromyographically in humans.

A size order of recruitment has been found to hold for motor neurons in the spinal cord.[59] Such a principle is believed to hold for extraocular muscles as well. The anatomic factor underlying the size principle is that motor units containing a small number of muscle fibers are served by smaller-diameter, slower-conducting axons. In the neuron the size of the perikaryon is proportional to the size of the axon. The smaller a neuron, the more easily it is recruited by the field potentials and summated activity of axons innervating the nucleus.[60] Thus, with increasing stimulation of a nucleus, the motor units are automatically recruited in sequence of size. As larger units are recruited, the increment of extra contractile force exerted by successively recruited units tends to stay a constant percentage of the level of force already in effect. Oculomotor units become active in the sequence of their recruitment thresholds, regardless of the type of movement being made. The small fibers in the orbital surface layer of muscle are constantly active, and the larger fibers of the orbital layer are recruited as required for a saccade or large version.

The extraocular muscles show reciprocal innervation of antagonists, as do skeletal muscles. This is known as Sherrington's law. Sherrington demonstrated inhibition to a lateral rectus by cutting the III and IV nerves on one side and then stimulating the cortex to obtain eye movements to the other side. The eye on the denervated side moved to primary position, demonstrating inhibition of the lateral rectus. In the spinal cord, stretch afferents from the agonist excite an inhibitory interneuron to the antagonist. Such an interneuron-mediated reflex mechanism of reciprocal innervation has not been demonstrated for the eye muscles. In Duane syndrome Sherrington's law is violated, owing to simultaneous contraction of antagonistic muscles[61] (Fig. 3.22).

Sherrington also observed that muscles that move the two eyes in the same direction receive similar innervations.[62] This principle usually goes under the name of Hering's law.[63] Hering regarded the two eyes as a single organ, a double eye. A pair of muscles, one for each eye, that move the eyes in the same direction (conjugate movement) are known as yoke muscles (e.g., right lateral rectus and left medial rectus). Hering's law says that both muscles of such a pair receive the same innervation. Because the eyes are approximately spherical, all the eye muscles have the same load and moment arm (distance from the center of rotation to the point of application of force on the surface of the globe). This uniformity in the mechanics allows the same innervation to move both eyes through the same rotation, preserving the alignment of both eyes onto the same target. This concept is very useful but in actuality is complicated by the fact that, except for the horizontal rectus muscles in horizontal gaze, none of the muscles produces a pure vertical, horizontal, or torsional rotation. Cross-coupling of muscle pull is very prominent among the vertical recti and obliques. Hering regarded them as a single group of muscles with varying interactions among them. Hering's law is violated during saccadic movements, in which frequently the two eyes receive slightly different innervation signals and typically monocular movements such as dynamic overshoot, glissades, or double saccades may occur.[64]

The three-dimensional cooperation of the extraocular muscles is in detail very complex. The actions of all the muscles must be taken into account at the same time, because as the eye moves away from primary position, the muscle actions change somewhat; secondary actions come into play, which then also cause further interactions among the various muscles.

Early mathematical models of the three-dimensional eye muscle interaction were developed by Krewson[65] and Boeder.[66] With the advent of digital computers, it has been possible to manage the extensive calculations required in modeling this system. Robinson introduced the most complete and accurate model, which takes into account the actual paths of the muscles along the surface of the globe and the innervation–length–tension relationship of a muscle.[67] His model has been further elaborated by Miller.[68]

The muscle innervation can be thought of in three components. A primary innervation places each muscle on a particular length-tension curve and determines to a first approximation what the eye position will be. In primary position, the force exerted by each horizontal rectus, vertical rectus, and oblique muscle is 8, 6, and 4 gram-force, respectively. This rises to approximately ten times as much at 40° into the fields of action of each muscle. A secondary innervation of about 0.5 gram-force/degree is required to balance out the passive tissue spring forces. It constitutes part of the agonist muscle's load. Tertiary innervations are adjustments required to allow for cross-coupling of muscle forces from one pair of muscles to another. For example, in elevation the obliques and vertical recti generate horizontal and torsional forces that must be counterbalanced, and the effectiveness of the vertical recti in producing elevation or torsion changes with direction of horizontal gaze. Another example of cross-coupling requiring a varying tertiary innervation is the adducting effect of the vertical recti, which varies with the direction of horizontal gaze.

Change in muscle action with change in direction of gaze is limited by the width of the muscle insertions. This was known to Helmholtz.[69] As the eye rotates in a direction orthogonal to the direction of action of a particular muscle, muscle fibers along one edge of the muscle are stretched out and

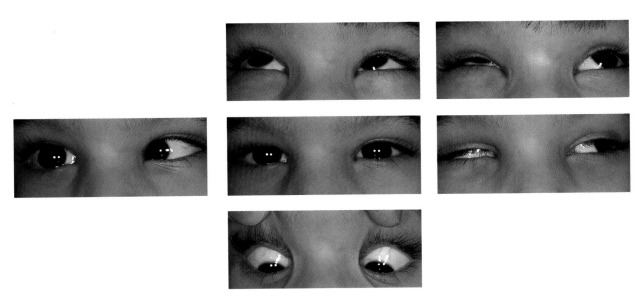

3.22 | Duane syndrome. On gaze to the left, the right medial and lateral rectus muscles both contract, resulting in enophthalmos and a narrow lid fissure. This violation of Sherrington's law of reciprocal innervation is due to anomalous innervation in which nerve fibers to the medial rectus also innervate the lateral rectus.

those on the opposite edge relaxed some. The net effect of this is to move the point of effective force application to the stretched side. The result is that the axis in the orbit, about which a given pair of muscles rotates the eye, tends to stay the same. The muscles also are anchored in place where they pass through Tenon's capsule and side slip is limited, thus minimizing changes in muscle action as the position changes.

It is possible to put the muscle fibers into a hypothetical scheme that shows why various types of fiber exist[70] (Fig. 3.23). The muscle fibers hypothetically are recruited in a sequence that optimizes the utilization of the red and white fibers and produces as fine a control of eye position as possible. The red fibers, capable of constant activity, would be recruited out of the field of action of the muscle, and the white fibers into the field of action. Because most saccades are within 15° of primary position, the most fatigable fibers (large, white, rapid twitch), recruited at maximum gaze effort, would be called upon infrequently. To produce fine control of fixation, the smoothly contracting tonic fibers would be recruited in the region about primary position. Above fusion frequency, the tonic multiinnervated fibers produce a smooth ripple-free contraction, minimizing mechanical jitter. The tonic units have the smallest innervation ratio (number of muscle cells per axon), making these motor units well suited for the fine gradation of contraction. The eye muscle twitch fibers have a low ratio of the single-twitch force to tetanic force (about 0.1). Individual motor units, firing asynchronously, disturb fixation less than with a higher ratio. These design considerations show how an engineer might go about constructing muscles that are very fast, fatigue resistant, and capable of controlling fixation to a few minutes of arc.

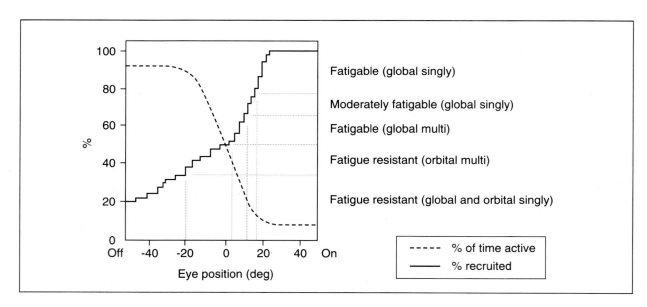

3.23 | Hypothetical arrangement of muscle fiber types. The more fatigable fibers are recruited into the field of action of the muscle. The fatigue-resistant fibers are more constantly active out of the field of action. The tonically contracting fibers, expected to produce lowest mechanical jitter, are recruited around primary position, where the eye must be as steady as possible.[70]

4 | EVALUATION OF OCULAR ALIGNMENT AND EYE MOVEMENTS

Howard M. Eggers

The exact characterization of eye position and movement is a difficult technical problem, and no single method is useful under all circumstances. The methods used are distinguished by whether physical contact is made with the eye and by resolution and dynamic range. The routinely used clinical methods involve no contact with the eye.

LABORATORY METHODS

In one group of research methods, an object such as a mirror or a coil of wire is placed on the eye and moves with it. The measurement system then uses the object riding with the eye to generate an electrical signal proportional to eye position. One of the most popular and exact methods is the eye coil, which contains several turns of insulated wire embedded in a silicone rubber annulus that rides at the limbus. The coil generates a current in response to a rotating or alternating magnetic field, which is then amplified and decoded to yield a direction value. This method is capable of resolution of a few minutes of arc and a dynamic range of 360°, but is limited, because of discomfort from the lead wires to the coil, to a maximum wearing time of less than 30 minutes. Through use of a special coil, changes in ocular torsion can be observed.

Another popular but less exact method is the EOG (named after the electro-oculogram, a test of retinal function). The standing electrical DC potential between the front and back of the eye is picked up by electrodes placed at the medial and lateral canthi for horizontal movements or above and below the superior and inferior orbital rim for vertical movements. The induced voltage is proportional to the eye position. This method suffers from difficulties in calibration, noise, stability, and drift.

A third group of methods uses the quantity of infrared light reflected by the junction of limbus and sclera as a measure of eye position. This method has a lower noise level but requires a stable positioning of the illumination and detection devices on the face, usually done by mounting the illumination and detection devices on an eyeglass frame.

CLINICAL METHODS

In the clinical examination of eye position, attention must be paid to the position of the head and eyelids in addition to the eyes. Head position can be a clue to strabismus: the head is usually positioned so as to minimize the deviation. For example, with a left lateral rectus weakness the minimal ocular deviation will be away from the field of action of the weak muscle. Gaze will be to the right and the head will be turned to the left. In superior oblique paresis, the head is tilted and rotated away from the side of the paresis to use gaze directions away from the field of action of the paretic muscle, and the chin is slightly depressed to avoid extreme downgaze. Alternatively, when single vision is not possible the head may be positioned to maximize the separation of the two images so that conflict between them is less confusing.

The eyelids can interfere with observation of the true position of the eyes and create the illusion of a deviation where none is present. This is frequently the case in infants. A wide nasal intercanthal distance creates the illusion of esotropia because less sclera than usual is visible nasally. This is called a pseudostrabismus.

The eye position cannot be determined solely by inspection because an eye may not actually be looking where it appears to be looking. This phenomenon is due to the angle between the optic axis of the eye and the visual axis. The literature is replete with various angles, carrying various names, all aimed at describing this effect. The initial problem is that the concept of an optic axis applies only to a centered optical system, and the eye is only approximately centered. The optic axis is best approximated by lining up the Purkinje images. This can be done with a small telescope and coaxial light (Tscherning's ophthalmophacometer).[1] The eye fixates a movable point on a scale reading out angle, and the position that most nearly superimposes the Purkinje images is taken as the angle kappa.

For the observer, the eye appears to be looking wherever the pupillary axis, a line through the center of the pupil and perpendicular to the cornea, is pointing (or the nearest approximation if such a line does not exist for a particular eye). The optic axis intersects the retina between the fovea and the optic disc and the pupillary axis lies very close to the optic axis. Therefore, outside the eye the visual axis is nasal to the pupillary axis by an angular amount named kappa. A positive angle kappa is defined by the visual axis being nasal to the optic axis, negative if it is temporal to the optic axis. A large positive angle kappa will create the appearance of an exotropia. A large negative angle kappa will simulate an esotropia. Donders[2] found that the average angle kappa is 5° in emmetropic eyes (range 3.5 to 6) and 7.5° in hyperopic eyes (range 6 to 9). Myopic eyes showed an average kappa of 2° but could sometimes be negative, creating a pseudoesotropia. A large positive angle kappa can result from temporal dragging of the retina in retinopathy of prematurity, creating a pseudoexotropia.

Clinically, a deviation of the eyes can be demonstrated by objective methods (e.g., corneal reflection methods, cover tests, haploscope) or by subjective methods (e.g., red glass, Lancaster red–green, Hess screen).

Objective tests do not require any psychophysical judgement or decision by the patient, and although they require cooperation by the patient they yield results of an accuracy unaffected by his or her psychophysical performance. Objective tests are useful in children and in adults who cannot make a definite observation or report it because of mental state or physical impairment.

In subjective tests, the patient reports the location in which he sees certain targets, from which eye position information can be derived. Subjective tests are potentially more accurate but may be tedious or tiring for the patient, with subsequent compromise of accuracy. Subjective tests lack any independent means of verifying that the results are accurate, and can yield inconsistent data if the patient does not understand clearly what to report or becomes confused about it.

The Hirschberg and Krimsky tests estimate the amount of eye rotation by the displacement of the corneal light reflection from a landmark, such as the center of the pupil. The original *Hirschberg method* involved the use of a candle and estimation of the position of the corneal reflection with respect to an assumed pupil size. Because the pupil is equal to the assumed size only by chance, strict adherence to this method yields only a rough estimate of the deviation. However, in an uncooperative child this may be the only measurement possible. To make the test more reproducible across multiple observations it is useful to note the pupil diameter as well as the decentration. It is also better to pay attention to the apparent position of the light reflection on the cornea, although this observation takes more time. Each millimeter of displacement across the cornea corresponds to approximately 15 prism diopters (PD) (7°) of deviation of the visual axis. With a 4-mm pupil a reflection at the edge of the pupil implies 2-mm decentration or 30 PD (15°). A reflection in mid-iris might be 3 mm decentered, or 45 PD. A reflection at the limbus implies 45° (90 PD).

The term "Hirschberg method" has come to be associated with any method that measures the position of the corneal reflection of a light source. Photographic methods refer the displacement to the frontal plane and yield a Hirschberg constant of 20 PD/mm.[3] The method, despite its potential accuracy, remains crude because of difficulties in determining exactly the position of the reflection. Visual estimation methods have limited accuracy, photographic methods are slow and cumbersome, and video methods usually lack resolution and require an array of computer equipment. Difficulties with the Hirschberg method include dimness of the reflection for distance measurements and lack of control of accommodation for near measurements, especially if the light that produces the reflection is also used as the fixation target. The way the test is usually described does not allow for the angle kappa, although it could be taken into account.

The *Krimsky methods*[4] improve on the Hirschberg method by quantifying the location of the reflection with prisms. The method is very useful with small children because minimal positioning or interaction with the patient is required. As originally described, prisms are placed in front of the fixating eye until the corneal reflection is centered in the deviating eye. The prism size is then taken as a measure of the angle of strabismus. Alternatively, the prisms can be placed in front of the deviating eye until the reflection in that eye is centered. The two methods differ by which eye is in primary position when the deviation is measured. If both a primary and a secondary deviation

OBJECTIVE METHODS
CORNEAL LIGHT REFLEX TESTS

exist (see below), these two procedures will provide different results. The method can be further improved if the angle kappa is known for each eye. This can be determined by having each eye fixate the light monocularly (if the eye is able to fixate centrally) and using the resulting position of the reflection as an endpoint to which the reflection is brought by the prisms. This allows for a different angle kappa in each eye and is more accurate than assuming that the reflection should be centered.

The *major amblyoscope* also can be used to generate the corneal reflection. A fixation target is required only on one side. The arms are positioned until the reflection in the nonfixating eye is centered. This is only an approximate method, and if the patient is cooperative enough to sit at the instrument it seems more appropriate to alternately illuminate a target on either side and thus perform the equivalent of a cover test. However, this Hirschberg method is useful when the patient is unable to fixate a target.

The *Maddox tangent scale* can be used to quantify the position of the corneal light reflex. This scale is labeled with degree or PD marks, arranged so that at the calibrated distance, usually 1 m or 5 m, the mark subtends the labeled angle. The patient is asked to look at successive marks until the corneal reflection of a light at the center of the scale is centered on the cornea.

COVER TESTS

The cover test, introduced by Donders,[2] is an easy, simple, and accurate way to assess any strabismus. Combined with prism measurements it provides the quantitative information required for diagnosis and follow-up care. A full assessment of strabismus with the cover test consists of three parts, named here cover test, uncover test, and alternate cover test, although the generic name for this entire group of test procedures is simply "cover test" (Figs. 4.1–4.7). All three tests require the ability and motivation of the subject to maintain fixation on a target specified by the observer. With this limitation, it is as useful for children as for adults. Frequently, motorized toys, movies, or videos are used to capture and hold a child's interest at distance. At near, little toys or pictures are used.

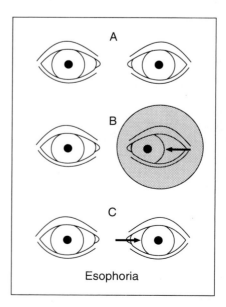

4.1 | Esophoria. *A:* With unobstructed binocular vision the eyes are straight, i.e., the image of the object of regard, or fixation target, falls on the fovea of each eye. Any muscle imbalance is controlled by fusional vergence. *B:* A cover placed in front of one eye disrupts the component of innervation due to binocular vision (fusional vergence) and the covered eye is free to deviate to a position of rest determined by the balance of forces exerted on the eyes by the extraocular muscles and the attached tissues (e.g., optic nerve, Tenon's capsule, conjunctiva). The fixating eye maintains fixation. *C:* With removal of the cover, binocular vision is restored and a change in muscle innervation, called fusional vergence, restores the eyes to bifoveal fixation.

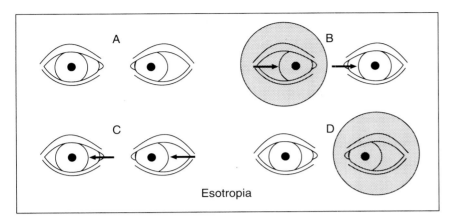

Esotropia

4.2 I Esotropia. *A:* One eye is used for fixation (usually the eye with better vision, or the "dominant" eye if vision is equal). *B:* A cover placed in front of the fixating eye produces a conjugate saccade, leading to fixation with the previously deviated eye. *C:* Removal of the cover leads to refixation with the preferred eye. *D:* Covering the deviated eye results either in no movement of the eyes or in an increase in the angle of deviation if there was partial control of the deviation through peripheral vision, i.e., a phoria component superimposed on the tropia or manifest deviation.

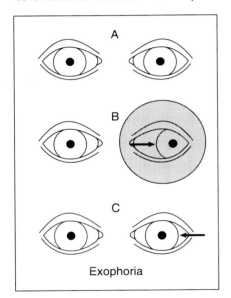

Exophoria

4.3 I Exophoria. *A:* Under binocular conditions the eyes are straight. *B:* An occluder allows a latent muscle imbalance to become manifest in the absence of binocular vision. *C:* Removal of the cover allows recovery of the original alignment.

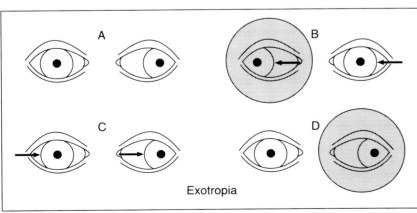

Exotropia

4.4 I Exotropia. *A:* The exotropic eye has a divergent position relative to the fixating, and, therefore, by definition, straight eye. *B:* With instructions to maintain fixation on a specific target, occlusion of the fixating eye leads to a refixation saccade in which the target is foveated by the originally deviated eye. *C:* Removal of the cover leads to a return saccade. If alternate fixation is present, fixation may remain with the originally deviated eye. *D:* Covering the deviated eye has no effect visible to the examiner on fixation with the fixating eye.

4.5 | Hyperphoria. *A:* No manifest deviation is present. *B:* The occluded eye deviates upwards if it has a vertical muscle imbalance (e.g., weakness of depressors relative to elevators). If the sound eye is occluded, vertical fusional vergence innervation is removed and, to maintain gaze on the target, greater downgaze innervation then goes to the fixating eye (which has the relative weakness of depressors), resulting in a greater downgaze response from the sound eye, which then becomes hypotropic. *C:* Restoration of binocular vision yields the original alignment.

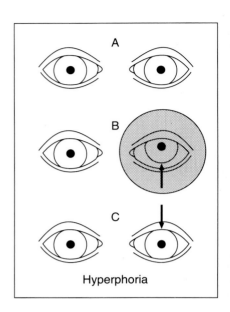

Hyperphoria

4.6 | Hypertropia. *A:* The hyperdeviated eye frequently shows a band of sclera between the iris and lower lid. *B:* Occlusion of the fixating eye leads to a conjugate downward saccade of both eyes. With large deviations the low eye may appear to have a blepharoptosis ("pseudoptosis"). *C:* Removal of the cover and return to the original position. *D:* No effect from covering the deviated eye.

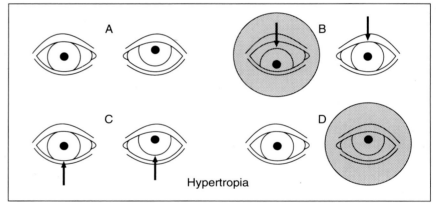

Hypertropia

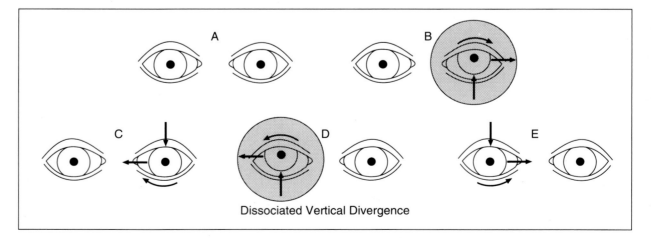

Dissociated Vertical Divergence

4.7 | Dissociated vertical divergence (DVD). *A:* Both eyes are straight under binocular conditions without cover. Usually, DVD is present with at least a small-angle strabismus, most commonly esotropia. *B,D:* Covering either eye results in an upward drift, accompanied by excyclotorsion, of the covered eye. *C,E:* After removal of the cover, the deviated eye returns to its unoccluded position. Sometimes the upward drift is accompanied by a horizontal divergence, i.e., a movement in the exo direction. In some subjects the nonfixating eye is hypodeviated. During occlusion it rises through primary position, returning to its low position on restoration of binocular vision.

In the *cover test,* as fixation is maintained on a target an opaque occluder is interposed over each eye in turn. The uncovered eye is observed for any movement. If this eye was not fixating the target, it will move to take up fixation. A manifest strabismus is then present (a heterotropia, or simply tropia). The direction of movement determines the kind of strabismus present (e.g., if the eye moves away from the nose the eye was deviated inwards and an esotropia exists). If the uncovered eye was already fixating the target, it will not move to take up fixation. The test is then performed on the other eye, because if the eye that was just covered was already deviated the fixating eye will not move, yet a strabismus is present. A complete cover test requires occluding each eye in turn. If no movement is elicited by cover of either eye, no manifest strabismus is present.

In the *uncover test,* the eye that was covered is observed as the cover is removed. If it had deviated as a result of the cover it will move to regain its alignment. This shows a latent deviation, one that is controlled by binocular vision. Such a deviation can be an intermittent deviation (e.g., intermittent exotropia), one that is controlled most of the time, or a muscle imbalance (heterophoria, or simply phoria), a deviation that is controlled all of the time. The movement to realign the eyes is *motor fusion.* The simultaneous binocular sensory perception, including singleness of vision, that results from having the eyes fixate the same target is *sensory fusion.*

For the *alternate cover test* the cover is alternately placed in front of either eye. This maneuver breaks up the vergence posture of the eyes and allows the observation of smaller and better controlled muscle imbalances. It brings out the total deviation, the manifest tropia plus any additional phoria.

Young children may not tolerate anything close to the face. The occluder may therefore have to be held some distance away from the face, thus occluding only the central portion of the visual field in one eye. This does not disrupt fusion as much as the complete field occlusion produced by a close cover but may be the best that can be done. Another alternative is to image the pupils with a mirror system and occlude the eyes remotely from the face, in the plane of this image.[5] Again, only the central visual field is occluded.

Covering an eye also can be useful in assessing the vision of a young child. If the vision in one eye is poor, covering the eye with better vision may elicit crying or efforts to remove the cover. The quality of monocular fixation in terms of steadiness or eccentric fixation can also be evaluated. Only extreme forms of eccentric fixation can be identified in this way, and definitive diagnosis requires the use of an ophthalmoscope that projects a fixation target onto the retina, so that the portion of the retina used for fixation can be directly observed.

PRISM MEASUREMENTS

Prisms are placed in front of one or both eyes to quantify the strabismus elicited by the cover tests (prism and cover measurements). A prism deflects a beam of light at each of its surfaces towards its base. Therefore, the apparent displacement of an object viewed through a prism is towards the apex of the prism. The strength of ophthalmic prisms is measured in units of prism diopters (PD). Prism strength in PD is equal to the deflection of a beam of light passing through the prism measured in centimeters at a distance of 1 meter. A 1-diopter prism will displace the light beam by 1 cm at 1 m. Thus, prism diopters are defined along a tangent scale and not along a circular arc the way degrees are defined. Prism diopters decrease in size the greater the angle. For small angles 1° is equal to 1.7 PD.

For quantitative work, accommodation must be controlled by use of a target containing small letters or pictures, and the subject is given a task that requires resolving the target. Unless accommodation is fairly exact for the target distance, these letters will not be resolved. A light should never be used as a fixation target for prism and cover measurements because it does not control accommodation, resulting in inexact and variable measurements. A light looks much the same whether it is in focus or out of focus on the retina.

When prism measurements are performed, one eye fixates a target in primary position (or whatever reference direction is being measured). The strength of the prism held before the other (deviated) eye is increased until the refixation movement made by each eye as the cover is moved to the opposite eye is just perceptibly reversed. This is a *prism and alternate cover* measurement. It measures the total deviation, consisting of the sum of the manifest deviation (tropia) plus any additional phoria component. In a *simultaneous prism and cover* measurement the cover is placed in front of the fixating eye and the prism in front of the deviated eye simultaneously. The prism strength is increased until the deviated eye makes a barely perceptible movement opposite to what is expected without any prism (e.g., moves further nasally in esotropia). This procedure measures only the manifest deviation. A commonly used convention is to consider that a 2-PD movement is just visible, so 2 then is subtracted from the measurement.[6]

It may be necessary to place the prisms in front of both eyes for large deviations; then neither eye will have been in primary position (or whatever the reference direction is) for that measurement. The prismatic effect of spectacle lenses can produce errors in the measurements. Spectacle lenses are centered on the assumption that the eyes are parallel for distance vision. In strabismus, the deviated eye has a prismatic effect that depends on the strength of the lenses and the size of the deviation. Prisms are manufactured to be used with their base parallel to the direction from the eye to the fixation target. This orients the prism near its position of minimal deviation. Stacking prisms in front of one eye violates this assumption and can lead to large measurement errors. However, vertical and horizontal prisms can be stacked with minimal error.[7]

Primary and secondary deviations result when the deviation is greater with one eye fixating in primary position than with the other eye fixating in the same position. The secondary deviation is the greater of the two. This situation is caused by a muscle paresis or by a mechanical restriction to globe rotation. The paretic muscle or restricted eye must therefore receive a higher level of innervation to reach the target. By Hering's law of equal innervation, the higher level of innervation goes to the yoke muscle in the normal eye, which responds by rotating further, and thus giving a greater deviation. Although they are usually measured for primary position, primary and secondary deviations can exist for any direction of gaze.

ROUTINE TESTING

Minimal routine testing for strabismus involves measurement of any deviation in primary position, at distance and near. The deviation for eyes down at near is important for reading. The near deviation also can be measured through +3.00 lenses or -3.00 lenses to determine the AC/A ratio (accommodative convergence/ accommodation) by the gradient method. In addition, the deviation can be measured (usually at distance) in the secondary eye positions: up, down, right, and left gaze. These measurements will show horizontal or vertical incomitance or an A or V pattern. Measurement in the tertiary positions (up and right, up and left, down and right, down and left) is usually done only at near, due to difficulties of positioning the head to allow gaze in these directions at distance without tilting the head, which can change the vertical deviation. The measurements in the tertiary positions are useful in evaluating vertical deviations. All these measurements are made in at least 25° to 30° of gaze away from primary position. The diagonal directions should have 25° to 30° of both vertical and horizontal gaze. Measurements made at even more extreme positions of eccentric gaze can be useful diagnostically, even though they may not reflect deviations that occur with normal eye movements. A deviometer is a device to accurately and reproducibly present a target in a certain direction of gaze for prism and cover measurements. It allows consistent positioning of targets on successive occasions. The combination of secondary and tertiary positions has been referred to as "cardinal positions" (eight positions), but the term is not consistently used this way. It is more frequently used for the six side positions, in which yoke pairs of muscles are active. The name "diagnostic positions" has been given to the combination of primary position plus secondary and tertiary positions of gaze (nine positions) (Fig. 4.8).

Figure 4.8. Gaze Directions

Name	Number of Directions	Directions
Primary	1	Straight ahead
Secondary	4	Directly
		Right
		Left
		Up
		Down
Tertiary	4	Diagonally
		Up and right
		Down and right
		Up and left
		Down and left
Midline	2	Straight up
		Straight down
Cardinal	6	Up and right
		Right
		Down and right
		Up and left
		Left
		Down and left
Diagnostic	9	Cardinal and primary
		and midline

In the head tilt test, any deviation is measured in primary position with the head tilted towards either shoulder (Fig. 4.9). The otolith reflex will attempt to change the torsional posture of the eyes in a direction appropriate to preserve the verticality of the retinal vertical meridians. When the head is tilted right, for example, the two vertical muscles on the superior surface of the right eye, which both intort the eye, will be activated. If the superior oblique muscle is paretic, the superior rectus will not have its elevating force opposed by the superior oblique's depressing force, and the eye will go high. Therefore, in a superior oblique paresis the hypertropia will be made worse by head tilt to the same side as the paretic muscle.

SUBJECTIVE TESTS
DIPLOPIA TESTS

These tests are subjective. The *red glass test* is done by placing a red glass in front of one eye, creating a red and white image of a fixation light. Horizontal and vertical prisms are placed in front of the eyes until the patient reports that the lights are superimposed. Alternatively, the Maddox tangent scale can be used with the red glass test. The patient reports the scale mark at which he sees the red light while the fixing eye is observing the white light.

The *Maddox rod* consists of an array of adjacent small glass cylinders. The refractive power of the cylinders is so great that a light source viewed through the array is blurred into a streak of light. The patient sees a streak with one eye and the point light source with the other. The streak is oriented vertically to measure horizontal deviations and horizontally to measure vertical deviations. Crossed or uncrossed diplopia is readily determined by asking if the point light is to the right or left of the vertical line (Fig. 4.10). To measure a deviation, a point source of light is viewed and prisms are placed horizontally or vertically (depending on the orientation of the Maddox rod) in front of either eye until the patient reports superimposition of the streak with the light. The Maddox rod precludes fusion and therefore cannot distinguish a phoria from a tropia, but it is not as effective at completely disrupting fusion as the opaque occluder used in the cover test. Phoria measurements made with a Maddox rod may therefore not be identical to those made with cover testing. A further defect with the method is that a point light source does not control accommodation (Fig. 4.11).

4.9 | The head tilt test is performed by tilting the head towards either shoulder and performing prism and cover measurements. The head must be tilted to both sides and the measurements compared. Note that the prism is tilted with the head. Any deviation is defined in coordinates relative to the head.

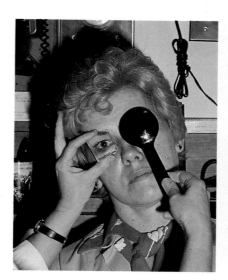
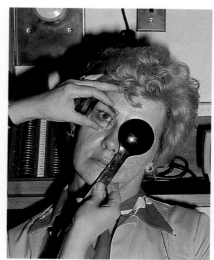

The *double Maddox rod test* is used to measure the torsional position of the eyes. A Maddox rod is placed before each eye in a trial frame. It is convenient if the rods are of different colors. The patient then rotates one of the rods until the two streaks are parallel. It is useful to have the first line positioned according to the patient's subjective impression of vertical or horizontal. This judgement is quite easy to make. Then the second streak is matched to that position. The second streak by itself then will also be horizontal or vertical. The angle of torsion can then be read off the angular scale used for cylinder axes, and the total degrees of torsion between the eyes calculated.

HAPLOSCOPIC TESTS

The haploscope presents each eye with a target identifiably different from the other. The common methods of identifying the images are by color, red–green goggles, and red–green lights (Lancaster red–green test, Hess screen), or with mirrors (Lee's screen, major amblyoscope).

The *Lancaster red–green test* uses a white screen ruled in 2° steps seen from the test distance (usually 7 cm spacing between the lines with no correction for the tangent error, to be observed from 2 m). Red–green goggles are worn. The examiner places a red or green line on the screen with a small projector and the patient then superimposes the other color line from

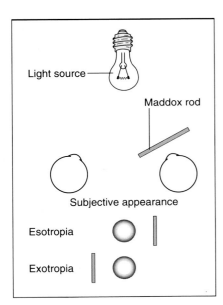

4.10 | In Maddox rod testing the subject looks at a light source. The Maddox rod in front of one eye blurs the point light source into a streak. The esotrope will see the streak on the same side as the Maddox rod, i.e., the patient will have homonymous diplopia. The exotrope will see the streak on the opposite side, indicating heteronymous diplopia. The streak may not be seen if suppression is too marked.

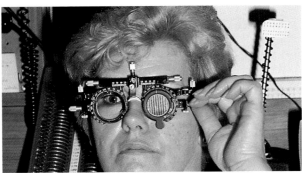

4.11 | The Maddox rod can be used to test for torsion in a variety of ways. The subject can rotate the rod to align the streak with a subjective sense of the horizon or with a visible line. A second Maddox rod of differing color can be placed before the second eye and both streaks aligned to the horizon or to each other. The angle of tilt is read off the axis scale of the trial frame. No single method has been accepted as standard, so the method used should be recorded with the measurement.

another projector. The position of the two lines is recorded. Each line represents the position of one of the foveas. An advantage of this method is that because it uses elongated targets it can give some indication of torsion.

The *Hess screen* uses a black screen containing red dots or LEDs at positions 15° and 30° away from fixation, vertically and horizontally. The patient superimposes a green pointer over the various red dots and the position of the pointer is recorded. The goggles are reversed to test the second eye. The test is usually performed at 0.5 m. It is particularly useful for analyzing possible paretic conditions (finding primary and secondary deviations).

The *Lee's screen* works in the same way as the Hess screen, except that the visual space of the eyes is separated with a mirror. A retroilluminated screen is used to present the stimuli on one screen and the patient responds by visually superimposing a pointer on the second screen (Fig. 4.12).

The *major amblyoscope* can be used to measure the angle of strabismus. In objective testing a fixation target is placed in each arm and the arms are alternately illuminated. The arms are positioned until no refixation eye movement occurs when the illumination alternates. Some models of amblyoscope allow the positioning of targets in torsion as well as horizontally and vertically.

EVALUATION OF DUCTIONS AND VERSIONS

A complete assessment of the ocular motility status requires, in addition to prism and cover measurements, an evaluation of the ductions and versions. The terminology of eye movements is summarized in Figure 4.13.

Ductions are movements of each eye considered by itself. Typically, the test is performed by having the eye follow a target into the extreme positions of gaze. The extent of adduction, abduction, elevation, and depression are noted, and the ductions in the two eyes are compared. Abduction should bring the lateral limbus to the lateral canthus. Adduction should bring the junction of the nasal and middle thirds of the cornea to a vertical line over the inferior lacrimal punctum. In this position very little sclera is visible nasally. The limbus test of Kestenbaum[8] is very useful in quantifying ductions. The movement of the limbus from primary position that results from an eye movement is measured with a millimeter rule. Abduction, adduction, and depression should all have 10 mm of rotation. Elevation is normal at 5 to 7 mm. Elevation and depression in adduction and abduction also should be examined and compared between the two eyes.

Versions are eye movements resulting from a change in the direction of gaze (elicited through any of the ocular motor control systems). When both eyes move in approximately the same direction this is a conjugate version. When the directions are different the movement is disjugate. The test is usu-

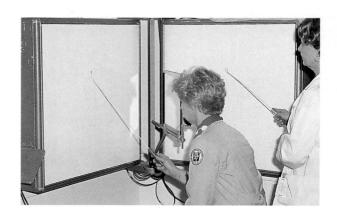

4.12 | The Lee's screen device is used to record primary and secondary deviations in strabismus. The visual fields of the two eyes are separated by a mirror. The subject superimposes a pointer, visible only to one eye, on the location of the examiner's pointer, viewed only by the other eye. Each eye in turn takes the role of viewing eye and answering eye.

ally performed by having the eyes follow a target into the various directions of gaze. Excessive or deficient movements are watched for. Gaze palsy will manifest as difficulty in achieving or in maintaining extreme gaze postures.

Quantification of the amplitude of versions or ductions can be performed on a Goldmann perimeter or tangent screen. An accommodative target

4.13. Eye Movement Nomenclature

DUCTION: UNIOCULAR EYE ROTATIONS; ONLY ONE EYE IS CONSIDERED

COMMON TERM	ALTERNATIVE TERMS	MOVEMENT
Adduction		Rotation towards the nose
Abduction		Rotation away from the nose
Elevation	Sursumduction Supraduction	Rotation upwards
Depression	Infraduction Deorsumduction	Rotation downwards
Intorsion	Incycloduction Conclination	Upper pole of cornea moves inwards
Extorsion	Excycloduction Disclination	Upper pole of cornea moves outwards
Dextrocycloduction		Upper pole of cornea moves to the right
Levocycloduction		Upper pole of cornea moves to the left

VERSION: CONJUGATE MOVEMENT OF BOTH EYES IN THE SAME DIRECTION

COMMON TERM	ALTERNATIVE TERMS	MOVEMENT
Right gaze	Dextroversion	Both eyes to the patient's right
Left gaze	Levoversion	Both eyes to the patient's left
Up gaze	Sursumversion Supraversion	Both eyes upwards
Down gaze	Deorsumversion Infraversion	Both eyes downwards
Dextrocycloversion		Upper pole of each cornea rotates to the right
Levocycloversion		Upper pole of each cornea rotates to the left

VERGENCE: DISJUGATE OF DISJUNCTIVE MOVEMENT OF THE EYES IN OPPOSITE DIRECTIONS

COMMON TERM	ALTERNATIVE TERMS	MOVEMENT
Convergence		Both eyes turn inwards
Divergence		Both eyes turn outwards
Positive vertical divergence	Supravergence Sursumvergence	Right eye higher than left eye
Negative vertical divergence	Infravergence Deorsumvergence	Right eye lower than left eye
Incyclovergence		Upper pole of each cornea moves inwards
Excyclovergence		Upper pole of each cornea moves outwards

with small letters is used to ensure foveal fixation. The target is moved through the cardinal directions into peripheral gaze. Beyond the limit of eye rotation foveation cannot be maintained and the letters can no longer be resolved. Rotation of 50° is normal. Older subjects have reduced elevation. The field of binocular vision can be similarly measured. For this a spot of light is used as the fixation target and the gaze angle at which diplopia begins is noted.

VERGENCES

Vergences are slow, disjunctive eye movements made in response to a change in innervation level (a step of innervation without the preceding pulse). They occur either as part of the near synkinesis or to achieve exact alignment of the eyes for sensory fusion. In natural use of the eyes, most vergence changes are made in conjunction with a saccadic shift in fixation to a target at a change in distance from the subject. Relative fusional divergence controls an esodeviation. Relative fusional convergence controls an exodeviation. By convention, the vertical vergence required to control a left hyperphoria is called a positive vertical vergence. A negative vertical vergence controls a right hyperphoria.

Fusional vergence amplitudes can be measured with an accommodative target (relative fusional vergences) or on a light (absolute fusional vergences). To measure relative fusional vergences, gaze is directed to an accommodative target and increasing prism is introduced in front of one eye, usually with a prism bar or a rotary prism (Fig. 4.14). The major amblyoscope can also be used to present targets in increasingly disparate directions as the arms are moved away from an orthotropic alignment. In either method the patient is asked to report when the object appears to be double. The prism power to reach this breakpoint is the vergence amplitude. The prism power is then reduced until fusion is regained. This is the recovery point. A full characterization of the relative fusional vergence amplitudes requires that both numbers be obtained. The recovery should be within 2 to 4 PD of the breakpoint. A greater difference indicates difficulty in recovering fusion once it is broken and can provide a source of visual symptoms. When convergence is being tested the patient may throw in accommodation to aid convergence. This will result in blurring of the accommodative target. The prismatic power at which blur occurs should also be recorded. At distance, normal fusional convergence is 14 PD, divergence 6 PD, and vertical 2.5 PD.[9,10] At 25 cm, convergence is 38 PD, divergence 16 PD, and vertical 2.5 PD. To test fusional convergence the prism is placed base in; to test fusional divergence the prism is placed base out. Positive vertical vergence is determined by placing an increasing amount of prism base down over the right eye and negative vertical vergence with the prism base up over the right eye (or the equivalent positions for the left eye).

Fusional vergence amplitudes may build up with time as a deviation progressively develops. This is commonly seen with congenital vertical deviations

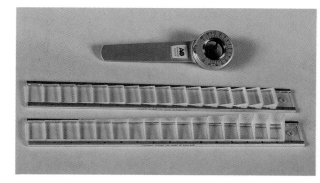

4.14 | Vergence amplitudes may be tested with either a rotary prism (top) or prism bars (bottom). The rotary prism has two vertical prisms mounted so that the vertical powers cancel out. When rotated in opposite directions the vertical components continue to neutralize each other, but the horizontal components add. The prism is held in front of one eye while gaze is maintained on an accommodative target. The horizontal prism power is then gradually increased until fusion can no longer be maintained. The prism bar presents prisms of increasing strength, in horizontal or vertical orientation, depending on the prism bar used. The small increase in power from one prism to the next makes no difference in the measured vergence amplitude.

and in intermittent exotropia. Orthoptic training can exercise the fusional mechanisms and lead to an increased vergence amplitude. Fusional vergence amplitudes may be reduced by poor visual acuity (on a refractive basis or due to amblyopia), fatigue, illness, or drugs (e.g., ethanol or tranquilizers).[11]

AC/A RATIO

The accommodative convergence to accommodation (AC/A) ratio is the change in convergence elicited by a change of accommodation. The convergence is usually measured in prism diopters and the accommodation in diopters. In the *gradient method* the accommodative fixation target is kept at a constant near distance and the stimulus to accommodation that the target provides is changed by interposing lenses (+1, +2, +3, -1,-2 -3) before both eyes. The deviation is measured for each test lens. Usually the test is abbreviated and only a +3 diopter lens is used. The calculation is made using the dioptric value of the stimulus to accommodation (stimulus AC/A ratio). If an optometer is available to measure the actual accommodation, a response AC/A ratio can be determined. In the *heterophoria method* the deviation is measured at distance and near, with only distance spectacle correction in place. A greater eso- or lesser exodeviation at near is considered a high AC/A ratio, and a lesser eso- or greater exodeviation at near is considered a low AC/A ratio.

The exact procedure to determine the AC/A ratio requires several steps. The accommodation of the eyes must be balanced so that each eye is accommodating equally, i.e., one eye must not be underplussed or overminused with respect to the other. A low plus lens is added over each eye for distance and additional plus added to each eye as needed until the 20/30 line is just blurred. The initial low plus blurring lenses for both eyes then are removed. The interpupillary distance (IPD) is measured for distance in centimeters. The phoria or tropia at distance and near are then measured by use of an accommodative target. The distance to the fixation target in diopters can be converted to the required amount of convergence in prism diopters by knowing the IPD.

$$\frac{100}{\text{Fixation distance (cm)}} = \frac{\text{PD of convergence}}{\text{IPD (cm)}}$$

The average patient is orthophoric at distance and mildly exophoric at near. For near fixation at 33.3 cm, with an AC/A of 4 PD/1D and an IPD of 6 cm, 18 PD of convergence are required (by the above formula). With the AC/A of 4, three diopters of accommodation will evoke 12 PD of convergence, leaving an exophoria of 6 PD. It follows that if the distance and near phoria measurements are the same the AC/A equals the IPD (see also Chapter 8, p.8).

A patient with an IPD of 6 cm shows orthophoria at distance and an esophoria at 33.3 cm of 8 PD. With a 6-cm IPD he must converge 18 PD at a distance of 33.3 cm. The near measurment is 8 esophoria, so the actual convergence is 18 + 8 = 26. The stimulus AC/A is then 26 PD/3 D, or $8^2/3/1$ D.

NPC

The near point of convergence (NPC) is measured to quantitatively evaluate convergence. A fixation target is placed 40 cm from the eyes in the midplane of the head and is brought progressively closer to the patient. When convergence can no longer be increased, one eye will deviate outwards. The distance from the lateral canthus to the target is taken as the near point of convergence. A normal NPC should be no greater than 10 cm. Deficient convergence is called convergence insufficiency. The eye that maintains fixation is usually considered to be the dominant eye, but several other tests exist for ocular dominance, such as sighting through a hole in a card.

SENSORY ADAPTATIONS IN STRABISMUS

Gary R. Diamond

VISUAL CONFUSION AND DIPLOPIA

If binocularity is established early in an infant's life it will be maintained unless sight is lost in either eye. When an individual develops strabismus, corresponding retinal elements in the two eyes are no longer similarly directed. This puts the individual at risk for developing two specific visual phenomena, both potentially quite uncomfortable: visual confusion and diplopia. These terms have specific meaning. Visual confusion is the simultaneous perception of dissimilar objects projecting on corresponding retinal elements (the two foveas, for example). Diplopia is the perception of one object projecting on two different (noncorresponding) retinal areas (Fig. 5.1). By considering the retina to be divided into a central, rod-free area roughly corresponding to the fovea (central 2.5 degrees), and a peripheral area, it is clear that the newly strabismic patient who has binocularity is confronted by four separate potential problems: central confusion; central diplopia; peripheral confusion; and peripheral diplopia.

Central confusion is immediately obviated in individuals of any age because the rod-free retinal areas cannot simultaneously perceive disparate targets. The fovea in the strabismic eye is immediately enveloped in a scotoma roughly 2.5 degrees in diameter.[1] This can be demonstrated in oneself by manually displacing one eye with a finger and noting the immediate decrease in visual acuity in that eye.

The onset of a new strabismus in children over the age of 7 to 9 years, and in all adults, will cause peripheral confusion, central diplopia, and central confusion unless it is successfully controlled by the fusional vergence system, by occluding one eye, or if severely decreased visual acuity is present in one eye. Even patients with acuity as low as 2/200 can experience severe symptoms resulting from visual confusion and diplopia.

SUPPRESSION AND ANOMALOUS RETINAL CORRESPONDENCE

Children under the age of 7 to 9 years are usually able to achieve the sensory adaptations of suppression and anomalous retinal correspondence (ARC).[2] These adaptations may develop rapidly or slowly after the appearance of strabismus, and usually occur together. Suppression scotomas obviate central diplopia by encompassing the retinal area on which the foveally viewed image in the aligned eye projects within a facultative, absolute scotoma (facultative, in that the scotoma is only present when that eye is strabismic, and absolute in that no image can be visualized within). When the strabismic eye fixes, the scotoma immediately disappears, only to reappear when the eye again is misaligned.

Interestingly, the shape and size of the suppression scotoma are different in an esotrope than in an exotrope.[3] An esotrope usually exhibits a small, round scotoma enveloping only the nasal retinal area within which the foveally viewed image in the aligned eye projects, although occasionally a

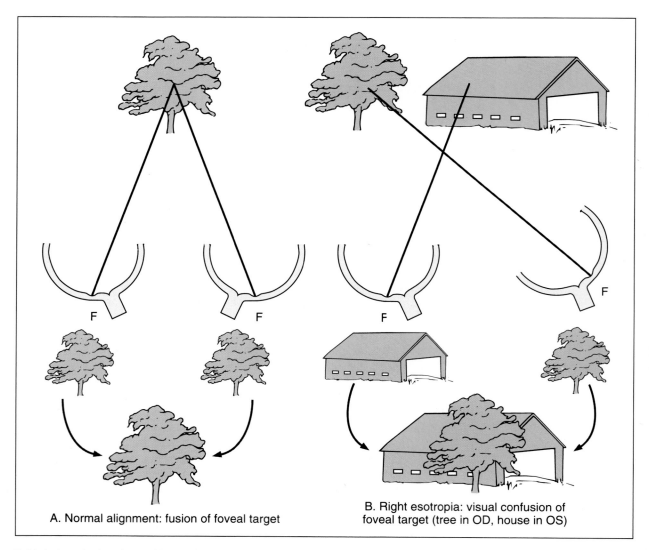

A. Normal alignment: fusion of foveal target

B. Right esotropia: visual confusion of foveal target (tree in OD, house in OS)

5.1 | *A:* A typical patient with straight eyes will fuse foveal targets. *B:* Binocular patient with right esotropia, with visual confusion of foveal targets. This does not exist clin-ically, as the fovea in the turned eye cannot accept an image disparate from that seen by the fovea in the straight, fixing eye.

somewhat larger suppressed retinal area can be demonstrated. An exotropic patient's suppression scotoma is much larger, encompassing the temporal retinal area on which the foveally viewed image in the aligned eye projects and, in addition, the entire area extending to a vertical line bisecting the fovea (Fig. 5.2). Postulated explanations for this difference include developmental and teleological differences between the nasal and temporal hemiretinas, the intermittent nature of many exodeviations, the constant nature of many esodeviations, and others, but no explanation is entirely convincing. Suppression scotomas can be demonstrated in patients who have strabismus by using testing techniques described in Chapter 6.

Peripheral visual confusion and peripheral diplopia are obviated in the newly strabismic child by the development of ARC, a reassignment of cortical directional values to "impose" comfortable, simultaneous perception on dissimilar retinal elements, essentially a "superimposition" of such dissimilar elements (Fig. 5.3). This reassignment of cortical directional values is quite flexible, enabling patients who have incomitant and intermittent forms of strabismus to maintain visual comfort despite varying deviation angles in different gaze positions. As described in Chapter 6, different sensory tests may demonstrate persistence of normal retinal correspondence (NRC) in certain patients who have known ARC and, conversely, persistence of ARC in

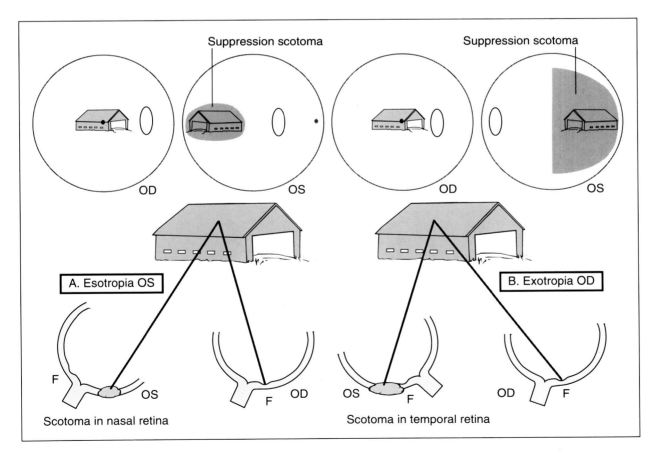

5.2 | *A:* Patient with esotropia in the left eye. A nasal retinal suppression scotoma obviates central diplopia.

B: Patient with exotropia in the left eye. A temporal retinal suppression scotoma obviates central diplopia.

patients who have realigned visual axes; thus, one must understand the limitations of the various sensory tests commonly used to diagnose ARC.

As ARC is infinitely flexible, fusional vergence is not required for visual comfort and, in fact, can rarely be demonstrated. Stereoptic appreciation, as demonstrated by readily available clinical testing, also is not found in patients with ARC, although specialized testing can demonstrate primitive stereoptic appreciation in some patients.

MONOFIXATION SYNDROME

Many binocular patients who have a small or absent tropia (up to 8 prism diopters eso or exo, and 4 vertically) and possible superimposed phoria exhibit monofixation syndrome (MS), a sensory state comprising features of both NRC and ARC (Fig. 5.4). Initially known by many terms, each explain-

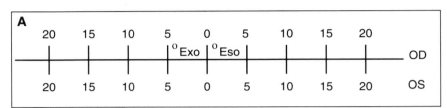

Normal retinal correspondence in aligned eyes

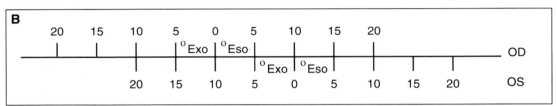

Objective and subjective cortical directional values 10° esotropia OD with normal retinal correspondence are identical. Resultant peripheral visual confusion and diplopia

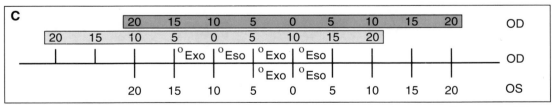

Objective (grey) eye alignment and subjective (red) cortical directional values 10° esotropia OD with anomalous retinal correspondence. Resultant single binocular vision and comfort

5.3 | *A:* Patient with aligned eyes. The visual cortex interprets the location of objects eccentric to fixation in each eye as coming from the same direction in space (noted as degrees from fixation). This is termed normal retinal correspondence. *B:* Patient with esotropia and normal retinal correspondence. The visual cortex receives images of two objects for each direction in space; this causes peripheral confusion. Also, each object in space will stimulate noncorresponding retinal elements in the eyes, leading to peripheral diplopia. *C:* Patient with esotropia and abnormal retinal correspondence. The visual cortex reassigns directional values to objects viewed with the deviating eye to correspond with those values in the aligned eye. These subjective directional values (shown in red) permit a form of comfortable single binocular vision by obviating peripheral confusion and peripheral diplopia. The objective alignment of the right eye appears 10 degrees esotropic to the examiner (gray values).

ing one sensory or motor component of the complete syndrome (Fig. 5.5), the generally accepted name MS emphasizes the essential feature of this syndrome, the presence of peripheral fusion without central fusion.[4] This means that only one rod-free retinal area (fovea) is viewing at a given time. Therefore, these patients will demonstrate an absolute, facultative central scotoma, usually measuring 2.5 to 3 degrees which, like a suppression scotoma seen in binocular patients who have childhood-onset strabismus and larger tropias, is present only when a given fovea is not fixing (Fig. 5.6). Precise terminology restricts the term *suppression scotoma* to that arising to obviate central diplopia. Because many patients with MS have no tropia, central diplopia presumably does not consistently occur. If the viewing foveas alternate freely in a young child, amblyopia will not occur; if one fovea is preferred, amblyopia can occur even in patients who do not have a demonstrably strabismic appearance, emphasizing the need for amblyopia screening in the young.

Peripheral fusion and demonstrable fusional vergence amplitudes (often of normal amount) usually are demonstrable in patients with MS and provide a generally stable alignment.[5] Presumably, the expanded nature of the peripheral Panum fusional area permits peripheral fusion to develop despite a small tropia (Fig. 5.7). Perhaps this reflects the greater than one-to-

Figure 5.4. Features of Monofixation Syndrome

CONSISTENT WITH NORMAL RETINAL CORRESPONDENCE

Presence of measurable fusional vergence amplitudes
Presence of stereopsis (to 67 arc seconds) in many
Relatively stable alignment
Demonstrable peripheral fusion
No measurable tropia in many

CONSISTENT WITH ANOMALOUS RETINAL CORRESPONDENCE

Small tropia in some
Lack of stereoptic appreciation in some

Figure 5.5. Older Terms for Monofixation Syndrome

Monofixational phoria
Microtropia
Microstrabismus
Eso flick strabismus
Small angle strabismus

one linkage between peripheral retinal photoreceptors and ganglion cells. Stereoscopic ability is often found, but it is rarely better than 67 arc seconds, as only one fovea is used in binocular viewing.[6] Note that the sensory status of patients with MS is the same whether or not a small tropia exists, although those who have large superimposed phorias may sometimes have asthenopic complaints.

Sensory testing will show peripheral without central fusion, possible stereoscopic appreciation (although never to normal limits), and generally normal fusional vergence amplitude. If the patient has a phoria superimposed on a small tropia, alternate cover testing will demonstrate larger strabismus than cover–uncover or simultaneous prism-and-cover testing.

Patients with MS exhibit sensory characteristics closer to NRC than ARC, i.e., the presence of fusional vergence amplitudes and possible gross stereoptic appreciation, although those who have a small tropia will not have precise alignment of corresponding retinal elements. Cover testing will show roughly 22% without phoria or tropia, 34% with phoria only, and 44% with a tropia and superimposed phoria, occasionally up to 20 prism diopters. Only MS permits the existence of a measurable tropia and superimposed phoria. Because of the absence of simultaneous foveal viewing, young patients are at risk for development of amblyopia, and approximately two thirds do become amblyopic, 90% if they also have a tropia. In the absence of anisometropia, three quarters of monofixating patients will be amblyopic

5.6 | Monofixation syndrome with no tropia. Note the central scotoma enveloping the area seen by the left fovea, but fusion of peripheral information.

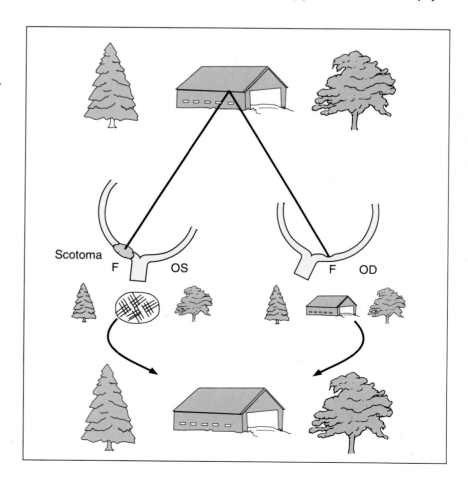

Of successfully aligned "congenital" esotropes who have monofixation syndrome, one third will be amblyopic. The amblyopia should be treated as described elsewhere, but once lost, central fusion (bifoveality) cannot be reestablished.

MS can develop spontaneously by unknown means, can be caused by anisometropia, is the best expected sensory state in patients who have "congenital" strabismus after successful surgical alignment, and is found in patients who have acquired unilateral organic foveal lesions (such as toxoplasmosis), although in the last instance the scotoma usually is larger.

Central fusion (bifoveal viewing with the possibility for superb stereoptic appreciation) can occur in the presence of very minimal deviation of the visual axes, less than that detectable by cover testing, and is termed *fixation disparity*; it measures roughly 14 minutes of arc (perhaps half a prism diopter) and is present in most individuals.[7] It should not be confused with MS.

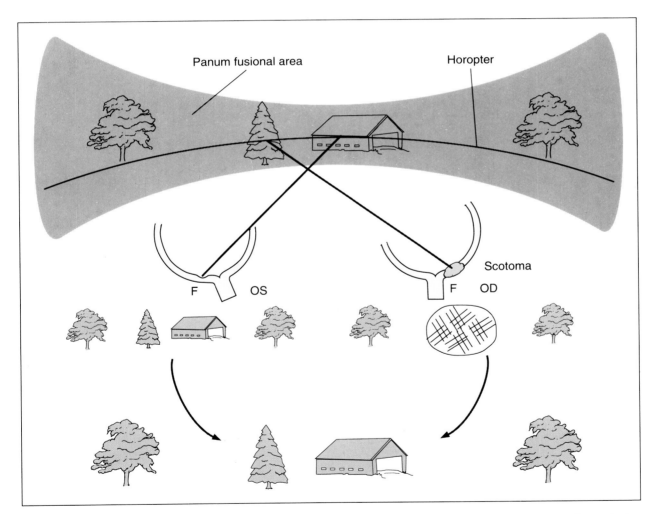

5.7 | Monofixation syndrome with 4 prism diopter right esotropia. Note the right central scotoma preventing perception of the central tree under binocular viewing conditions, but fusion of peripheral information (trees). The horopter is an infinitely thin surface in space containing all object points projecting to corresponding retinal points. It is surrounded by the Panum fusional area, within which objects in space can be fused even though projecting on noncorresponding retinal points.

6

EVALUATION OF SENSORY STATUS IN STRABISMUS

Howard M. Eggers

Evaluation of the binocular sensory status in strabismus involves the determination of visual functions other than visual acuity. Some of the visual capabilities acquired through simultaneous perception by the two eyes are perception of movement in depth, binocular summation, and stereopsis. Perturbations of simultaneous binocular vision lead either to the loss of these capabilities or to diplopia, which can require occlusion of an eye for relief.

Singleness of vision involves an integration of the differences in the patterns of retinal stimulation so that a single percept is formed. Stereopsis requires the discrimination of differences between the patterns of stimulation on the two retinas, in terms of parallax geometry, and the construction of a unique, new percept (binocular depth).

PHYSIOLOGY
BINOCULAR SINGLE VISION AND STEREOPSIS

From the standpoint of visual physiology, vision through two eyes requires explanation of singleness of vision and of stereopsis. The term *fusion* is used to describe the single impression wherein the dissimilarity between the images in the two eyes is not observed in the presence of simultaneous perception (i.e., there is not singleness because one image is not perceived, which is called supression). This is *sensory* fusion. The term fusion is also used to describe fusional vergences, i.e., the eye movements that serve to align the eyes so that single vision can occur, better termed *motor* fusion. Sufficiently dissimilar stimuli presented to the two eyes may not be fusible. Retinal rivalry is the result of such a situation; superimposed, unfusible portions of the two images are seen in alternation. Examples of rivalrous stimuli are red and green versions of the same object, each seen by only one eye, or lines seen vertically by one eye and horizontally by the other (Fig. 6.1). Motor fusion and stereopsis may be produced by rivalrous stimuli, so the occurrence of sensory fusion is not a prerequisite for these other physiologic functions.

Stimulation of a small area of the retina with light results in a sensation of light in a particular direction. Such a small patch of retina and its associated direction value is termed a *retinal element*. The fovea of each eye represents the subjective straight-ahead position. Whatever is imaged on the fovea is experienced by the subject as being straight ahead (Hering's *principal visual direction*) (Fig. 6.2). The other retinal elements outside the fovea have direction values that can be assigned coordinates on the basis of direction and angular distance into the periphery, in a pattern depending on direction and distance from the fovea. A fundamental of *binocular* direction localization is that both foveas carry the subjective straight-ahead localization (Hering's law of *identical visual direction*). Corresponding points are a pair of retinal elements, one from each eye, that have the same primary subjective directions (primary in the sense that the directions are those that occur in the absence of sensory fusion). Single vision is thus explained by the fact that objects in the binocular field of vision are seen singly because they stimulate corresponding points.

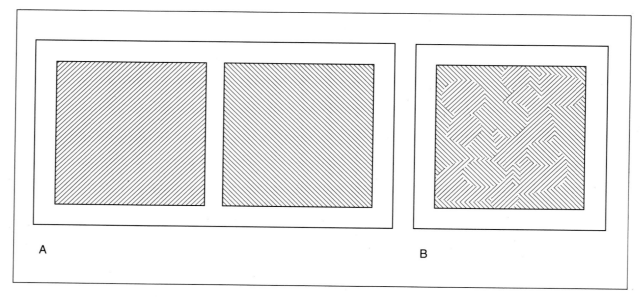

A

B

6.1 | Binocular rivalry occurs when the patterns of stimulation in the two eyes are sufficiently dissimilar that fusion is not possible. *A:* Stereogram consisting of lines oriented orthogonally between the two eyes. *B:* In the resulting binocular percept, the visual input to either eye at times dominates in any portion of the visual field, and the input from the other eye is suppressed.

The idea of corresponding points shows that no difference exists between the stimuli received in the two eyes, and therefore there is no mystery as to why vision with two eyes is single. The locus in physical space of the intersection of the two sets of monocular lines of common visual direction (i.e., corresponding points) is known as the horopter. The location of objects on the horopter explains why those objects are seen as single. The concept of the horopter exists to explain singleness of vision.

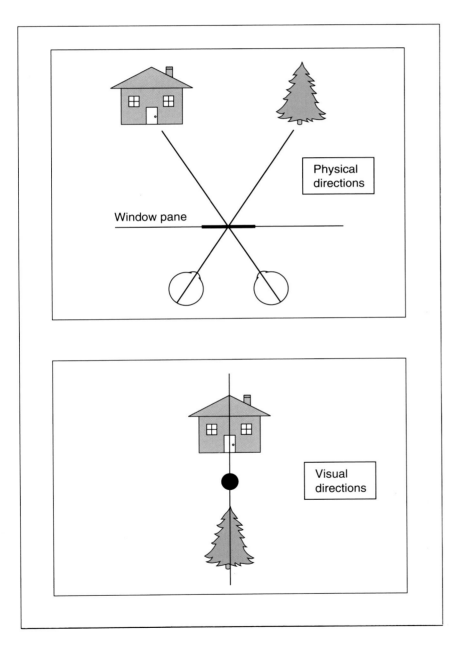

6.2 | Demonstration of Hering's law of the identical visual direction of the two foveas. Whatever is imaged on the fovea is seen as being in the straight-ahead direction. The two eyes fixate a mark on the window pane. In one eye the tree and in the other eye the house have visual directions identical to the window mark and thus are seen to be superimposed, regardless of the true geometry. Seeing two objects in the same location is called visual confusion. Objects remote from the plane of fixation are seen in physiologic diplopia. Therefore, the house and the tree will also be seen diplopically.

In 1838, Wheatstone discovered the adequate stimulus for stereopsis and demonstrated it with his stereoscope[1] (Fig. 6.3). The stimulus for stereopsis originates in the difference in vantage point between the two eyes. Objects, edges, or contours nearer or farther away than the fixation point are displaced, relative to the fixation point, differently in the two eyes (Fig. 6.4). This geometric disparity in position of binocularly observed contours, expressed as an angle, is the feature responsible for eliciting stereopsis. Therefore, no exact stimulation of corresponding points by objects can occur in three-dimensional space.

In actuality, however, for a retinal element in one eye a range of elements exists around the exactly corresponding point in the second eye, any one of which also can fuse with the element in the first eye. This area is called Panum's fusional area (Fig. 6.5). The range of possible fusion thus extends beyond exact correspondence and, in the presence of fusion, the direction values of the fused retinal elements in one or both eyes is modified to accommodate the retinal disparity. The binocularly perceived object that is imaged on noncorresponding retinal loci, but fused within Panum's area, is seen as having only one primary subjective visual direction.

For a stimulus at a fixed retinal locus in one eye, the area of retina in the other eye over which the same stimulus can be displaced and still be seen singly is the definition of Panum's area. It is a retinal threshold for diplopia. During attempted binocular fixation on a stationary target the eyes drift in alignment and small saccades and drifts occur. The vergence posture can change by as much as 5 min arc over a period of a few seconds. This inexactness in the oculomotor system produces variations in the disparity of stimulation at any single retinal location. Under these conditions, Panum's area has a size and shape that depend on the temporal and spatial frequency of the disparity modulation. Under 120 msec flash exposure conditions, Panum's area in the fovea has been found across several subjects to be circular with a mean diameter of 14 min arc.[2,3,] The size of Panum's area increases in the periphery. At 0.5° retinal eccentricity the horizontal extent of Panum's area decreases from 20 min arc at low temporal (0.1 Hz) and spatial (0.125

6.3 | Wheatstone's stereoscope. The visual spaces of the two eyes are separated with mirrors and an independent pattern of stimulation is presented to each eye on a flat surface without depth. A perception of depth is created by the horizontal disparities present between the two stimuli.

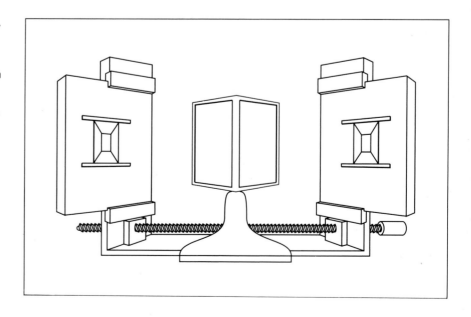

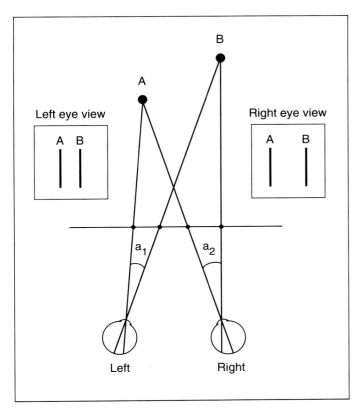

6.4 | Geometrical disparity. The difference in angular separation of objects A and B subtended at the eyes is the geometrical disparity n = a1-a2, expressed in minutes or seconds of arc. The direction of each object can be recorded on a plane interposed between the eye and the object. The separation of the objects as represented on the plane is different in the view of each eye because of the different location of the vantage point of each eye. A perception of depth will be elicited merely by viewing the cards representing the view of each eye. Such a pair of views is a stereogram.

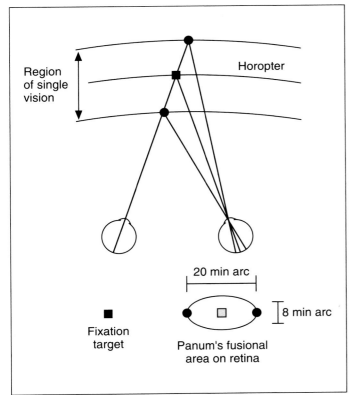

6.5 | Panum's fusional area. As one eye fixates a target (square), a search object is moved in depth. The corresponding point in the second eye is indicated by the gray square, but the fixation target is not visible to the second eye. The ellipse of retinal area, for which typical dimensions are given for 0.5° away from the fovea, is Panum's area, within which diplopia is not appreciated. It allows single vision in a depth of space surrounding the horopter. The depth is grossly exaggerated for clarity.

cyc/°) frequencies to 1.5 min arc at a temporal frequency of 5Hz and spatial frequency of 2 cyc/°. As temporal and spatial frequency increase, the shape changes from a horizontal ellipse, with a width to height ratio of 2.5:1, to a circle[4] (Fig. 6.6).

The geometric disparity produced by the occurrence of objects in depth requires that noncorresponding points be fusible (Panum's area), thus giving the horopter thickness. However, corresponding points do not have to fuse, and in the presence of stereopsis, for sufficient depths, fusion of rather remote, noncorresponding retinal elements may occur[5] (Fig. 6.7). Stereopsis does not require fusion, and objects seen diplopically or with rivalry can create the sensation of depth. Singleness of vision and stereopsis are different neurophysiologic processes. Scatter in the receptive field locations in the two eyes of binocularly responding neurons in the visual cortex allows the selective response of cortical units that have both the appropriate location in the visual field and a disparity in location between the two eyes.

Objects sufficiently far behind or in front of the horopter are seen in physiologic diplopia. Under ordinary circumstances this diplopia is not

6.6 | The size and shape of Panum's area depend on the temporal and spatial frequency of the disparate stimuli. These results were obtained using a line stimulus, offset 0.5° from the fovea, which was modulated in depth in time and along its length in depth for spatial frequency. The horizontal but not the vertical diameter of Panum's area decreases with an increase in temporal frequency of the stimulus. Both the vertical and horizontal diameters decrease with an increase in the spatial frequency. At sufficiently high temporal and spatial frequencies, Panum's area is circular. These results indicate a minimum area determined by spatial frequency and an extension of the horizontal size at low temporal frequencies. Scale mark 10 min arc. (Adapted from Schor CE, Tyler CW: Spatio-temporal properties of Panum's fusional area. *Vis Res 1981;21:683–692.*)

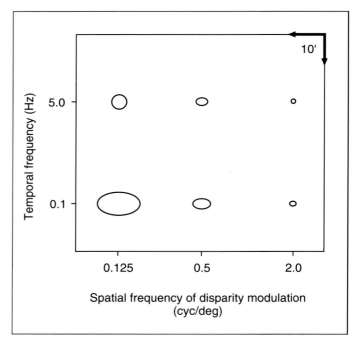

6.7 | Wheatstone's demonstration that, in the presence of stereopsis, corresponding points need not be fused and noncorresponding points may fuse. This stereogram pair is seen stereoscopically as a thin vertical line with a thick line protruding towards the viewer in depth.

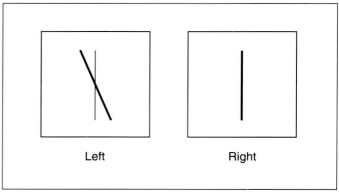

noticed. Physiologic disparity, not to be confused with geometric disparity, is the difference in the visual directions of an object seen diplopically (according to Hering's law of identical visual direction). Such diplopia can be a stimulus for fusional vergence movements of the eyes.

The horopter is the locus of the best depth discrimination and of single vision. For binocular vision, the superior quality of binocular function present on the horopter is analogous to the superior function of the fovea for monocular vision.

A theoretical horopter can be calculated as the locus in space of points having zero retinal disparity relative to the fixation point. Simplifying assumptions are that the eyes are spherical, that the center of rotation is at the nodal point, and that the optics are centered and spherical. The horopter for a horizontal plane containing the fixation point, the nodal points of the eyes, and the foveas is the Vieth–Müller circle (Fig. 6.8). All these assumptions, however, do not hold, and the empirically determined horopter is flatter than the Vieth–Müller circle (the Hering–Hillebrand horopter deviation).[6]

Several criteria can be used to specify the horopter. With the eyes steadily directed to a fixed point, other points can be positioned to elicit identical primary subjective visual directions; appear to lie in a frontoparallel plane; lie in the center of the region of binocular single vision; maximize stereoscopic sensitivity to change in position; and provide no stimulus for a fusional movement of the eyes.

These criteria also define the physiologic significance of the horopter. Many methods exist to determine the empirical horopter. Two of the more

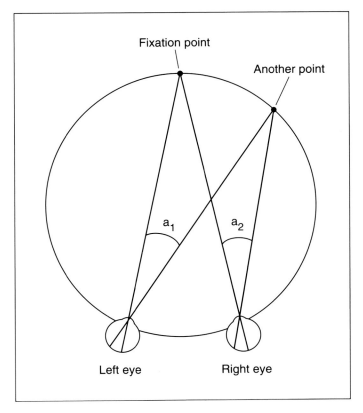

6.8 | The Vieth–Müller circle. If the eyes are assumed to be spherical, with the center of rotation at the nodal point, all points in space with a zero disparity will fall on this circle. This is the same as saying that this circle is the locus of intersection of the projected direction values of corresponding points. Angle a1=a2, by virtue of a theorem in plane geometry that states that all triangles erected on a common chord in a circle (the interocular axis) and having their apex on the circle will have equal apex angles. Therefore, it is assumed that equal retinal distances map into equal angles in space.

commonly implemented criteria are identical visual direction,[7] which specifies the nonius horopter (Fig. 6.9), and the apparent frontoparallel plane.

The apparent frontoparallel plane is determined by presenting the observer with an array of vertical rods, each independently adjustable in depth (Fig. 6.10). While the central rod is observed, the other rods are positioned to lie in the subjectively perceived frontoparallel plane. However, ambiguity exists in the criterion the subject will use—i.e., equidistant from the ego center or truly frontoparallel—and reason to believe that the zero-disparity points should lie on a circle. Meridional magnification of the hori-

6.9 | A horopter determined with the nonius method. The abscissa is the angular distance from the fixation point. The ordinate is the depth from the observer in millimeters. Fixation distance is 40 cm. The actual horopter is flatter than the Veith–Müller circle, and the exact shape depends on the fixation distance. An esophoria is demonstrated by the position of the horopter closer to the observer than the fixation point. In exophoria the horopter is further away than the fixation point. (Reproduced from Ogle KN: *Researches in Binocular Vision.* Philadelphia: WB Saunders, 1950.)

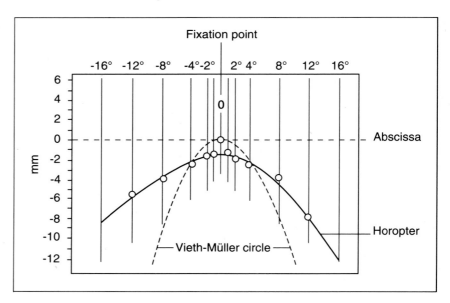

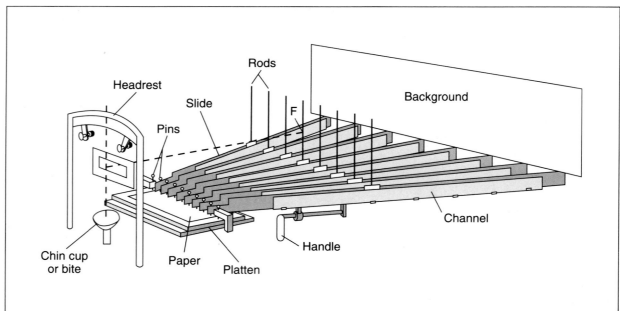

6.10 | Apparatus to determine the apparent frontoparallel plane. The central rod F is fixed. While gaze is maintained on F the peripheral rods are moved to lie at the same subjectively perceived distance. (Reproduced from Ogle KN: *Researches in Binocular Vision.* Philadelphia: WB Saunders, 1950.)

zontal distances in one eye leads to a rotation of the apparent frontoparallel plane around a vertical axis (Fig. 6.11). In the nonius method, the oculocentric visual directions of the two eyes are equated without the possibility of fusion of the stimuli in the two eyes (Fig. 6.12).

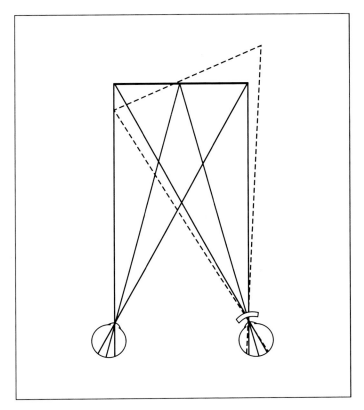

6.11 | Horizontal meridional magnification of the image of one eye, by producing the disparities that would truly result from a rotated plane, causes an apparent rotation of the frontoparallel plane.

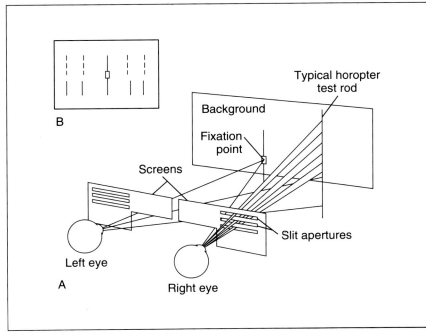

6.12 | The grid–nonius apparatus for determining the horopter. *A:* The central rod is visible to both eyes. The test rod is visible at its bottom to one eye only, and at its top to the other eye only. The masking apertures make the top portion of the test rod appear interrupted to one eye. The task is to position the test rod in distance so that the two halves appear continuous. The nonius horopter is the locus of aligned test rods. *B:* Illustration of the appearance of the rods to the observer. (Reproduced from Ogle KN: *Researches in Binocular Vision.* Philadelphia: WB Saunders, 1950.)

The shape of the horopter in a vertical dimension has been much less investigated than its shape in a horizontal plane of gaze. It tilts away from the observer, the inclination of the tilt being a function of the fixation distance. The tilt derives from the torsional posture of the eyes, the amount of extorsion depending on the fixation distance. The tilt carries the bottom of the horopter to ground level under the eyes (for a standing observer). Determinations of the vertical horopter using the criterion of equidistance[8] (Fig. 6.13) and a nonius method[9] (Fig. 6.14) give qualitatively similar results. A consequence of the tilt of the vertical horopter is that a line must be tilted away from the observer at its top to be seen as truly vertical.

PHYSIOLOGY OF STEREOPSIS

Cues to the perception of depth can be observed either monocularly or binocularly. Monocularly perceivable cues include: the apparent size of objects of known size; interposition of a near object on a more distant one; linear perspective (e.g., converging railroad tracks); aerial perspective, or the loss of contrast in distant objects; monocular movement parallax; effects of light and shade; and gradients of texture (the fading of texture with distance). Except for motion parallax, these cues all can be incorporated into paintings, which represent a view of the world from one vantage point (i.e., monocular).

6.13 | A vertical horopter determined by judgements of equal distance from the observer. The outer surfaces represent the extent of one standard deviation. The plane of equidistance tilts away from the observer. The fixation point is at the waist of the figure. Above and below the fixation point the judgements become increasingly variable. (Reproduced from Amigo G: A vertical horopter. *Optica Acta 1974;21:277–292.*)

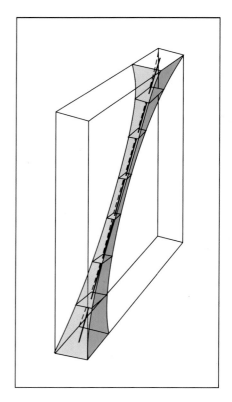

Stereopsis is one of the forms of depth perception. It is a unique sensation, elaborated under conditions of simultaneous binocular vision. It is based on the differences in the horizontal positions of visual contours, nearer or farther away than the fixation point, relative to each other when observed from the vantage point of each eye in three-dimensional space. Wheatstone demonstrated with his stereoscope that horizontal disparity is the adequate stimulus for stereopsis (see Fig. 6.3). Visual features in depth are seen as horizontally displaced relative to the fixation point by different amounts in the two eyes (see Fig. 6.4). This geometric disparity is conventionally expressed as an angle (see Fig. 6.4). The Wheatstone stereoscope presents the appropriate disparity to each eye on a flat card, and a perception of depth results from the disparity. Objects nearer than the fixation point give bitemporal retinal stimulation. Any resulting diplopia would be crossed, and the disparity is said to be crossed or convergent. Objects more distant than the fixation point give binasal retinal stimulation. Any resulting diplopia would be uncrossed, and the disparity is said to be uncrossed or divergent. This nomenclature can be more easily remembered if the reader notes that fixation of a crossed stimulus requires "crossing" of the eyes, and fixation of an uncrossed stimulus requires "uncrossing" of the eyes.

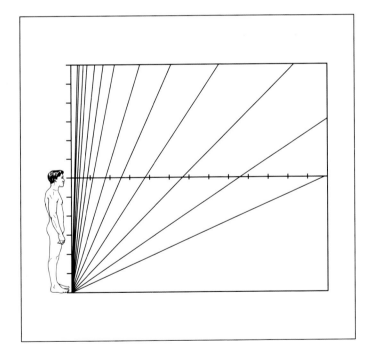

6.14 | The vertical horopter is straight and passes through the fixation point and a point on the ground directly under the eyes (nonius method). (Reproduced from Nakayama K: Geometrical and physiological aspects of depth perception, in Benton S (ed): *Three Dimensional Imaging. [Proc Soc Photo-Optical Instrument Engineers 1977;120:2–9.]*)

With gaze on a fixation point, relative depth (d) to another point depends on a difference of vergence angles (α-β) required to fixate the two points (Fig. 6.15). The required convergence in turn varies with the interpupillary distance (IPD). Thus,

$$d = \frac{IPD}{2\,[\,1/\tan(\alpha/2) - 1/\tan(\beta/2)\,]}$$

expresses depth as a function of IPD and the convergence angles. Then an approximation for disparity (in radians) as a function of relative depth d and distance D is

$$\delta = \frac{IPD \times d}{D^2 + dD}.$$

For small depths at large distances, disparity is proportional to depth.

Vertical disparities naturally occur due to slight torsional or vertical misalignment of the eyes. They also arise from objects off the midline and closer to one eye than the other, requiring slightly unequal angles of vertical gaze. A natural aniseikonia occurs owing to the larger image size resulting from a closer object. Because the two eyes are horizontally separated in the head, stereoscopic mechanisms analyze the horizontal disparity. The tolerance for vertical disparity appears to serve the role of allowing the horizontal mechanisms to work when a slight vertical disparity also exists.

Julesz has shown that a visual contour is not even required, and disparities can be stimulated with a field of random dots, showing that stereopsis

6.15 | *A:* Retinal disparity. The observer fixates at a far point (F). The nearer point (N) is at a distance (d) closer. The difference in vergence angles required to fixate the two points (α-β) is the retinal disparity. It is equal to the sum of the displacements in retinal location of N_R and N_L from F_R and F_L, respectively, on the retina in units of visual angle. *B:* Stereogram of the same near and far objects. *C:* In the retinal image, bifoveal fixation of point F superimposes F_R and F_L. The distance between N_R and N_L is the (crossed) disparity in units of visual angle.

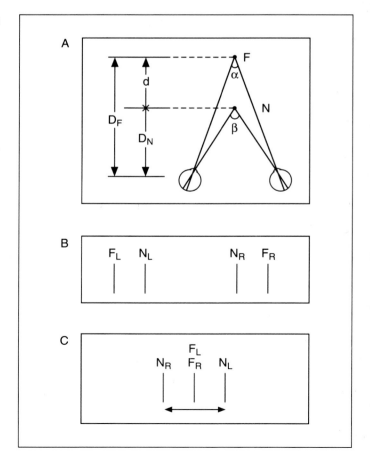

occurs independent of form perception[10,11] (Fig. 6.16). Stereopsis may also arise from rivalrous or nonfusable stimuli (Fig. 6.17).

Stereoacuity is the disparity threshold at which a difference in depth is appreciated. Stereoacuity is best at the fovea and drops off rapidly into the peripheral field and with distance in depth away from the fixation point.

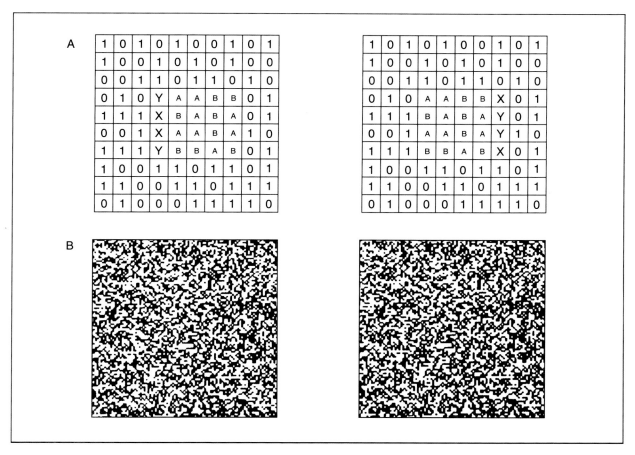

6.16 | Random-dot stereograms. *A:* Construction of a random-dot stereogram. A block of dots is horizontally displaced by an amount equal to the desired disparity. The resulting unmatched patterns are filled up with new random patterns. *B:* A finer-grained stereogram of a square floating above the background. (Reproduced from Julesz B: *Foundations of Cyclopean Perception.* Chicago: University of Chicago Press, 1971.)

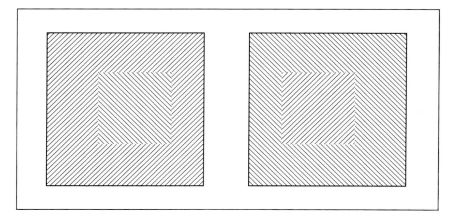

6.17 | A stereogram showing stereopsis produced by nonfusible and rivalrous stimuli. (Reproduced from Kaufman L: On the nature of binocular disparity. *Am J Psychol 1964; 77:398–401.*)

Under optimal conditions the foveal stereoscopic threshold is 10 sec arc, corresponding at arm's length to a depth difference of 0.2 mm. Stereopsis takes some time to develop, and a maximal response requires up to 3 sec. At small displacements in depth from the fixation point, the perception of depth is proportional to the disparity, a relationship termed *patent stereopsis*. At greater disparities, the disparity–depth relationship is lost and localization can reliably be said only to be nearer or farther than the fixation point (*qualitative stereopsis*).[12] In the center of the visual field, up to 7° of convergent (crossed) disparity can be correctly localized in depth, as nearer or farther than the fixation target, before chance levels of performance are reached. Up to 12° of divergent (uncrossed) disparity can be correctly localized under the same conditions.[13,14] Still larger disparities are recognizable in the peripheral visual field. These dimensions are more than an order of magnitude larger than Panum's area and show that stereopsis is not dependent on fusion of the targets.

6.18 I Stereoscopic threshold disparity for peripheral angles of 10°, 5°, and 0° are shown in *A, B,* and *C*, respectively. Fixation distance 43.7 cm. The ordinate is logarithmic. Open and closed symbols represent the data of two subjects. The lines are best fits to the data (least-squares method). (Reproduced from Blakemeore C: The range and scope of binocular depth discrimination in man. *J Physiol (Lond) 1970;211:599–622.*)

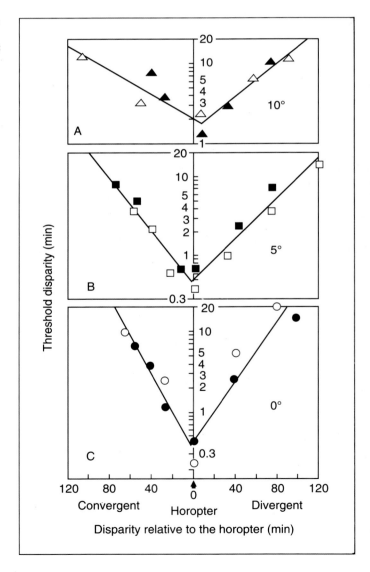

For displacements in depth away from the horopter, the stereothreshold increases exponentially with distance, but less rapidly in the periphery[15] (Fig. 6.18). As targets are moved horizontally along the horopter into the peripheral visual field, the stereothreshold gradually increases[16] (Fig. 6.19). The lowest stereothreshold is at the horopter (Fig. 6.20). The best relative depth discrimination (lowest threshold for difference in depth of targets away from the horopter) is at 5° into the periphery. At the fovea, the more rapid decline of depth discrimination with distance from the horopter may be due to the limits of bilateral cortical representation. The split-brain human cannot see disparities in the middle of his visual field at all, although stereo performance in the periphery is normal.[17] The threshold to detect an

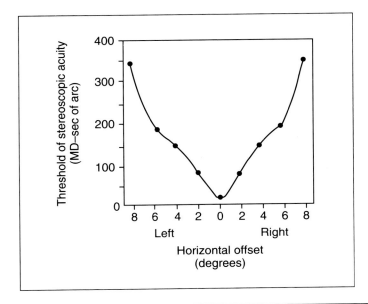

6.19 | Threshold stereoacuity as a function of horizontal angular distance from fixation. (Reproduced from Rawlings SC, Shipley T: Stereoscopic acuity and horizontal angular distance from fixation. *J Opt Soc Am 1969;59:991–993.*)

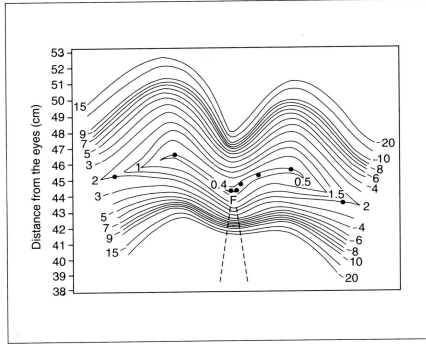

6.20 | Isothreshold disparity contours. The linear scale is approximate for both directions. The black dots represent the nonius horopter determined at fixation and up to 10° to both sides. F = fixation point. The magnitude of the threshold for each contour line is labeled at either end in min arc. Observe that greater sensitivity to a difference in depth occurs at 5° away from fixation than at the fixation point itself. (Reproduced from Blakemeore C: The range and scope of binocular depth discrimination in man. *J Physiol (Lond) 1970;211: 599–622.*)

increment of horizontal disparity on a standing disparity depends on the length of presentation. For 1,000 msec presentations, the threshold is about 5.5%, roughly twice the threshold for judging the change in width for the same displacement in depth. In the presence of stereopsis the monocular width information is not available.[18]

The neurophysiologic theory of stereopsis depends on having a population of cells that exhibit a range of receptive field position disparities.[19,20] Furthermore, each cell must be able to discriminate disparities within its receptive field.[21] Superimposed on the topographic representation of the visual field on the striate cortex is a scatter of monocular receptive field locations (Fig. 6.21) The binocular scatter is built up of the two monocular scatters. The receptive field scatter maps into a block of space surrounding the horopter in which a range of cortical units is responsive to the range of disparities in depth. Small vertical disparities occur in the position distribution of cortical receptive fields and allow for the naturally occuring vertical disparities.

In the alert, behaving monkey, six kinds of depth sensitivity have been described in striate cortex (V1, area 17) and in extrastriate cortical areas V2 through V5[22,23] (Fig. 6.22). Tuned zero cells give maximal response at zero disparity, i.e., on the horopter. Tuned inhibitory cells respond with maximal inhibition at zero disparity. Tuned near cells and tuned far cells respond over a small range of disparity to stimuli just in front or just behind the fixation

6.21 | Scattergram of receptive field locations for cells in the cat striate cortex, within 4° of retinal eccentricity. The centers of the receptive fields for one eye have been moved to a common point, and the resulting scatter in position in the second eye has been plotted. Scatter within the inner circle is caused by experimental error; the radius equals one standard deviation. The distribution approximates a two-dimensional Gaussian. (Reproduced from Bishop PO: Stereopsis and the random element in the organization of the striate cortex. *Proc R Soc Lond [B] 1979;204:415–434.*)

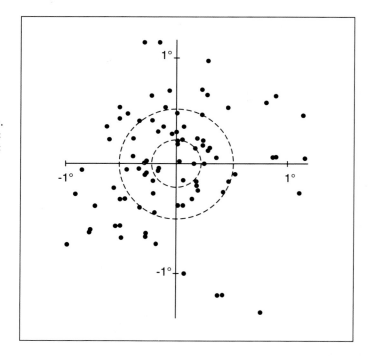

point. Near and far cells are more broadly tuned and respond over a greater range of disparities. In fact, a continuum of responses may occur between the tuned near and the near cells, the tuned far and the far cells. In the cat, striate cortical units have been found to be exquisitely sensitive to the relative position of stimuli within the receptive field.[24]

The three classes of cortical neurons imply the operation of three mechanisms in stereoscopic depth perception. Stereoanomalous humans differentiate among disparities only over limited regions of the normal range. Clinical testing of such individuals with coarse stereoscopic stimuli (0.5° to 4° of disparity) shows deficits that sort into three groups: poor response to crossed (near) stimuli, poor response to uncrossed (far) stimuli, and a third group that does not perceive disparities near zero.[25–27] A subject in the third group might refer all near zero stimuli to far and all crossed and uncrossed disparities to near, thus losing the sign of the disparity but not the magnitude. A 30% chance of lacking one of these depth mechanisms exists in one cerebral hemisphere. Subjects who lack a coarse stereo mechanism still show normal fine stereopsis.

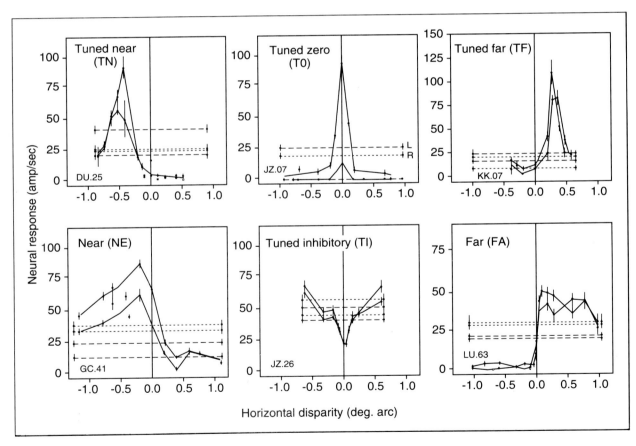

6.22 | Disparity sensitivity profiles of neurons in monkey visual cortical areas V1, V2, V3, and V3A. Two examples are shown for each cell class. (Reproduced from Poggio GF, Fischer B: Binocular interaction and depth sensitivity in striate and prestriate cortex of behaving rhesus monkey. *J Neurophysiol 1977;40:1392–1405.*)

Disparity also can be a stimulus to vergence movements of the eyes.[28] If the stimuli are similar enough to allow sensory fusion, the vergence response is maintained. Stimuli that are too dissimilar to fuse still elicit a transient fusional movement. Anomalies of transient vergence in response to short-duration disparate stimuli have been shown to fall into groups that lack either convergence or divergence (Fig. 6.23), implying a deficit in one of the groups of cells that give rise to coarse stereopsis.

Binocular perception of position in depth is mediated either through classic (Wheatstone) stereopsis or through daVinci stereopsis.[29] The visual system can recover information about depth, contour, and surface from occlusive relations in the real world. DaVinci stereopsis arises from the occlusion of distant surfaces, to differing extents in the two eyes, by near surfaces containing vertical contours. The unpaired image points, visible in one eye and not the other, are perceived in increasing depth in proportion to angular separation from a fused edge (up to 40 min arc). Unpaired image points also give rise to the subjective perception of an occluding contour (when no occluding surface is actually present). Neurophysiologic recordings in visual cortical area V2 in alert, behaving monkeys show responses to such contours.

MOTION IN DEPTH

Stereopsis detects position in depth on the basis of subtle geometric cues. Psychophysical evidence occurs in humans, and supporting neurophysiologic evidence in animals, that the visual system contains separate information processing channels for velocity in depth.[30] Instead of computing the trajectory of a moving object from a sequence of positions in depth, the human visual pathway directly analyzes the directions and speeds of motion in the two retinal images.

When an object's trajectory passes wide of the head, the retinal images move in the same direction, although at different speeds. Objects whose trajectory passes between the eyes have retinal image motions in opposite directions. Persistent viewing of binocularly fused targets oscillating in depth leads to a reduction in sensitivity to perception of these oscillations (adaptation). Directionally specific adaptation to motion in depth is the principal evidence for these channels. Four underlying curves of sensitivity versus trajectory direction can be found: two tuned to objects passing between the eyes, either to the right or left of the midline, and two widely tuned curves for objects that miss the head (right and left).

The ability to see motion in depth has been mapped across the visual field. In clinically normal subjects, areas can exist in the binocular visual field where motion in depth is not seen. The defects can be in different areas, depending on whether the oscillating search target is presented in crossed or uncrossed disparity (i.e., closer or farther away than the fixation point). Defects that depend on disparity in this way occur after the images from the two eyes have been combined and are therefore said to be cyclopean. Perimetry to motion in depth is a research tool and is not usually performed clinically.

BINOCULAR SUMMATION

For many visual tasks, the simultaneous use of two eyes gives better performance than one eye.[31] Such tasks include detection of a dim flash of light, increment thresholds (detection of an increment of light flashed on an illuminated background), and threshold detection of flicker and contrast. The improvements in performance vary from subject to subject and tend to be small. As a quantitative example, the detection of contrast in grating stimuli shows a binocular to monocular sensitivity ratio of 1.4 ($\sqrt{2}$). Suprathreshold tasks of acuity, reaction time, and form recognition accuracy also show an improvement when performed binocularly.[32,33]

The basis of the binocular improvement is due either to the summation of neural signals or to probability summation, or to both. An improve-

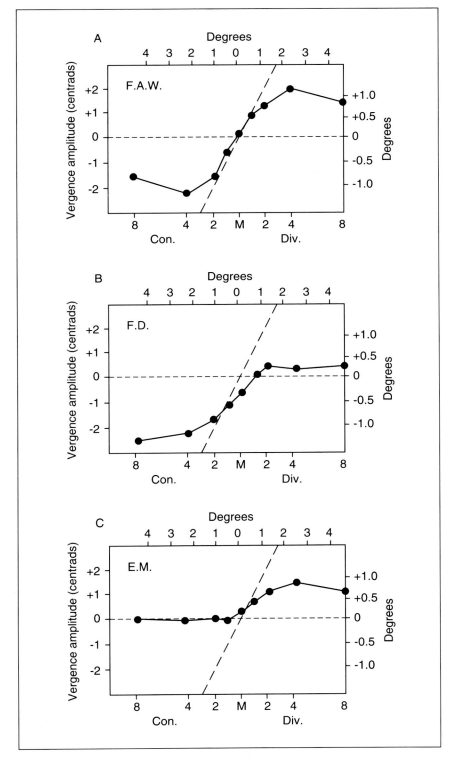

6.23 | Vergence responses plotted as a function of stimulus disparity in degrees, convergent or divergent. *A:* Normal response. *B:* Lack of divergence responses. *C:* Lack of convergent responses. (Reproduced from Jones R: Anomalies of disparity detection in the human visual system. *J Physiol (Lond)* 1977; 264:621–640.)

ment from neural summation requires the convergence of monocular signal pathways onto binocular pathways before the decision process. The binocular pathway may then have greater responses when fed from the two monocular sources. The monocular inputs must be adequately similar to stimulate the same pathways in the two eyes.

The binocular advantage called *probability summation* stems from the application of the independence theorem of probability theory. The assumptions are that the observer as a whole detects an event when either eye detects it, and that the two eyes act independently. Then, under binocular conditions, two chances will occur, instead of one, to detect the stimulus event. These two chances lead to improved performance.

CLINICAL TESTING

Clinical sensory evaluation in strabismus is a matter of testing *binocular* visual function. Examination answers the following questions: Are both eyes working at the same time (simultaneous perception)? Do the retinal elements of both eyes have the same direction values? How good is stereoscopic function? Lack of simultaneous perception is called *suppression*. Lack of identical direction values is called *anomalous retinal correspondence*. Stereopsis is degraded by suppression and by even small angles of strabismus.

TESTS OF SIMULTANEOUS PERCEPTION

In strabismus, under binocular viewing conditions, locations may exist within the visual field at which simultaneous perception in the two eyes does not occur. Such locations are said to show suppression. Testing for suppression is a matter of testing for simultaneous perception throughout the visual field. This can be done in a straightforward manner by doing binocular perimetry or by using red and green filters or a mirror to separate the visual fields of the two eyes.[34] In practice, binocular perimetry is very tedious and requires constant checking to see that the angle of strabismus has not changed during the test. Over time, the typical patterns of suppression have become known and the simpler tests described below are usually sufficient for normal clinical purposes.

DIPLOPIA (RED GLASS) TEST

Diplopia is the seeing of one object in two different locations. Binocular diplopia is caused by the image of the object falling on noncorresponding retinal elements in the two eyes, so that it is seen in a different direction by each eye. Monocular diplopia is caused by the production of two spatially separated images by the refractive media of the eye. It is usually resolved by a pinhole. *Confusion* is the seeing of two different objects in the same location. Confusion and binocular diplopia can exist simultaneously, and the content of the symptomatic complaint depends on whether the patient's attention is directed to the object (which is double) or to the location (which has two different objects).

A red glass held in front of one eye labels with a red color everything seen through that eye. A fixation light, seen double, appears as a white light and a red light. If one or the other of the two lights is not observed, suppression is present. In the presence of normal retinal correspondence, if the laterality of the image and the eye seeing that image are the same (e.g., right image with right eye) the diplopia is said to be homonymous or uncrossed. This pattern is characteristic of esotropia. Heteronymous or crossed diplopia is characteristic of exotropia. For vertical diplopia the high eye sees the low image.

Vectographic displays contain a composite of two orthogonal directions of Polaroid® material, arranged so that the dark lines are polarized in either one or both of the directions. Glasses with Polaroid filters therefore allow each eye to see only the correspondingly polarized lines. This method has been used to make Project-O-Chart® slides in which certain letters in each line are visible only to one eye. If amblyopia is present, letters large enough to be visible to the amblyopic eye must be used. As lines are read, letters visible only to one eye may not be seen. This is due to suppression, a lack of simultaneous perception. The unseen letters fall within a suppression scotoma surrounding the fovea. After occlusion of the eye that did see its letters, the suppressed eye will see its letters if its visual acuity is sufficient. This is because suppression is present only under binocular viewing conditions. The monocular performance of each eye can be perfectly normal, yet suppression occurs in the binocular state.

The Worth four-dot test uses red and green glasses to dissociate stimuli to the two eyes (Fig. 6.24). The stimulus contains four spots of light in a square pattern: two green, a red, and a white. The two green and the white are visible to the eye behind the green filter (the "green" eye). The red and the white are visible to the eye behind the red filter (the "red" eye). The patient is asked how many lights are seen. The patient will report two for the "red" eye, three for the "green" eye, four if both eyes are perceiving and the eyes are straight, and five if both are perceiving but the eyes are not straight. Asking the color of the lights sometimes leads to confusion, especially with younger children, and should be considered a supplementary or confirmatory question. The test is relatively crude in that duration of presentation

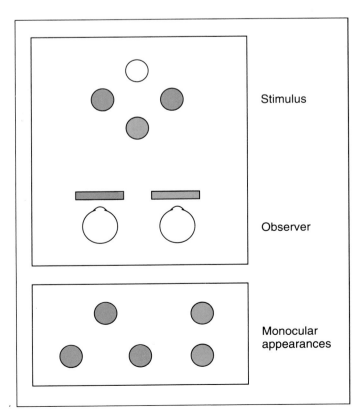

Stimulus

Observer

Monocular appearances

6.24 | Worth four-dot test. The stimulus contains white, red, and green spots. Visibility of these spots is controlled to the two eyes by red and green plano power filters mounted in a spectacle frame that is superimposed over the subject's glasses. The lights seen indicate the state of binocular perception under these conditions.

and fixation location are not controlled. For example, if the subject looks at each light in succession, a suppression scotoma could be moved away from the lights visible to the other eye, enabling them to be seen in the presence of suppression. The test can be made somewhat quantitative if the distance to the flashlight target is measured. The angular size subtended by the outside edges of the lights must then be calculated. Lack of perception of both pairs of lights then can be interpreted as a suppression scotoma of an angular size at least big enough to extend beyond the lights. Moving the light closer will then produce a larger angle between the lights, and at some distance both pairs may be seen. The angular size inside the lights is therefore the size of the suppression scotoma.

Apparatus for the Worth four-dot test comes as a wall-mounted box and as flashlights in various sizes for use at closer distances (Fig. 6.25).

BAGOLINI LENS TEST

The Bagolini striated lens contains tiny grooves or scratches that create a streak appearance to point light sources. It is dissimilar to a Maddox rod constructed of microscopic cylinders, because vision is otherwise clear. The Maddox rod has an occluding effect, in which very little besides the streak of light radiating out from the point light sources is visible. The Bagolini lens thus labels the image in each eye by a streak in an orientation that depends on the orientation of the lens before that eye, but does not disrupt vision in any other way except for a mild softening of contrast, which is taken as being negligible. It thus shows the sensory status under natural viewing conditions that are undisturbed by the test itself. The test is used for suppression by asking if lines radiating in both directions from the light are seen. Some observers with suppression can identify a portion of one line that is missing, constituting the portion of the line falling on the suppression scotoma. The test is most useful for anomalous retinal correspondence.

FOUR-DIOPTER BASE OUT PRISM TEST

This test demonstrates a suppression scotoma in one eye under binocular viewing conditions. While fixation is maintained on a target, a four-diopter prism is placed in front of one eye (Fig. 6.26). It is best for the examiner not

6.25 | Worth flashlights come in various sizes. The angular subtense of the spots is different in the small and large lights.

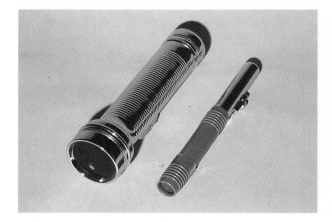

to look through the prism but rather beside it, otherwise the time delay to make a saccade may lead to missing the patient's eye movement. The base can be placed in any direction, but usually a base out position is used. A typical result is that if the tested eye was fixating, the four-PD jump in target position will be observed through that eye and a saccade made to the new target position (in the direction of the apex of the prism). The saccade is then followed on a slower time scale by a fusional vergence movement of the other eye. If the tested eye has a scotoma, or if a strabismus exists and the tested eye is not being used for fixation at the moment of the test, the displacement in the target will not be perceived (because its image is displaced into a non-seeing area of retina) and only the fusional vergence movement occurs in that eye. The companion, fixating eye does not move. If neither eye moves, it sometimes helps to ask the subject to look at the target if he/she sees it jump (not everyone automatically looks at the jump of the target). Both eyes must be tested with the prism. The essential finding is a difference in the response between the eyes. An eye that makes a saccade in response to the prism was not suppressed at the moment the prism was inserted. A vergence response is usually seen in the eye behind the prism if suppression occurs when the prism was inserted, or in response to the prism being placed in front of the other eye. Some subjects make only vergence responses and no saccade with either eye. Such a result cannot be taken as evidence of suppression. Occasionally, responses are not consistent and the test cannot be interpreted.

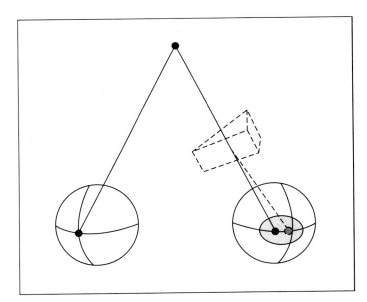

6.26 | Four-diopter base out prism test. The insertion of the prism before the eye displaces the image of the target. If it falls within a suppression scotoma the jump will not be perceived and a saccade will not be generated.

MAJOR AMBLYOSCOPE

The major amblyoscope is a haploscope, i.e., a device that separates the visual spaces of the eyes and allows presentation of stimuli separately to each eye (Fig. 6.27). If the stimuli are to be presented to the macula of each eye, each arm of the device must be positioned so that the fovea is lined up with the fixation point in that arm. Pictures then are presented to the two eyes (e.g., a lion to one eye and a cage to the other). If the lion is suppressed the cage will be seen as empty. Another approach is to show the same image to both eyes, but differing in a detail that acts as a check mark for perception occurring in each eye. For example, a man can be wearing a hat in one picture and be holding a stick in the other. A subject who does not suppress will see a man with a hat and a stick. Suppression may come and go, depending on whether strabismus is present. Thus, presentation of stimuli to the two maculas simulates the condition of no strabismus. Suppression elicited under these conditions is considered to be deeply ingrained, because it is present when no conflict or rivalry exists between the stimuli. Under natural viewing conditions, the same stimulus will be presented to the fixating eye and a point on the retina of the deviating eye that is displaced from the fovea by the angle of the deviation. To simulate this condition the arms of the amblyoscope should remain straight.

DEPTH OF
SUPPRESSION

No easy way exists to determine the depth of suppression. What must be done is to weaken the stimulus to the fixating eye—e.g., a reduction in the luminance of a fixation light or the contrast of a grating—until perception switches to the formerly suppressed eye. The results depend on the exact testing conditions. Bagolini introduced a red filter ladder to occlude the fixating eye with red filters of increasing density.[35] In practice, the ladder has nonuniform steps of density and color and fades with time.

TESTS OF RETINAL
CORRESPONDENCE

A *retinal element* is the retinocerebral apparatus engaged in elaborating a sensation in response to stimulation of a small area of retina. Such a sensation is perceived as having a direction in space relative to straight ahead. Stimula-

6.27 | The amblyoscope separates the visual space of the two eyes and allows the presentation of different targets. It can be used to perform a cover test and thus to measure the angle of deviation, including torsion, and to test for suppression, stereopsis, and ARC.

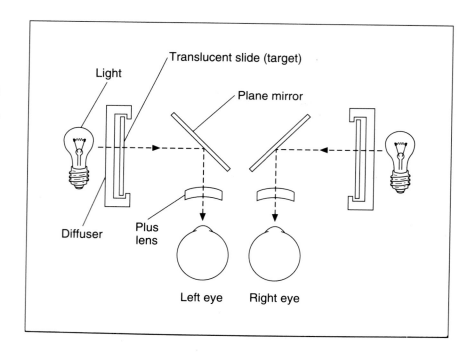

tion of the fovea results in a perception of straight ahead. Corresponding retinal elements or points refer to the identical perceived direction resulting from stimulation of a pair of retinal elements, one in each eye, each displaced from the fovea by an equal angle in space. In normal retinal correspondence these perceived direction values are the same for the two eyes. In anomalous retinal correspondence (ARC) the direction values in the deviated eye have shifted horizontally by an amount equal to the deviation (harmonious ARC) or less than the deviation (unharmonious ARC). The effect of ARC is to change direction values in the deviated eye to what they should be to give both eyes the same localization in space. Objects that are perceived in the same direction do not need to be suppressed. In strabismus acquired early enough in childhood, the typical findings are suppression of the central retina and ARC in the periphery.

ARC occurs under binocular viewing conditions. Various sensory tests, to the extent that they fail to reproduce natural binocular seeing conditions, may change the result they are to measure. Stimulation of the two retinas under conditions that are not identical, or possibly even simultaneous, is said to dissociate the two eyes. The most dissociating test is the after-image test. Less dissociating are the haploscopic tests, and least dissociating is the Bagolini striated lens test.

DIPLOPIA TEST

After objective measurement of the deviation with prism and cover, a red glass is placed in front of the deviated eye and the location of the red light reported on a Maddox cross. The subjectively observed position is compared with the objectively determined position. For this test to work, the suppression scotoma must be lessened by alternately covering the eyes. On removal of the cover transiently less suppression may occur, enabling both lights to be seen. Alternatively, a vertical prism can be used along with the red glass to displace the image out of the suppression scotoma.

HAPLOSCOPES

The arms of the major amblyoscope are set to the objective angle of deviation, so that the targets are imaged on both foveas. If the targets are seen as superimposed, normal retinal correspondence exists. If the targets are diplopic, crossed diplopia will occur with esotropia and uncrossed diplopia with exotropia. The angle of anomaly is measured by having the patient move the arms of the amblyoscope until the targets are superimposed (subjective angle). When this angle equals the objective angle, the ARC is harmonious. When the angle is different, the ARC is unharmonious.

The Lancaster red–green apparatus can be used to determine retinal correspondence. The concept is the same as for the major amblyoscope. The visual spaces are separated by the colored goggles.

In the phase-difference haploscope, the visual space of the two eyes is separated by rapidly spinning, occluding disks that alternately allow each eye to view a scene along with a pointer that is visible only to that eye.[36] With a manifest strabismus and harmonious ARC, the patient will superimpose the pointers. A lack of superimposition indicates unharmonious ARC. The phase-difference haploscope is the least dissociating of the haploscopic devices.

AFTER-IMAGE TEST

In this test an after-image is imprinted on each retina with a photoflash unit. The flash area is masked except for a slit through which the light is visible. The center of the slit is covered with a fixation mark. The resulting area of unstimulated retina protects the fovea from an after-image. Under monocular conditions, with the nonfixating eye carefully covered, a flash is delivered to one eye with the slit vertically oriented and to the other eye with the slit horizontally oriented. A positive after-image is then seen in each eye if the ambient light is dim, or a negative after-image if the room lights are bright. Because the fovea of each eye carries the straight-ahead direction, a cross should be seen under these binocular conditions (Fig. 6.28). If ARC is present the after-images will not align at the central blank fixation spot but will be shifted horizontally. A crossed (heteronymous) localization pattern occurs in esotropia because the straight-ahead direction value is now in the nasal retina in the deviated eye. Because the primary, straight-ahead direction value has shifted nasally, the foveal location of the flash is seen by retina that now has the direction values of temporal retina, which gives crossed diplopia. By a similar argument, it can be seen that ARC in exotropia will yield (homonymous) uncrossed diplopia. As the deviation changes from moment to moment, with incomitancy or intermittency, the direction of the after-image may change.

FOVEO–FOVEAL TEST OF CÜPPERS

If amblyopia exists in one eye sufficiently deep to produce eccentric fixation, the fovea probably will not be used for fixation under the test conditions. Under these circumstances, it is possible to place a stimulus on the retina with an ophthalmoscope while the other eye fixates a light.[37] The relative location of the stimuli is then reported by the patient. Alternatively, a vertical after-image can be placed in the better eye and the location of the fovea in the amblyopic eye marked with Haidinger's brushes. *Haidinger's brushes* is an entoptic phenomenon elicited by viewing a homogeneous blue field through a rotating Polaroid filter. A rotating brush- or hourglass-shaped spot is seen at the location of the fovea. The phenomenon is thought to be caused by differential absorption of light by the yellow macular pigment in the area of radiating Henle fibers around the fovea. Haidinger brush attachments are available for major amblyoscopes, and this variant of the test is best done with this instrument.

6.28 | After-image test. The vertical after-image is imprinted on one eye and the horizontal on the other. R = right eye after-image; L = left eye after-image. *A:* Normal retinal correspondence. *B:* Anomalous crossed localization in esotropia. *C:* Anomalous uncrossed localization in exotropia.

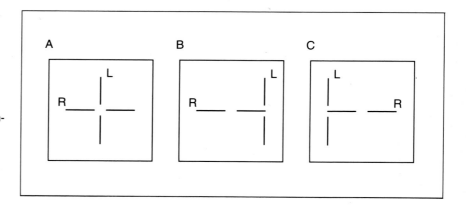

The use of the Bagolini striated lenses to examine for suppression is described above. When these are used to test for ARC the position of the eyes must be known. The test cannot be interpreted accurately unless it is known whether or not strabismus is present. A point light is viewed by the subject wearing the striated lenses. In the presence of orthophoria, one fixation light will be seen and both streaks will pass through that light (Fig. 6.29). In the presence of a manifest deviation, diplopia on the light implies no suppression and no diplopia implies suppression. If both streaks pass through the light, ARC is present. Occasionally, the subject may notice a gap in one of the streaks. This results from a suppression scotoma; however, if the suppression area is large the second streak may not be seen. These breaks in the streak lead to verbal ambiguities, because what is intended is to ask whether the light lies on the line, or where the line would be, if it were not suppressed in a particular segment. It is sometimes helpful to have the patient draw what is seen.

BAGOLINI STRIATED GLASSES

Practical clinical stereopsis testing involves the administration of an established test. The most commonly performed clinical tests superimpose the targets for the two eyes and control the visibility of the appropriate target to each

STEREOPSIS TESTING

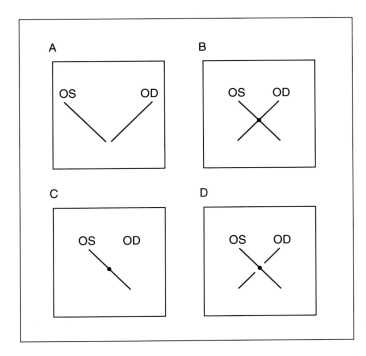

6.29 | Bagolini striated lens test. The diagrams represent the appearance to the subject. *A:* Diplopia with esotropia. *B:* Crossing of the lines through the light indicates NRC if no deviation occurs, and ARC if a deviation occurs. *C:* Suppression of one entire image. *D:* Small scotoma around the fixation point and either orthophoria with NRC or manifest deviation with ARC.

eye with Polaroid filters (Randot) (Fig. 6.30) or colored, anaglyphic glasses (TNO) (Fig. 6.31). Clinical testing does not control important parameters that are specififed in research work, such as location of fixation, duration of presentation, luminance, and adaptation effects, so results are only approximate.

The Titmus stereotest has been a clinical standard for many years. The largest disparity is a photograph of a large housefly (3,000 sec arc at 40 cm testing distance). A child is asked to grasp the wing. Reaching above the plate is taken as a correct response. An adult is asked whether the wing appears to be above the plate. Smaller disparities (400, 200, and 100 sec arc) are presented as rows of five animals, only one of which floats above the surface of the plate. Circles, arranged as four alternative choices, present disparities from 800 sec arc down to 40 sec arc. The child is asked to touch the one that pops up closer to him/her. Some of the larger disparities in the circles can be detected by monocularly perceivable cues. To solve this problem, a similar test has been devised in which the stimuli are embedded as random dot stereograms (Randot test). To avoid the need for wearing Polaroid spectacles, sometimes a problem in young children, the

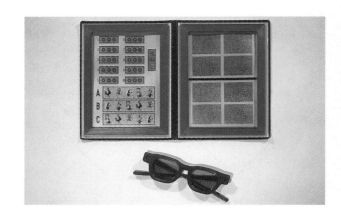

6.30 | Randot stereotest manufactured by Titmus Optical Co. The images are dissociated with Polaroid filters.

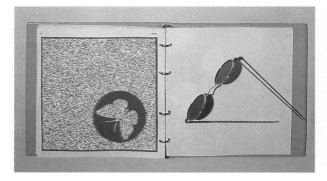

6.31 | TNO stereotest. The images are dissociated with red–green glasses.

random-dot stereogram can be presented through a cylinder grating (Lang stereotest)[38] (Fig. 6.32).

The TNO stereotest (Fig. 6.31) uses random-dot stereograms and separates the images to the two eyes with red–green glasses. It contains disparities from 480 to 15 sec arc.

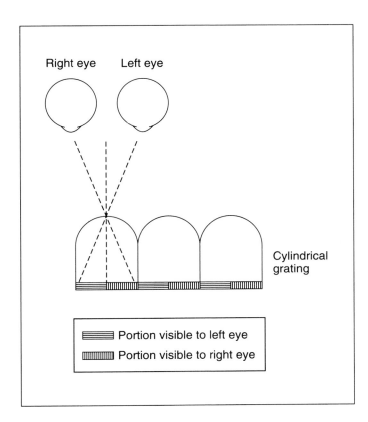

6.32 | The Lang stereotest is based on viewing random dot stereograms through cylindrical gratings. Each random-dot element is projected into a portion of space by an immediately overlying cylindrical lens of short focal length. Both halves of the stereogram are combined next to each other in the display, dot by dot, and the grating controls visibility of the dots to the two eyes. The entire assembly of grating and random-dot display is approximately 2 mm thick. Observers with sufficient stereoacuity can perceive objects, such as a cat or a star, composed of random dots floating over the background. The display is useful for testing young children because no goggles are required. The display must be held approximately perpendicular to the line of sight so that each eye can see the appropriate dot. Diagram not to scale.

7 | EXOTROPIA

Howard M. Eggers

Exodeviation refers to a latent or manifest divergence of the visual axes. An *exophoria* is a latent deviation held in check by the fusional mechanisms that work under binocular viewing conditions. An *intermittent exotropia* is controlled by fusional mechanisms only part of the time. An *exotropia* is not controlled by fusion and is present all the time under binocular viewing conditions (called a *constant* exotropia when it is being specifically distinguished from intermittent exotropia).

Exotropia is diagnosed by cover testing. Unlike most pseudoesotropia, which is due to the configuration of the eyelids, pseudoexotropia results from a large positive angle kappa, i.e., from the anatomic configuration of the eyes and not the lids (Fig. 7.1). The term pseudoexotropia carries no implication as to

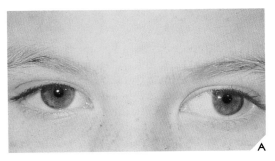

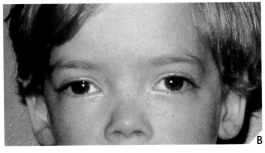

7.1 | Pseudoexotropia. *A:* Exotropia. *B:* Pseudo-exotropia from large positive angle kappa. This appears to be an exotropia due to one's expectations about the size of angle kappa. Smaller angles of exotropia may not be diagnosed accurately by inspection. Cover testing is required to diagnose any strabismus.

the normality of the eyes. Temporal dragging of the retina in retinopathy of prematurity leads to a large positive angle kappa and the appearance of exotropia. The eyes may be demonstrated to be straight by cover testing or an additional true exotropia may exist if the vision is poor. Such a case could be construed as having a real exotropia superimposed on an original pseudoexotropia.

PRIMARY EXOTROPIA

The eyes are maintained in exact registration by fusional mechanisms: tonic and fusional vergences. *Tonic* (nonretinal) vergence refers to the basic tonus of the eye muscles. It is characterized by the alteration in eye position produced by changing from sleep or anesthesia to the waking state (measured in the absence of sensory fusion). Because so little is known about tonic mechanisms (e.g., whether they are even organized into opposing convergent and divergent directions), it is perhaps better to think of the tonic forces as providing a posture for the eye from which fusional mechanisms operate.

Minor differences in such factors as orbital mechanics, size of the muscles, and force developed by the muscles cause the two eyes not to have exactly the same direction in space. *Fusional* vergence is the name given to the adjustments that are made in the muscle innervation to achieve exact alignment. This motor fusional output brings the eyes into exact registration to allow binocular sensory fusion. Accommodative convergence, along with accommodation of the lens and miosis of the pupil, constitutes the near triad of responses to a near target. Accommodative esotropia can result from the function of this near synkinesis. Esotropia occurs when convergence exceeds the relative fusional divergence. There is no equivalent physiologic mechanism of accommodative divergence, merely a relaxation of convergence.[1] Accommodative convergence can serve the role of masking an exotropia, and deficiencies of accommodative convergence can lead to exodeviations at near.

In most cases the fundamental cause of exotropia is unknown. Ascribing the deviation to the wrong amount of underlying muscle tonus does not provide much understanding and is largely descriptive. In some cases a family pedigree implies a genetic basis. Exotropes have a distribution of refractive errors representative of the general population. Women comprise 60% to 70% of exotropes.[2,3]

Exotropia is classified by the magnitude of the deviation under prism and cover measurements according to a system introduced by Duane.[4] For purposes of classification, the deviations in primary position at distance and near are said to be different if the measurements differ by at least 10 PD. Measurement at 30 m instead of the usual 6 m significantly increases the distance deviation in about one third of patients.[5] The classification type is based on the distance at which the deviation is greatest: distance *(divergence excess)*, near *(convergence insufficiency)*, or equal at distance and near *(basic exodeviation)*. Duane's terms are now regarded as being purely descriptive and carry no necessary implications about pathophysiology. The physiology of the change in deviation with distance is presently understood in terms of the accommodative convergence/accommodation (AC/A) ratio.

A further type, *simulated divergence excess*, has a deviation larger at distance than at near, but the near deviation can be increased to equal or exceed the distance deviation by special manipulations. Burian occluded one eye for 30 to 45 minutes and then performed prism and cover measurements without allowing any intervening binocular vision.[6] He found that most cases of divergence excess showed an increase in near deviation after occlusion to amounts similar to the distance deviation. Of 237 patients, only 10 had true divergence excess after this procedure. Another manipulation is to relax accommodation at near with +3.00-D-sph lenses. The higher the AC/A ratio, the greater will be the effect on the deviation. The near deviation will increase, sometimes to as much as that at distance. In these patients, accommodative convergence has masked the near exodeviation (Figure 7.2).

The symptoms experienced by the exotrope depend on the age at which the exotropia began. If it begins before the age of 8 years, suppression is probably present. Suppression attenuates binocular vision and thus many of the symptoms of exotropia. If the visual acuity is the same in both eyes, the eye used for fixation may sometimes alternate. However, alternation of fixation can cause difficulty in reading (the reading place in the text is lost) and occasionally causes dizziness. The exodeviated position can lead to sensations of physical discomfort or even, rarely, pain. Social interactions can be disturbed because it is not possible to tell where or at whom the patient is looking.

Exotropia acquired after age 8, when suppresssion can no longer be developed, produces visual symptoms that usually derive either from diplopia or from the struggle to maintain binocular vision. These latter syptoms, as described by the patient, can include blurry vision; intermittent diplopia; headache; a vague, nonspecific difficulty in reading (especially for prolonged periods); stress, pressure, or pain about the eyes; and a panoply of other vague symptoms that go by the name of "eye strain." Binocular asthenopia is a general term for symptoms caused by trying to maintain binocular vision. Exotropia, through loss of binocularity, further interferes with other binocular functions such as stereopsis, motion in depth, and binocular summation. Patients unsophisticated in visual science seldom verbalize the loss of these capabilities, at least not without a detailed history of symptoms, but frequently notice their return after the eyes are straightened.

Intermittent exotropia has an additional symptom of photophobia. A child with intermittent exotropia often squeezes one eye shut in bright sunlight. The functional reason for this (e.g., whether to avoid diplopia or to dim the subjective sensation of brightness) is not known. Bright light has

Figure 7.2. Classification of Exotropia

AC/A	DUANE CLASSIFICATION		EXAMPLE
Low	Convergence insufficiency		XT 10 XT' 35
Normal	Basic		XT 35 XT' 35
High	Divergence excess		XT 35 X' 5
		+3.00	X' 5
High	Pseudodivergence excess		XT 35 X' 5
		+3.00	XT' 35

been shown to reduce the amplitude of fusional convergence in patients who show a well-controlled intermittent exotropia.[7] Exophoric patients do not show this effect.

The common idea that the deviated eye does not participate in vision and that the exotropic patient is effectively monocular is erroneous. The sensory adaptations of suppression and anomalous correspondence develop when exotropia begins early enough in life that binocular physiology is still modifiable by visual experience. This is probably by age 8 in most people. Exotropia beginning after age 8 results in diplopia.

The binocular sensory physiology of exotropia is somewhat variable, depending on the presence or absence of concomitant amblyopia, and the results of sensory testing can depend on the exact conditions. The traditional thought is that the exodeviated eye is suppressed in an area of the retina from the fovea to the temporal periphery (hemiretinal suppression), or even that the entire retina is suppressed (found under red glass testing).[8,9] Under stimulus conditions that are more natural (Bagolini striated lenses), the suppression scotoma can be shown to extend into the nasal retina.[10,11]

In subjects who have alternating fixation, suppression of the deviated eye is most intense in a retinal region corresponding to the direction in space of the fovea of the fixating eye, but is reduced or absent in the periphery.[12] The fixating eye also experiences suppression from the deviated eye, in a peripheral area corresponding to the fovea of the deviated eye. Thus each eye suppresses the other, although to unequal extents. The vision of the fixating eye is therefore not fully normal. Furthermore, a binocular interaction occurs between the eyes, wherein the binocular grating acuity in the peripheral retina of the fixating eye is better than normal at a location corresponding to the fovea of the deviated eye. Extensive peripheral areas of the binocular visual field, away from the fovea of the deviated eye, also can show binocular depth perception (detection of motion in depth).

INTERMITTENT EXOTROPIA

In children, exotropia usually begins with an exophoria. With time this deteriorates into an intermittent exotropia and later becomes a constant exotropia (Fig. 7.3). The exodeviation is initially greater at distance and with time increases at near. The intermittent deviation can be re-fused either spontaneously without shift of gaze, concurrently with a shift of gaze, which usually involves a shift in vergence posture as well, or with a shift to near gaze. Suppression develops along with the deterioration into a constant-

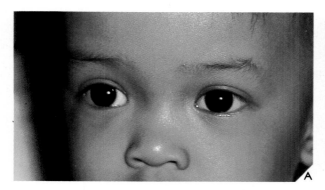
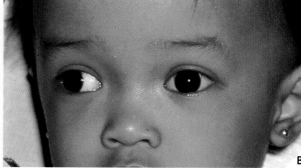

7.3 | Intermittent exotropia. *A:* Eyes straight. *B:* A few moments later, the exotropia has become manifest.

angle exotropia, and the development of suppression probably contributes to further deterioration. Presumably, as suppression becomes deeper any visual cue to the presence of exotropia is lost, and the eye remains in its deviated position for longer periods of time. One can speculate about other changes that may take place over time: muscle tone, tonic convergence, the function of central fusional mechanisms, and reduction in accommodative capabilites.

Intermittent exotropes are often noted to be sensitive to bright light, which triggers the deviation. Sunglasses and a hat with visor should be worn in the summertime.

INFANTILE EXOTROPIA

Exotropia at or near birth is often secondary to other congenital defects, such as craniofacial anomalies, neurologic disease, marked anisometropia, restrictive syndromes, or eye diseases resulting in poor vision.

Constant exotropia presenting in the first 9 months of life usually shows an average deviation of 35 to 40 PD.[13] With time the deviation tends to increase. Other typical features are approximate equality at distance and near, alternation of fixation, unremarkable refractive error, a dissociated vertical divergence, and normal versions and ductions. Other less constant features are a head tilt and an A pattern. Fusion is not established on surgical correction. In contrast, infants who first exhibit only an intermittent deviation are much more likely to regain some degree of fusion after the eyes are straightened surgically.

CONVERGENCE INSUFFICIENCY

Convergence insufficiency is characterized by a variety of symptoms that accompany near visual tasks: blurred or doubled vision, fatigue, a sensation of tension about the eyes, and headaches. Sometimes one eye is covered. Frequently no obvious cause exists.

Convergence insufficiency can be associated with defects of accommodation.[14] Lack of use of accommodation may occur in myopes, who do not need to accommodate, and in hyperopes of 6 D or more, who may not accommodate much at all because of the great effort required. Early presbyopes may control a convergence insufficiency through increased exertion of the near synkinesis. The lens progressively fails to respond but convergence is improved. A reading correction may bring out the underlying convergence insufficiency. Convergence insufficiency with reduced NPA may be seen in Adie syndrome and after head trauma. Impaired accommodation without convergence insufficiency also may occur after head trauma.

Convergence insufficiency associated with reduced accommodative capacity has been described after systemic illnesses such as encephalitis, diphtheria, mononucleosis, and streptococcal throat infections. A group of young adults has been identified that is characterized by a gradual onset of convergence insufficiency, but also a remote near point of accommodation and a very low AC/A ratio. The latter finding implies that stimulating accommodation will do nothing to improve the convergence in this group. The treatment is prisms and a near add.

The diagnostic findings are a poor near point of convergence and poor relative fusional convergence at near. Typically, a small phoria occurs at distance and an exophoria or intermittent exotropia at near, although orthophoria or even esophoria also may occur at near. On rare occasions the effort to fuse may result in accommodative spasm. An exotropia should not exist at near, since this implies an absence of fusional effort and no symptoms should be expected in the absence of such an effort. The difficulty in recovering fusion, once broken, may be striking. Relative fusional divergence should be normal, and the near point of accommodation should be appropriate for age. An associated reduced amplitude of accommodation and remote near point of accommodation may occur, especially with presbyopia. However, convergence insufficiency is not characteristic of presbyopia.

Visual comfort requires that not more than one third of the maximal possible convergence be exerted for sustained near tasks. Thus, for near work at 33 cm the NPC should be no farther than 11 cm from the interocular baseline or center of rotation of the eye (clinically approximated by measuring from the lateral canthus).

NONSURGICAL TREATMENT

Asymptomatic exophoria requires no treatment. Symptomatic exophoria and intermittent and constant exotropia can be treated with optical devices, with exercises, or surgically.

Obstacles to the function of the patient's normal fusional mechanisms should be removed if possible. Amblyopia must be treated at responsive ages. Significant refractive errors must be corrected (astigmatism, anisometropia, myopia). With a sufficiently high AC/A ratio, minus lenses may help to control an exodeviation in patients young enough to respond to the greater accommodative load. They will be of most benefit if fusion is enabled. Partial reduction in the exodeviation is of no lasting value, and the deviation may change as the patient makes or does not make the accommodative efforts required by the minus lenses. The appropriateness of correction of hyperopia depends on age, magnitude of the hyperopia, and the AC/A ratio. By lessening accommodative requirements, the exotropia could be made worse. However, if the vision is made clearer (e.g., through the partial correction of high hyperopia), then the exodeviation could be better controlled through fusional vergence. The prescription of plus power for presbyopia may exacerbate a preexisting exodeviation and lead to symptoms from the exotropia. If surgery is planned, full plus should be given to maximize the deviation before surgery.

Base-in prism may be prescribed in permanent spectacles if fusion will be made possible. As little prism as possible should be given to allow some continuing activity of the patient's natural convergence mechanisms. Plastic Fresnel prisms are useful for trial purposes to determine how much prism power is needed, but much less prism can be ground permanently into lenses than can be obtained with Fresnel prisms.

For convergence insufficiency the initial treatment is usually orthoptic exercises. With adequate refraction and attention to relief of presbyopia, near vision will be clear. Myopes should be corrected fully and hyperopes undercorrected if possible. A trial of patching should then relieve symtoms if the struggle to maintain binocular vision (e.g., from convergence insufficiency) was the cause of the symptoms. Under these conditions orthoptic exercises are worthwhile.

Orthoptic exercises fall into two groups, distinguished by the stimulus to convergence: prism and near point exercises. Either type of exercise can be prescribed with either an accommodative or a nonaccommodative target. Exercises can be directed at building up either relative fusional convergence or voluntary convergence, the latter through exercise of the near synkinesis.

Relative fusional vergence is exercised by use of a target that requires a specific level of accommodation for the details in the target to be visible (an accommodative target). Absolute fusional convergence can be exercised with a light or pencil as a target. An exact level of accommodation is not required by these targets, and voluntary activation of the near synkinesis can assist convergence onto these targets, but at the cost of inexact accommodation. The patient may not be aware of using the near synkinesis to fuse. The innapropriate accommodation can result in blurry vision. The habit of converging by activating the near synkinesis can also lead to poor results after surgery, should surgery be necessary.

Relative fusional convergence is exercised by fixating a near accommodative target and then introducing a base-out prism in front of one eye. After each prism the patient must re-fuse the target. The prism can be increased up to 30 or 40 PD.

Near point exercises require maintaining fixation on a approaching target. The target is brought to the break point and then backed off slightly. Fusion is maintained and then the target approached closer again, etc. Near point work is often done with a nonaccommodative target (pencil, finger, or light), although an accommodative target can also be used. A stereogram is an excellent accommodative fixation target. Loss of fusion is recognized readily with a stereogram, and the spatial extent of the stimulus allows participation of more peripheral retinal areas.

In another method, a red filter is placed over one eye and a penlight is used as the fixation target. Physiologic diplopia will demonstrate to the patient that convergence is inadequate. This method is useful in the presence of suppression because the light and the red filter may allow the recognition of diplopia. Convergence then is exercised by prisms or by near point work.

Botulinum toxin has been used for exotropia. The lateral rectus muscle is injected with a dose that depends on the magnitude of the deviation. The results are poorer than for esotropia, and the exotropia usually recurs (Fig. 7.4).

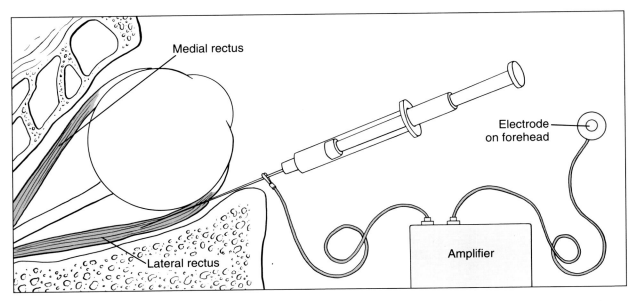

7.4 | Botulinum toxin injection. The dose to be delivered to the muscle is diluted in 0.1 ml of preservative-free saline. Under topical anesthesia, a long, teflon-coated 26-gauge needle is introduced into the muscle under guidance of an electromyographic amplifier and audio monitor. The needle is entirely insulated except for its tip. The injection should be performed in the region of the neuromuscular junctions. When the needle tip is in the muscle, recruitment of muscle units can be heard on the audio monitor as the muscle contracts .

SURGICAL TREATMENT

Although useful in some patients, and especially for convergence insufficiency, orthoptics is not a substitute for surgery. Few patients have the determination to continue exercises daily for the rest of their lives, and younger children do not have the concentration or discipline to do them for very long, if at all.

The indications for surgery are symptoms or the presence of the deformity of exotropia. If it can be proven that the patient was exotropic from birth, it is unlikely that much binocular sensory function will be present once the eyes are straight. Usually, however, this information is lacking. Some binocular sensory function often returns after surgery. The patient is not always subjectively aware of this, and it may manifest as, for example, a phoria component of the postoperative deviation. Symptoms that are subjective (e.g., eye strain) and are not direct manifestations of binocular visual physiology (e.g., diplopia) may not be reliably improved with surgery, and caution should be exercised in predicting specific sensory benefits.

Intermittency per se is not necessarily an indication for surgery. One can also evaluate whether the intermittent deviation is interfering with the use of the eyes. In the visually immature child (under 8 years), an increase in difficulty of controlling an intermittent exotropia (shown by the frequency or duration, or both, of the deviation) is an indication for surgery, because this implies that the depth of suppression is increasing.[15] Firmly ingrained suppression can limit the ability of binocular sensory mechanisms and fusion to function or to stabilize the eye position postoperatively. Alternatively, one must keep in mind that normal development of binocular sensory function is good for the child and that it is possible, by obtaining an overcorrection, to disrupt this process. A small-angle esotropia with some suppression, limitation of stereopsis, and risk of amblyopia could be the result. Patients with intermittent exotropia often exhibit a variety of minor sensory defects after surgery, including suppression, reduced stereopsis, and microexotropia. One sixth of patients appear to end up with completely intact binocular sensory function. The defects in the others presumably existed before surgery and may have played a role in producing the intermittent exotropia in the first place.[16]

The goals of exotropia surgery are alignment of the eyes and restoration of as much normal binocular function as possible. The benefit may be limited to relief of diplopia by alignment of a suppression scotoma in the deviated eye with the fovea of the fixating eye. In exotropia there is a strong tendency for the eyes to rediverge after surgery, and the aligned state is best achieved by a temporary period of overcorrection. If the postoperative esotropia causes diplopia that is symptomatically disturbing, Fresnel prisms or occlusion should be used. Both the response of exotropes to surgery and the shift in postoperative alignment are more variable than in esotropia. The trick is to produce an amount of overcorrection that will simply wear off within a few months after surgery, but this amount cannot be known in advance. Some patients will tolerate no diplopia postoperatively. For such patients a lesser amount of surgery is indicated.

The choice of surgical procedure depends on the deviation. A common practice is to recess both lateral recti for the divergence excess type of exotropia.[17] For basic exotropia and the simulated divergence excess type, the procedure is either recession of both lateral recti or monocular resection of one medial rectus and recession of the lateral rectus.[18] A large deviation may require bilateral resection and recession. The presence of less exotropia in lateral gaze predisposes to postoperative overcorrections, especially after bilateral lateral rectus recessions.[19] In such cases monocular surgery should be done and the use of adjustable sutures would be especially advantageous.

For convergence insufficiency associated with a large exophoria at near, surgery also can be done as a last resort. Both medial rectus muscles are resected. Postoperatively, an esotropia at distance should be produced. Prisms on the upper portion of spectacles will most likely be required for relief of diplopia. Over several weeks or months the prism power can be reduced and single vision finally obtained at distance. Occasionally diplopia from esotropia remains in lateral gaze. With time the exotropia at near recurs; however, it does not seem to be as symptomatically annoying to the patient as before surgery.[20]

Undercorrection of exotropia appears to predispose towards recurrence. If relief of symptoms depends on exact alignment, a prism may help. Undercorrection is common in intermittent exotropia, especially by several months after surgery. A small residual deviation can require no treatment. Larger deviations can be given Fresnel prisms to permit binocular function, stabilize the deviation, and improve fusional vergence amplitudes. A second operation may eventually become necessary.

Overcorrection of exotropia is desirable for a few weeks after surgery. A postoperative esotropia of 10 to 15 PD frequently is recommended. A large overcorrection with limitation of eye rotations indicates that too much surgery was done, or possibly that a muscle has slipped off its attachment to the globe. Immediate reoperation is desirable in this situation. A small overcorrection may be tolerated symptomatically (esophoria). If diplopia results, a prism or occlusion may be required. The surgical production of incomitance can result in esotropia in lateral gaze and persisting diplopia, sometimes intolerable for the patient even though elicited only in far lateral gaze. After a few weeks, miotics or hyperopic refractive correction may be required. Adults should have been wearing full hyperopic correction before surgery. Small overcorrections may be correctable nonsurgically with botulinum toxin injections. Duction exercises, in which the patient forcibly abducts an eye that has restricted abduction after surgery, can be helpful. Reoperation is best delayed until the deviation has stopped changing.

SECONDARY EXOTROPIA

Exotropia can be caused by longstanding poor vision, as occurs with amblyopia, or by anisometropia, uncorrected unilateral aphakia, and various diseases of the eyes that impair vision (sensory exotropia). Among patients under the age of 5 years, poor vision leads to approximately equal numbers of estropes and exotropes. After the age of 5, exotropia predominates.

Secondary exotropia can also be caused by mechanical factors, such as weakness of the medial rectus muscle or scarring after trauma (Fig. 7.5). Paresis of the third nerve due to intracranial causes usually involves the medial rectus muscle as well as the other muscles innervated by this nerve. Isolated inferior division paresis (inferior rectus and inferior oblique) is possible with damage to the orbital floor, sparing the medial rectus. The medial rectus can be damaged in isolation during ethmoid sinus surgery.

Pseudoexotropia results from a large, positive angle kappa. This can occur with or without other ocular anomalies. A disease that commonly produces a large positive angle kappa is retinopathy of prematurity, in which the retina can be dragged temporally by vasoproliferative tissue. In addition, a wide interpupillary distance tends to give the appearance of exotropia.

Exotropia may be associated with craniofacial anomalies that feature a divergence of the orbits: Crouzon syndrome and Apert syndrome. If major craniofacial surgery is to be done, the exotropia should be surgically corrected after the facial surgery.

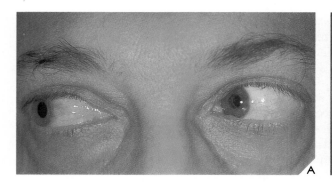

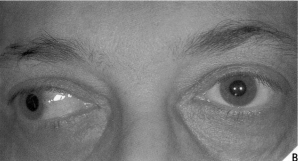

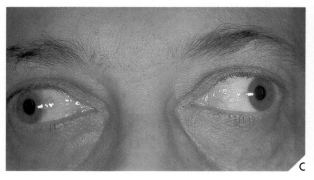

7.5 | Exotropia from trauma to the right medial rectus muscle during ethmoid surgery. *A:* Rightgaze. *B:* Primary position. *C:* Leftgaze. The right eye does not move at all. The right medial rectus was severed close to its origin and applies no adducting torque to the eye. In a paresis, inhibition of the antagonist allows the eye to return close to primary position in extreme gaze effort to the paretic side. Here, even the spring force of a paretic muscle is lacking and the eye does not move.

Consecutive exotropia refers to the development of exotropia in a formerly esotropic patient. This can occur either spontaneously, with associated poor vision, with accommodative esotropia from high hyperopia, or after surgical weakening of the medial rectus muscles in surgery for esotropia, at any time interval from immediate to many years.

CONVERGENCE PARALYSIS

Convergence paralysis is an inability to converge through either accommodative or fusional convergence. A severely reduced convergence exists to near targets and a horizontally comitant exotropia occurs at near, often with the sudden onset of crossed diplopia. If there is a preexisting exophoria, diplopia will also be present at distance. The pupillary light reflex and adduction are normal. The near triad should be normal except for convergence. In many cases of so-called convergence paralysis, however, the entire near synkinesis is affected. Accommodation is usually reduced or even absent, and pupillary miosis to accommodation may be reduced or absent (the reverse of an Argyll–Robertson pupil). To distinguish properly convergence paralysis from a reduction of the entire near synkinesis, pupillary miosis and lens accommodation must be demonstrable on efforts to fixate a near target at the same time that convergence does not occur; otherwise, it has not been established that the patient attempted to accommodate (the distinction of an organic defect from a functional one).

Fusional convergence may be absent. Binocular fusion is first established, either at a distance great enough that no exotropia occurs or with the help of prisms. Base-out prisms of increasing strength are introduced. In convergence paralysis no fusional convergence exists and diplopia will result immediately. In those patients who have convergence but make no effort to converge, fusional vergence will operate reflexly for small introduced prisms and no diplopia occurs.

Convergence paralysis nearly always indicates an intracranial lesion. In Parinaud syndrome,[21] convergence paralysis is associated with upgaze paralysis. The lesion responsible is near the quadrigeminal plate or the third nerve nucleus (rostral midbrain). Other causes of convergence paralysis are multiple sclerosis, encephalitis, and neurosyphilis.

Treatment of the visual symptoms is prisms and a near add, depending on accommodative function.

DUANE SYNDROME

Duane syndrome is defined as a limitation of abduction, adduction or both due to a specific pathophysiology (co-contraction of the medial and lateral recti).[22] The clinical manifestation is retraction of the globe on attempted adduction (with concomitant narrowing of the lid fissure). Variable features include: eso- or exotropia, sometimes present only in lateral gaze to one side;

head turn (to achieve binocular vision); sursum or deorsumduction of the adducted affected eye (possibly also present in abduction); and A, V, or X pattern (Fig. 7.6).

Electromyography of the extraocular muscles has shown that anomalous innervation patterns explain the co-contraction.[23] In all variants of Duane syndrome EMG recordings show the medial rectus to have a normal innervation pattern. The lateral rectus always receives some component of medial rectus signal, and a variable amount of lateral rectus signal, depending on the individual case. EMG recordings of the lateral rectus in cases with limitation of abduction (Huber's Duane Type I) show a minimum of innervation on attempted abduction (there is no normal lateral rectus innervation signal) and a peak of innervation on attempted adduction (i.e., the lateral rectus receives an innervation similar to the medial rectus). Abduction is deficient because abduction innervation is lacking. In cases with limitation of adduction (Huber's Duane Type II), the lateral rectus shows the innervation pattern of both medial and lateral recti. Adduction is deficient due to co-contraction of the lateral rectus when it should be inhibited. In cases exhibiting deficient abduction and adduction (Huber's Duane Type III), the lateral rectus receives an innervation signal identical to that of the medial rectus and no abduction signal, and both horizontal recti contract as one muscle.

Esotropia is more common in Types I and III and exotropia in Type II. In cases with an A, V, or X pattern, the lateral rectus receives the innervation signal of either the inferior rectus, the superior rectus, or both. In many cases the lateral rectus is found to be inelastic on traction testing. The upshoot or downshoot in adduction may be due either to sideslip of the tight, fibrotic lateral rectus[24] or to an innervation anomaly in which the superior or inferior rectus muscle receives the medial rectus innervation signal.[25] Widespread brainstem abnormalities have been found in Duane syndrome.[26-28]

Appropriate surgery depends on the exact pathophysiology of the particular case at hand, and each case must therefore be analyzed individually. Possible goals for surgery are repositioning of the field of binocular single vision to alleviate a head turn, treatment of a strabismus, or reduction of retraction and the vertical deviations in adduction. Resection of co-contracting muscles can make the retraction worse. Sideslip of the lateral rectus, when it occurs, may be improved by a posterior fixation suture. Because of the limited range of rotation of the affected eye, postoperative diplopia can be a complication if no suppression pattern is established for the new alignment.

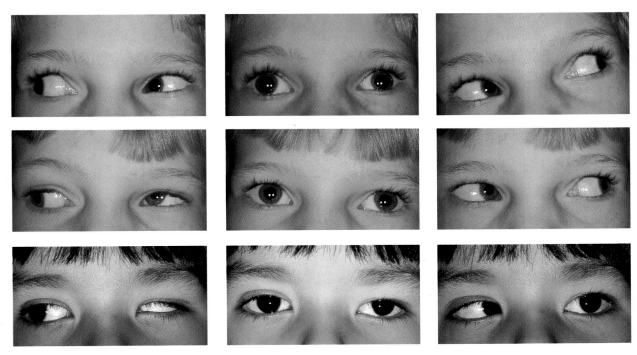

7.6 | Exotropia with Duane syndrome. Three cases, increasing in severity of retraction from top to bottom. All have exotropia in primary position. The top two cases have full abduction but limited adduction. Retraction and elevation in adduction are very mild in the top and moderate in the middle. The bottom case has limited abduction, severe retraction, and marked upshoot on adduction.

Gary R. Diamond

Esotropias represent the most common form of strabismus and include congenital, accommodative, cyclic, and nonaccommodative forms. They are also seen in some patients who have the Duane or the Möbius syndrome.

CONGENITAL ESOTROPIA

The most common form of esotropia is "congenital" esotropia, somewhat arbitrarily defined as esotropia presenting before 6 months of age (Fig. 8.1). Recent work has demonstrated that many infants begin life with a moderate exodeviation, which disappears between 2 and 4 months of age; prospective studies have determined that this is the age at which "congenital" esotropia is first noted. It could not be predicted at a younger age which children would develop congenital esotropia at age 2 to 4 months.[1] These very important observations suggest that the causes of "congenital" strabismus are neither purely motor nor purely sensory in most cases, but rather represent a difficulty in coupling the two systems.

The incidence of congenital esotropia is roughly 1% in most series, and may be more common in children who have neurological disorders.[2] The term *congenital esotropia* is so

8.1 | Congenital esotropia with decentered light reflex in the left eye. (From Cheng KP, Biglan AW, Hiles DA: Pediatric ophthalmology, in Zitelli BJ, Davis HW (eds): *Atlas of Pediatric Physical Diagnosis*, ed 2. New York: Gower Medical Publishing, 1992, 19.6.)

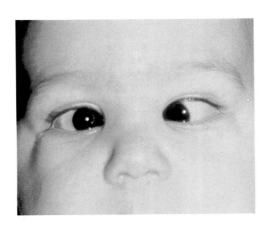

widely used that it should be retained despite evidence that very few, if any, children are truly esotropic from birth. Sex and racial distributions are equal. Concordance in one series was 81% in monozygous twins, and 9% in dizygous twins.[3] It is common to find accommodative esotropia or other cases of congenital esotropia in the proband's family.

PRESENTATION

Amblyopia occurs in between 25% and 40% of patients but the majority "cross-fixate," using the right eye to fix across the nose to view objects to the left of the patient, and vice versa (Fig. 8.2).[4] A child who does not have amblyopia should switch fixation at the midline as an object is brought from one side to the other rather than maintaining fixation and adopting a progressive head turn. As a rule, the deviation is equal to or larger than 35 prism diopters and is comitant, measuring roughly the same in all gaze positions, distance and near. Cover test measurements may be difficult in very young children, and variations of the light reflex test with the deviation neutralized by prisms held apex-to-apex before both eyes may be required. The deviation tends to be constant but may vary; rarely, spontaneous resolution occurs over a 3- to 4-year period. Refractive errors tend to be similar to those of normal children of the same age.

Inferior oblique overaction is noted in up to 75% of such patients, with onset most frequent during the second year of life; it can be unilateral or bilateral[5] (Fig. 8.3). Early surgical correction of the esotropia does not decrease the incidence of later development of inferior oblique overaction. This must be differentiated from dissociated vertical deviation (DVD) which also occurs in roughly 75% of these patients and has similar onset patterns[6] (Fig. 8.4). DVD may be manifest or latent, very asymmetric, and may present as any combination of elevation, abduction, and excyclotorsion (Fig. 8.5).

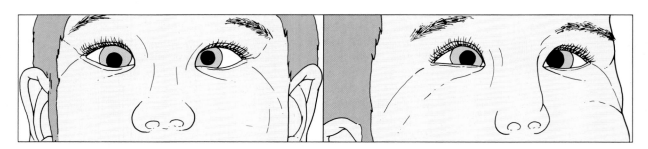

8.2 | *A,B:* Infant with congenital esotropia and cross-fixation using the right eye to view left and vice versa. Doll's-head maneuver will show full abduction.

8.3 | Overelevation in adduction of the left eye due to inferior oblique overaction in a patient with esotropia. This must be distinguished from dissociated vertical deviation, which also may cause overelevation in adduction. (From Cheng KP, Biglan AW, Hiles DA: Pediatric Ophthalmology, in Zitelli BJ, Davis HW (eds): *Atlas of Pediatric Physical Diagnosis,* ed 2. New York: Gower Medical Publishing, 1992, 19.6.)

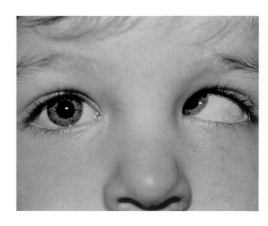

Although its cause is unknown, it may represent a primitive eye movement pattern in the presence of deficient fusion, perhaps caused by momentary loss of tone in the superior oblique muscle.

Nystagmus can manifest in both rotary and latent horizontal forms. The former is uncommon and tends to diminish during the first decade of life. Latent nystagmus with fast phase towards the unoccluded eye is present in approximately 50% of patients, and may confound attempts at monocular acuity measurement; fogging one eye with plus lenses or the use of anaglyph (red–green) lenses may provide a more accurate acuity measurement in the presence of latent nystagmus.

Roughly half of the children referred by pediatricians to ophthalmologists for esotropia at a young age have pseudostrabismus, an illusion caused by a wide nasal bridge, epicanthal folds, and the ability of young children to converge accommodatively to very close distances (Fig. 8.6). Side-gaze observations by nonophthalmologists can be particularly deceiving, as the adducted eye is easily buried under the skin fold. Hirschberg light reflexes can demonstrate alignment to the parents, as can elevation of nasal bridge skin away from the face to alter the facial appearance temporarily.

Figure 8.4. Dissociated Vertical Deviation Compared with Inferior Oblique Overaction

DISSOCIATED VERTICAL DEVIATION	INFERIOR OBLIQUE OVERACTION
Present in all gaze positions	Present in adduction only
Does not obey the Hering law	Obeys the Hering law
Slow floating abduction, elevation, excyclotorsion movement	Rapid elevation, abduction movement
Not associated with A or V pattern	Often associated with V pattern
Proportional to ambient illumination in fixing eye	Not proportional to illumination in fixing eye

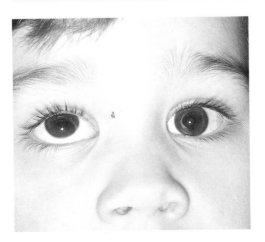

8.5 | Dissociated vertical deviation in the right eye. If the patient were fixing with the right eye, no hypodeviation would be seen in the left. Therefore, DVD does not obey the Hering law. (From Cheng KP, Biglan AW, Hiles DA: Pediatric Ophthalmology, in Zitelli BJ, Davis HW (eds): *Atlas of Pediatric Physical Diagnosis*, ed 2. New York: Gower Medical Publishing, 1992, 19.7.)

DIFFERENTIAL DIAGNOSIS OF CONGENITAL ESOTROPIA

The differential diagnosis of congenital esotropia (Fig. 8.7) includes entities discussed in detail below. Mention should be made of nystagmus blockage (compensation) syndrome which, in the opinion of some, comprises a significant segment of the young population who have large-angle, early-onset esotropia.[7] These patients have a large esotropia and nystagmus at a young age; the nystagmus is of minimal amplitude in adduction and maximal in abduction. Therefore, they make a continuous effort to maintain both eyes in adduction through the use of convergence, and it may be impossible to neutralize the esodeviation with prisms held before one or both eyes. Although nystagmus may be observed in patients with the common form of congenital esotropia, it is equally present in all gaze positions. Various series have described the incidence of nystagmus blockage syndrome as affecting 10% or 12% of esotropic patients, but many feel it is much less common.

TREATMENT

The theoretical goals of treatment include excellent visual acuity in each eye, perfect single binocular vision in all gaze positions at distance and near, and a normal esthetic appearance. All are obtainable except for perfect single binocular vision because, with very rare exceptions, these patients, even with early treatment, do not view with both foveas simultaneously. However, as discussed below, most will obtain peripheral fusion and the monofixation syndrome, and generally stable alignment. Other reported benefits of successful surgical alignment include improvement in fine motor skills and heightened bonding of parents and child.

Amblyopia is traditionally treated preoperatively, because compliance is usually better, acuity can be more easily evaluated (the eye moves to take up fixation in the presence of a large strabismus), and amblyopia responds more quickly in younger children. A common approach is to occlude the better-sighted eye during all waking hours and to evaluate the child at intervals related to age. Thus, a 1-year-old child would be evaluated 1 week after onset of occlusion, a 2-year-old after 2 weeks, and a 6-month-old 3 days after the onset of occlusion. After acuity is equalized, the duration of patching can be decreased to approximately 2 hours per day with good assurance that amblyopia will not return; in compliant families, patching can be discontinued with a 50% or better assurance that amblyopia will not return. Others have cyclopleged the better-sighted eye, if hyperopic, with atropine, or have occluded the better-sighted eye with an opaque contact lens, with success.

The impact of treatment of refractive errors of less than +2.00 is usually variable and minimal. Larger refractive errors should be corrected and the

8.6 | Pseudostrabismus caused by a flat nasal bridge, wide epicanthal folds, and small interpupillary distance. (From Cheng KP, Biglan AW, Hiles DA: Pediatric Ophthalmology, in Zitelli BJ, Davis HW (eds): *Atlas of Pediatric Physical Diagnosis*, ed 2. New York: Gower Medical Publishing, 1992, 19.9.)

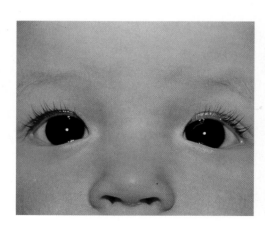

deviation remeasured, as postoperative exotropia can occur if surgery is performed on uncorrected, highly hyperopic eyes. An occasional patient responds to miotic treatment, but these patients usually have an intermittent deviation and probably have an early-onset accommodative esotropia.

Patients with congenital esotropia, when left untreated, do not display binocular vision of any variety when they become old enough to cooperate in tests of their visual sensory status; the primary goal of surgical treatment is to align the eyes sufficiently so as to stimulate the development of binocularity. This binocularity will usually fulfill the definition of the monofixation syndrome as delineated by Parks, and is a generally stable alignment.

The mainstay of therapy for this form of strabismus is surgery. Ing found that surgical alignment before the age of 24 months resulted in peripheral fusion in 93% of patients; surgery after 24 months resulted in similar results in only 31% of patients.[8] However, no available data exist to suggest that surgery at 6 months of age is more effective that that performed 1 year later. Advocates of surgery after the age of 2 years are concerned about later development of inferior oblique overaction and DVD requiring separate surgical procedures, the difficulty in measuring acuity in children who have aligned visual axes, and are unconvinced of the benefits of the monofixation syndrome (peripheral fusion without central fusion). Given reproducible strabismus measurements, informed and supportive parents, the availability of safe pediatric anesthesia, and absence of amblyopia, most strabismus surgeons in North America would opt for achievement of horizontal alignment by the age of 2 years.

The two major surgical options for correction are symmetric medial rectus recessions on both eyes (possibly adding a monocular or binocular lateral rectus resection) and a recession of one medial rectus combined with resection of the opponent lateral rectus on the same eye (see Chapter 15). Some surgeons prefer a limbal incision, claiming ease of access and orientation as well as the ability to recede contracted conjunctiva and thus augment the effect of the medial rectus recession. Many prefer the fornix approach popularized by Parks, because it often does not require suture closure and avoids proximity to the cornea, permitting rapid patient mobilization.

Whatever the approach, a recent tendency towards larger medial rectus recessions has significantly improved the surgical success rate. Recent series

Figure 8.7. Differential Diagnosis of Congenital Esotropia

Early-onset accommodative esotropia

Nystagmus blockage (compensation) syndrome

Möbius syndrome

Duane syndrome

Cyclic esotropia

Esotropia associated with visual loss in one eye, neurological impairment, or increased intracranial pressure

Strabismus fixus and other fibrosis syndromes

have quoted rates of alignment within 10 prism diopters of perfect alignment as high as 90%. Some surgeons prefer to perform recessions measured from the limbus rather than from the original muscle insertion, claiming increased uniformity and better results. A common protocol for surgical treatment is shown in Figure 8.8.

A novel approach to congenital esotropia is the use of botulinum toxin, originally popularized by Scott and studied further by Magoon.[9] He injected one medial rectus in 15 children and found excellent results, stable for at least 1 year. Most children required ketamine sedation, and many required more than one injection.

Because of instability of postoperative alignment, children who undergo surgery for congenital esotropia require long-term follow-up. Residual esotropia of greater than 10 prism diopters observed 4 to 6 weeks after initial surgery may respond to antiaccommodative measures if the patient is significantly hyperopic, but probably will require a second surgical procedure. This might be bilateral lateral rectus resection for those who initially underwent bilateral medial rectus recessions, and a recess–resect procedure on the unoperated eye for those who underwent a unilateral procedure. A significant fraction of patients initially aligned later develop accommodative esotropia and require treatment with glasses or miotics.[10]

Because patients with DVD usually exhibit no binocularity when the DVD is present, they are asymptomatic; the major reason to consider treatment for the DVD is esthetic. If the DVD is monocular or highly asymmetric, optic means may permit the switching of fixation to the eye with the DVD,

Figure 8.8.

Symmetric Surgery for Congenital Esotropia

DEVIATION (PRISM DIOPTERS)	RECESS MEDIAL RECTUS OU (MM)
35	5.0
40 or 45	5.5
50 or 55	6.0
60 or 65	6.5
70 or greater	7.0

Asymmetric Surgery for Congenital Esotropia

DEVIATION (PRISM DIOPTERS)	RECESS MR (MM)	RESECT LR (MM)
35	5.0	8.0
40 or 45	5.5	9.0
50 or 55	6.0	10.0
60 or 65	6.5	10.0
70 or greater	7.0	10.0

thus rendering it entirely latent. Usually, however, surgical treatment is necessary. This can be symmetric or asymmetric and may involve significant recessions of the superior rectus muscle(s) or resection of the inferior rectus muscle(s). Some surgeons combine the former with a posterior fixation suture, which alone is ineffective. It is crucial to dissect the intermuscular septum from the vertical recti so as not to affect lid position.

Inferior oblique overaction often is primarily esthetic but may also interfere with binocular function if elevation of the adducted eye occurs close to fixation and if it is bilateral. Because of the frequency of increased overaction in an unoperated, overactive oblique muscle after the other is weakened, unilateral surgery should be reserved for cases that are clearly unilateral. Traditional weakening procedures include disinsertion, myectomy, denervation and extirpation, and measured recession. Anteriorization of the oblique insertion to the margin of the inferior rectus significantly weakens the muscle and may serve as effective treatment for simultaneous DVD. Clear separation between DVD and inferior oblique overaction is necessary, as weakening of a normally functioning inferior oblique can lead to limitation of elevation in adduction, head postures, and all the signs and symptoms of cyclovertical muscle palsy.

ACCOMMODATIVE ESOTROPIA

Accommodative esotropia is characterized by two mechanisms that may occur in varying proportions in the same individual. The first cause is high hyperopia, averaging +4.50, and the second is a larger eso tendency at near fixation than can be comfortably controlled by fusional divergence.

Patients with high hyperopia must generate large accommodative input to see clearly at near fixation, thus stressing fusional divergence amplitudes. They may choose blurred vision and maintain comfortable single binocular vision, or may choose clear vision and risk asthenopia or esotropia. Patients with high hyperopia who do not develop esotropia, yet who maintain excellent acuity, often have low ratios of accommodative convergence to accommodation.

Patients with typical hyperopia (average +2.25) or myopia who develop an eso deviation greater at distance than near have an overactive convergence response to a given accommodation requirement, a "high AC/A ratio." This ratio can be calculated by two methods, the heterophoria method and the gradient method, as described in Figure 8.9. Some patients have mildly high hyperopia and mildly high AC/A ratios, and therefore have a mixed mechanism of accommodative esotropia. In all cases, however, the patient's fusional divergence amplitudes are insufficient to control the eso tendency.

PRESENTATION

The typical history is of intermittent esotropias' appearing between 6 months and 7 years of age (average 30 months) towards the end of the day or when the child is very tired, ill, or daydreaming, especially at near fixation distances such as across the dinner table. At onset, the child may experience asthenopia, as fusional divergence amplitudes are stressed, and may rub the eyes or squint; an older child may complain of headaches or diplopia. As the esotropia becomes more frequent, ARC and suppression, when available, relieve asthenopic symptoms at the possible expense of fusional divergence amplitudes. Some children maintain intermittent esotropia for long periods of time, whereas others progress quickly to constant esotropia, especially at near fixation.

The ophthalmologist should be alert to historical clues, should evaluate the AC/A ratio and, if possible, should measure fusional divergence amplitudes at distance and near fixation. Historically, atropine has been considered essential for obtaining the maximal hyperopic refractive error; however, its use requires a return visit and its cycloplegic effect is prolonged. The office use of cyclopentolate and tropicamide permits immediate treatment and, in most patients, obtains within +0.50 diopter of the refractive error obtained with atropine, although a few will have greater uncovered hyperopia.

It is important to recognize that most individuals without strabismus have flexible AC/A ratios that adjust to the changes in refractive error over the person's lifetime; patients with accommodative esotropia, on the other hand, often have a rigid AC/A ratio that inflexibly responds to changes in refractive correction. This fact can be used to the patient's benefit, by prescription of a hyperopic correction.

In older patients the fusional divergence amplitudes can be measured, and these will prove to be deficient. As successful treatment proceeds, normal fusional measurements will be obtained.

Figure 8.9. AC/A Ratio Calculations

HETEROPHORIA METHOD

Determine phoria by prism and alternate cover test at optical infinity and 1/3 meter distances. Control accommodation and correct acuity to 20/30 with least plus lens.

$$AC/A = IPD (cm) + \frac{\Delta_2 - \Delta_1}{F}$$

Δ_1 = distance phoria
Δ_2 = near phoria (eso is +, exo is -)
F = near fixation distance in diopters of vergence

Example: IPD = 60 mm or 6 cm
Δ_1 = 4 eso
Δ_2 = 30 eso
F = 1/33 cm = 3 diopters

$$AC/A = 6 + \frac{30-4}{3} = about\ 15/1$$

GRADIENT METHOD

Determine phoria by prism and alternate cover test at a fixed distance, generally 1/3 meter. Control accommodation and correct acuity to 20/30 with least plus lens. Vary lens power held before eyes and remeasure alignment.

$$AC/A = \frac{\Delta_2 - \Delta_1}{D}$$

Δ_1 = original phoria in diopters
Δ_2 = new phoria with new lens
D = power of lens

Example: Δ_2 = 2 eso
Δ_1 = 6 eso
D = +1.00

$$AC/A = \frac{6 - 2}{1} = 4/1$$

If the eso deviation cannot be found on initial attempts, occlusion of one eye for 45 minutes to 3 hours can be performed, or the patient can be cyclopleged and cover testing performed with suitably large targets after cycloplegia. An eso deviation after cycloplegia provides strong confirmation of parental observations and may be sufficient evidence to indicate the necessity for treatment.

Differential diagnosis includes variable esotropia accompanied by normal AC/A ratios and refractive errors; these uncommon patients exhibit fusional divergence amplitudes equally deficient at distance and near. Some of these patients respond to antiaccommodative measures and others do not. Another group of patients have a V-pattern esotropia with greater deviation in downgaze. It is important to measure near deviations in primary position to avoid confusing this group with accommodative esotropes.

DIFFERENTIAL DIAGNOSIS OF ACCOMMODATIVE ESOTROPIA

Treatment consists of antiaccommodative measures, primarily the prescription of much or all of the patient's hyperopic refractive error (to "do the focusing for the child" so as not to stimulate accommodation, and thus convergence) (Fig. 8.10). In very young children or myopes, the uncoupling of accommodation from convergence with miotics can be considered.

Glasses are a problem in children under approximately 1 year of age because their weight and flat nasal bridge, lack of cooperation, and small face make fitting difficult. Treatment of accommodative esotropia in this group is often better initiated with miotics such as phospholine iodide 0.125% used every evening for 2 weeks. If successful, less frequent administration can be attempted. Because of the risk of pupillary margin cysts, phenylephrine 2.5% can be added 2 weeks after miotic initiation to maintain pupillary dilatation and avoid these cysts. Because phospholine is a true cholinesterase inhibitor that has potential systemic effects, parents should be warned to alert all physicians to the child's use of this drug, especially when general anesthesia is indicated; nondepolarizing agents can then be used to avoid prolonged anesthesia reversal. Despite years of experience with this drug in the treatment of accommodative esotropia, when it is used at this frequency and strength in children no cases of cataract or retinal detachment have been described. Because older children may complain of brow ache and miotic spasm, an attempt is made to

TREATMENT

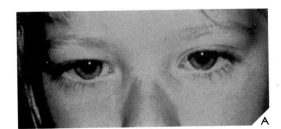

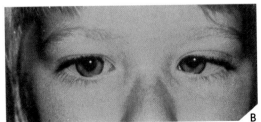

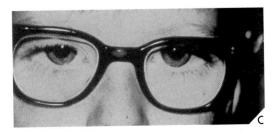

8.10 | This hyperopic child with left esotropia only at near fixation responds to full hyperopic glasses correction with no residual esotropia. The accommodative esotropia is fully corrected by single-vision lenses. (From Fells P, Lee JP: Strabismus, in Spalton DJ, Hitchings RA, Hunter PA (eds): *Atlas of Clinical Ophthalmology*. London, New York: Gower Medical Publishing, 1984, 18.7.)

switch patients to glasses at the age of 1 year when possible; however, many parents wish to remain with the miotic because it has no esthetic disadvantages, works constantly, and does not demand the child's cooperation.

In children from 1 to 4 years, the full cycloplegic refraction is given and the child is reevaluated after a month's full-time wear of the prescription. If the distance and near esodeviations are reduced to within monofixational range (8 prism diopters of esotropia or less) and the child is without asthenopic signs or symptoms and with a comfortably controlled phoria, the treatment is considered initially successful and the patient is reevaluated in 3 to 6 months' time, depending on age. At every visit, visual acuity at distance and near, alignment at distance and near, and sensory testing are performed. Cycloplegic refractions are repeated every 6 months. If the distance tropia is greater than the above limits, the cycloplegic refraction is repeated, and if it remains so with the new refraction or if no change has occurred in the refraction, the patient becomes a surgical candidate. If the distance deviation is controlled but an esotropia greater than the above limits is present at near fixation, or if a symptomatic phoria at near fixation persists, the patient should be fitted with bifocal glasses (Fig. 8.11). It is important to warn parents that a newly fitted child will exhibit larger and more frequent esodeviations when the glasses are removed.

The bifocals should be prescribed high enough to split the pupil in primary position; strengths above +1.00 can be prescribed as executive style, but lower strengths often can only be ground as a large flattop style. The ini-

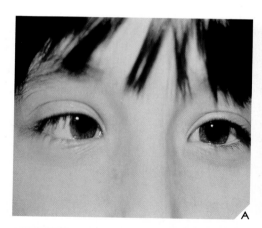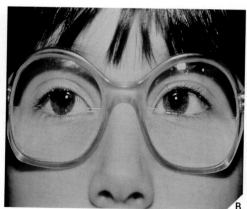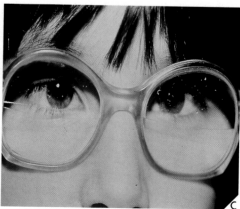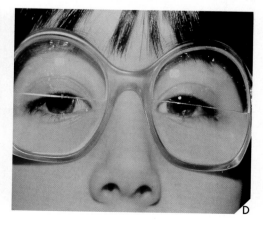

8.11 | This hyperopic child with right esotropia greater at near fixation (*A*) than distance had aligned eyes only at distance fixation (*B,C*) with single-vision lenses. A bifocal was prescribed, which aligned her eyes at near fixation (*D*). (From Cheng KP, Biglan AW, Hiles DA: Pediatric Ophthalmology, in Zitelli BJ, Davis HW (eds): *Atlas of Pediatric Physical Diagnosis,* ed 2. New York: Gower Medical Publishing, 1992, 19.8.)

tial bifocal strength can be estimated by measuring the near eso deviation with various strengths of trial frame lenses, or can be arbitrarily given as +2.50 to +3.00. The patient is asked to wear the bifocals for a month and then to return for reevaluation; rarely, except for a V-pattern esotropia, will the near deviation not respond to bifocal prescription if the distance deviation is controlled with full cyloplegic refraction. Patients who have V-pattern accommodative esotropia may require miotics alone or in addition to single-vision glasses, as bifocals require downgaze fixation and the deviation is largest in downgaze in such patients.

As a rule, glasses and miotics represent equally effective treatments and it is rare for a patient respond to one but not the other; conversely, both together will rarely salvage a patient who does not respond to one or the other. An intellectual preference exists for refractive treatment for the highly hyperopic "refractive" accommodative esotrope, and miotic treatment for the patient who has a high AC/A ratio.

At about 5 years of age the parents of the successfully treated child will note less eso deviation without glasses; at about 6 years of age the glasses can be progressively weakened, roughly 0.50 to 0.75 diopters every 6 months, beginning with the bifocal. A common practice is to place the weaker correction in a trial frame and perform cover testing; occasionally, a patient will appear aligned during this office evaluation but will develop a significant eso deviation, asthenopic symptoms, or both, when wearing the weaker correction. This latter group must return to the previous stronger prescription. It is often possible to rid children of their bifocals by 8 or 9 years of age and of their mild to moderate hyperopic correction by the early teens. Patients who have high hyperopia, significant astigmatism, or anisometropia may require optical correction for acuity purposes after their accommodative esotropia has resolved; some can be treated with contact lenses.

Patients whose treatment is initiated between 4 and 8 years of age may not accept their full hyperopic correction without a period of cycloplegia. Ideally, the minimal correction necessary to provide and maintain comfortable single binocular vision and (in the case of high hyperopia) good visual acuity is prescribed. After age 6 the AC/A ratio tends to normalize, but the hyperopia may increase. Initiation of treatment in children older than 9 years is difficult but is similar to that described above; some of these older patients may respond to miotics.

At any time after a period of successful antiaccommodative treatment, a patient may develop an esotropia not controlled with glasses or miotics.[11] Repeat refraction should be performed, and if greater hyperopia is found additional correction should be prescribed. It is difficult to predict the effect of even as little as +0.50 additional correction on a decompensated accommodative esotrope. If no effect is obtained after a few weeks' trial, the patient should undergo strabismus surgery. The contribution of high hyperopia, a high AC/A ratio, progressively increasing hyperopia, undercorrection of hyperopia, and overactive inferior obliques to decompensation of accommodative esotropia is still somewhat unclear. The clinical experience of this author is that significant inferior oblique overaction implies less likelihood that weaning from glasses can be achieved, and a greater incidence of decompensation; the same is true of decreased interpupillary distance.

Strabismus surgery classically is directed only towards the nonaccommodative component of the distance eso deviation, with an arbitrary addition (1 mm additional recession per medial rectus) for a high AC/A ratio.

Cautiously, more extensive surgery may be performed in highly hyperopic patients to ease them postoperatively into weaker glasses. Some feel that posterior fixation sutures combined with medial rectus recessions benefit patients with a high AC/A ratio. Parents should be warned of the continuing need for antiaccommodative treatment even after strabismus surgery.

A difficult group of patients are those teenagers who are well controlled in bifocals or high hyperopic correction who have esthetic concerns. Switching to contact lenses will place less accommodative demand on the patient and may permit comfortable single binocular vision at near fixation without the need for separate reading glasses. Bifocal contact lenses may be tolerable to some; few will be satisfied with "monovision" fitting of one lens for distance needs and the other for near. Blended bifocals may be tolerated by some teenagers and may permit persistent bifocal treatment without the dysesthetic impact of a bifocal line. Some teenagers will accept miotics in addition to single-vision glasses to avoid the bifocal. Finally, cautious single medial rectus recession or small bimedial rectus recession can be performed in patients who fuse at distance when wearing single-vision lenses and who wish to be rid of their bifocal.

The effective management of accommodative esotropia demands a long period of cooperation among patient, physician, and parents, and is as much art as science. Nowhere else in strabismus management are communication skills as important.

CYCLIC ESOTROPIA

First reported by Burian in 1958,[12] this curious condition most commonly presents as alternating 24-hour periods of perfect alignment followed by constant, usually large-angled (30 to 40 prism diopter) esotropia. The age of onset is usually 3 to 4 years. Other cycles of alternation, often 12 or 36 hours, are described.[13] When the eyes are aligned, excellent fusional abilities and steropsis are found; when esotropia is present, patients exhibit ARC and suppression. Some patients with cyclic esotropia display irritability and emotional withdrawal during the strabismic period. The incidence has been estimated at 1 in 5,000 cases of strabismus (roughly 150 cases appear in the literature). Aids to diagnosis include a strong suspicion and a log of the strabismus periods kept by the parents. This condition differs from intermittent esotropia because during the aligned periods little or no strabismus can be elicited despite prolonged occlusion.

The cause is unknown but may be related to the "biological clock" phenomenon popularized by Richter.[14] Some patients develop a cyclic esotropia after head trauma, a neurosurgical procedure, strabismus surgery, or infection. The course is usually stable, but some patients decompensate to a persistent strabismus.

Antiaccommodative meaures are usually of little effect during the periods of strabismus and are not needed during the aligned periods. Surgical treatment carries a typical success rate whether performed during aligned or strabismic periods.

MÖBIUS SYNDROME

Möbius syndrome consists, in its full presentation, of bilateral abduction limitation, with or without esotropia; upper motor neuron VII nerve palsies; and XII nerve palsy with atrophy of the tongue.[15] Some patients have difficulty suckling as young infants, as well as abnormal phonation. Close inspection of the tongue reveals atrophy of its terminal third. The upper motor neuron

VII nerve palsies cause smooth facies, absent nasolabial folds, a round mouth and decreased facial emotional responses. Lid closure is variable. Patients with esotropia (38%) usually have tight medial recti on forced duction testing;[16] those with gaze palsy and straight eyes do not. The esotropia, when present, is quite large, and the patients cross-fixate similar to congenital esotropes; as a rule, however, abduction to the midline cannot be performed.

The syndrome is not strictly defined; some patients are included who also have vertical gaze palsies and lower motor neuron VII nerve palsies. The cause of the esotropia may include both involvement of the VI nerve fascicles and nuclei and aberrant medial rectus insertion, as some patients are found to have medial recti that insert quite close to the limbus. No treatment is necessary or successful in patients who have gaze palsies alone; those with esotropia and inability to abduct to the midline require medial rectus recessions. These recessions may be technically quite challenging because the muscles are very tight and difficult to hook, suture, and safely detach from the globe; double-overlapping marginal myotomies may be safer in some situations. Resections of the nonfunctioning lateral recti should be avoided as fruitless.

Systemic associations include mental retardation, polydactyly, syndactyly, brachydactyly, clubbed feet, peroneal muscular atrophy, and a peculiar gait.[17] Brainstem auditory evoked responses are often abnormal.

DUANE SYNDROME

Duane syndrome, comprising 1% of all strabismus, is a congenital miswiring of the medial and lateral rectus muscles such that globe retraction on attempted adduction occurs, as well as limitation of adduction, abduction, or both. Its most common variant (Type I; 85% of cases) presents more commonly (60%) in the left eye and more commonly (60%) in girls as severely limited or absent abduction (Figs. 8.12 and 8.13). Neuropathologically, this has been shown to be caused by an absent VI nerve nucleus and nerve and innervation of the lateral rectus by a branch from the inferior division of the III nerve.[18] Thus, classical electromyographic findings of absent lateral rectus firing on attempted abduction, and firing of both horizontal recti on attempted adduction, can be explained.[19] No mechanism exists to improve the abduction limitation. About 40% of patients develop esotropia and tight medial rectus muscles, adopting a head turn towards the same eye to maintain single binocular vision, or they maintain a straight head but accept esotropia, ARC, and suppression, if available.[20] Recession of the medial rectus in the involved eye will align the eye but will not improve abduction beyond primary position. Rarely, very large weakening procedures performed on the medial rectus will lead to consecutive exotropia by way of poorly understood mechanisms. A small medial rectus recession in the opposite eye will help stabilize the pathologic eye in primary position by application of the Hering law; resection of the lateral rectus is avoided, as it will increase retraction and not improve abduction.

Duane syndrome is bilateral in roughly 20% of cases; the sex and eye predominance pertain only to the Type I described above. Less common forms include Type II (14%), with limitation of adduction and a tendency towards exotropia, and Type III (1%), with limitation of both abduction and adduction and any form of horizontal strabismus. Often associated is a "tether" phenomenon consisting of overelevation, overdepression, or both, in adduction as the retracted globe escapes from its horizontal rectus restrictions. This can be surgically improved with horizontal rectus posterior fixa-

8.12 | Head posture in a child with left Duane syndrome Type I shows a face turn to the left to compensate for deficient abduction in the left eye. (From Fells P, Lee JP: Strabismus, in Spalton DJ, Hitchings RA, Hunter PA (eds): *Atlas of Clinical Ophthalmology.* London, New York: Gower Medical Publishing, 1984, 18.13.)

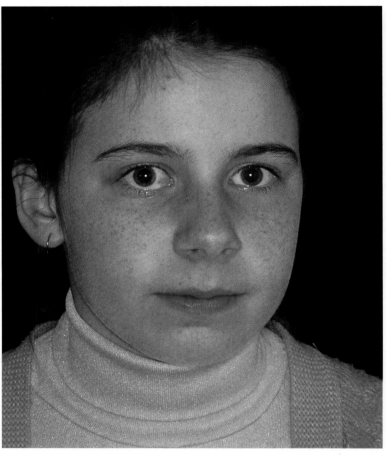

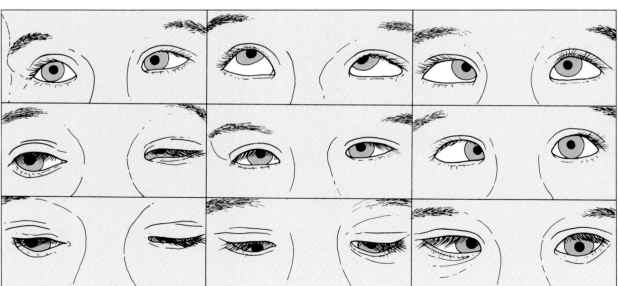

8.13 | Versions in a child with left Duane syndrome Type I shows no abduction beyond the midline, with retraction of the left eye and narrowing of the left lid fissure on adduction.

tion sutures or by horizontal splitting of the lateral rectus into a "Y" structure, with resuturing of the muscle above and below the axis of the lateral rectus. If extreme retraction with pseudoptosis is dysesthetic, both horizontal recti can be receded to relieve the retraction.

Systemic associations in 30% include: Goldenhar syndrome; Klippel–Feil anomalad; a rare autosomal dominant form; and the Wildervanck association of Duane syndrome, Klippel–Feil anomalad, and congenital labyrinthine deafness. Pairs of identical twins who have mirror-image Duane syndrome have been described.

Brainstem auditory evoked responses are occasionally abnormal, suggesting widespread neurological abnormalities.

STRABISMUS FIXUS

This very rare congenital, stationary, very large-angle esotropia of unknown cause may represent a form of congenital fibrosis of the medial rectus muscles. No abduction is usually possible, and strabismus surgery on these very tight muscles is often of little benefit.

ESOTROPIA IN THE NEUROLOGICALLY IMPAIRED

The incidence of strabismus is higher in neurologically impaired children than in the general population. In addition to the above categories, children with neurologic impairment may have a variable intermittent esotropia that is unresponsive to antiaccommodative measures. This may be stable, may worsen to a constant tropia, or may disappear with maturity. Surgery should be avoided unless measurements of the deviation are reproducible, the patient is intellectually capable of benefiting from improved binocular function, and the effects of any neurotropic medications are understood. Surgical outcome may be less successful in these patients, but antiaccommodative measures may be helpful. In addition, a patient under significant emotional stress will occasionally present with a temporary esotropia, sometimes related to accommodative spasm.

ESOTROPIA ASSOCIATED WITH VISUAL DEFICIT

Children who have impaired vision in one or both eyes are at risk for developing strabismus. Esotropia will develop in a high incidence of infants under 2 years of age who have decreased acuity secondary to congenital cataract, corneal opacity, retinal pathology, or other devastating media clarity impairments. The prognosis for development of stable single binocular vision with early treatment of the media pathology and surgical alignment is poor; therefore, in most cases surgical treatment is performed primarily for esthetic improvement.

9 | OBLIQUE MUSCLE DYSFUNCTIONS

Gary R. Diamond

Overactions and underactions of both oblique muscles are well recognized. Often, the prefix "primary" is used to indicate ignorance of the cause of the dysfunction and the prefix "secondary" is appended when the dysfunction is caused by a known dysfunction of another cyclovertical muscle. Gobin suggested that many oblique dysfunctions are caused by a mismatch between the course of the inferior oblique muscle and the superior oblique tendon.[1] If the trochlea were positioned anterior to the bony origin of the inferior oblique when viewed coronally, a mechanical advantage would accrue to the former; conversely, if the trochlea were positioned behind the inferior oblique origin, the inferior oblique would obtain mechanical advantage (Fig. 9.1). The former situation is seen in some patients who have midface retrusion or hydrocephalus (Fig. 9.2), and the latter in some patients with orbital roof retrusion. However, many patients with oblique muscle dysfunction have normal orbital anatomy and as yet unknown reasons for the dysfunction.

PRIMARY INFERIOR OBLIQUE OVERACTION

Overelevation in adduction caused by inferior oblique overaction develops in about 72% of congenital esotropes, 34% of accommodative esotropes, and 32% of intermittent exotropes who are followed for more than 5 years.[2] In this study the incidence of inferior oblique overaction in patients with congenital esotropia was not related to age of strabismus onset, time from onset to surgery for the esotropia, age at first surgery, or decompensation of horizontal alignment; it was, however, related to the number of surgical procedures necessary to align the eyes horizontally. The mean age of onset was 3.6 years.

Primary inferior oblique overaction is usually asymmetric and may be unilateral at onset (23%). Frequently, the second eye will become involved soon after unilateral surgery for infe-

9.1 | Posterior displacement of the left trochlea may give mechanical advantage to the left inferior oblique.

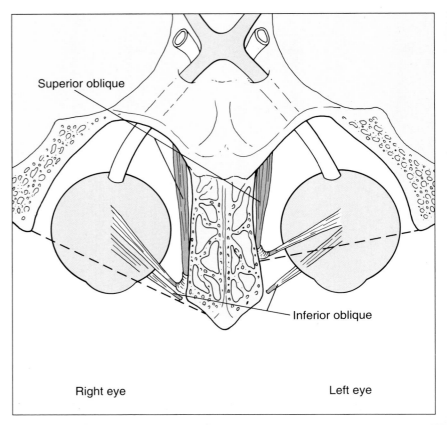

Superior oblique

Inferior oblique

Right eye

Left eye

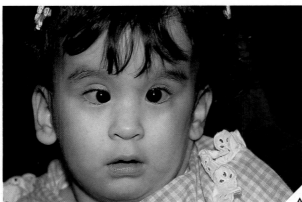

A

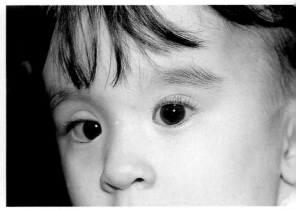

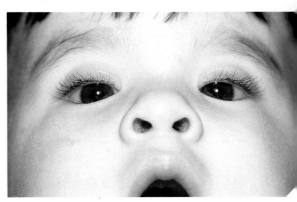

9.2 | Hydrocephalus and frontal bossing. As the frontal fossa floor advances, it pulls the trochlea forward. This trochlear advance is postulated to give mechanical advantage to the superior oblique muscles, with resultant overdepression in adduction (*B*) and an A-pattern strabismus. Note greater esotropia in primary position (*A*) than downgaze (*C*).

rior oblique weakening. Occasionally, inferior oblique overaction may occur without simultaneous horizontal strabismus.

The hyperdeviation in the affected eye can present a few degrees in adduction, in full adduction only, or only in the field of action of the inferior oblique (Fig. 9.3). Several grading systems have been derived for this overaction, none of them ideal (Fig. 9.4). If extreme bilateral overaction is present, the patient has only a narrow range of comfortable single binocular vision to either side of primary position.

A V-pattern strabismus is often associated with inferior oblique overaction and yields greater exo deviation in upgaze than downgaze. This can be easily explained by the tertiary abducting ability of the inferior oblique muscles in upgaze, but it is unclear why all patients with inferior oblique overaction do not develop a V-pattern strabismus. Vertical strabismus in primary position is quite uncommon despite asymmetry of overaction.

Patients with primary inferior oblique overaction exhibit no subjective symptoms of ocular torsion, but do have objective evidence of excyclotorsion of the involved globes. The Parks–Bielschowsky three-step test is negative, and no torsion is admitted by the patient on Maddox rod, Bagolini lens, or Lancaster red–green testing. However, examination of the fundus shows the fovea to be located below its normal position of 0.3 disc diameters below a horizontal line extending from the center of the disc (inverted, of course, by indirect ophthalmoscopy). Forced duction testing shows the inferior oblique muscles to be tighter than normal. Presumably, for patients with primary inferior oblique overactions sensory adaptations are available to reconcile globe excyclotorsion and thus to maintain comfortable single binocular vision without adoption of a head posture.

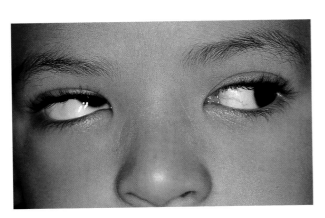

9.3 | This child has inferior oblique overaction in the right eye and overelevation in adduction.

FIGURE 9.4. Grading of Hyperdeviation

GRADE	ELEVATION OR DEPRESSION IN ADDUCTION
Trace	5 Δ
1 +	10 Δ
2 +	20 Δ
3 +	30 Δ
4 +	45 Δ

The differential diagnosis of primary inferior oblique overaction is listed in Figure 9.5. Dissociated vertical deviation often coexists with inferior oblique overaction, especially in patients with congenital esotropia. A form of pseudo-inferior oblique overaction has been presented by Capo and Guyton[3] which may explain normalization of oblique function after exotropia surgery.

Although treatment of primary inferior oblique overaction is usually performed for esthetic purposes, it often provides a functional benefit as well, because duction normalization permits a wider range of single binocular vision. Commonly performed procedures include myectomy, graded recessions, and disinsertion. More recent procedures include anteriorization[4] and denervation with extirpation.[5] Care should be taken to include the entire muscle in the procedure; in addition, direct visualization of the muscle should prevent possible rupture of a vortex vein or violation of the Tenon capsule. The latter may lead to fibrofatty proliferation of orbital fat on the sclera and to an adherence syndrome of progressive hypotropia, abduction, and excyclotropia with duction limitation. Excessive traction on the inferior oblique muscle may traumatize parasympathetic fibers of the ciliary ganglion, resulting in (usually transient) pupillary dilatation and decreased accommodative tone. Postoperatively, patients with primary inferior oblique overaction do not usually complain of torsional diplopia, and horizontal or vertical alignment in primary position is not affected.

SECONDARY INFERIOR OBLIQUE OVERACTION

Secondary inferior oblique overaction is usually caused by paresis of the antagonist superior oblique with contracture, but may occasionally be associated with superior rectus palsy in the opposite eye. Patients with secondary overaction often have a vertical strabismus in primary position. Adult patients with recent onset of palsy may complain of vertical and torsional diplopia and may also have a positive Parks–Bielschowsky three-step test. Of course, these patients also have the objective signs of oblique dysfunction mentioned above: excyclotorsion of the fovea around the optic nerve and

FIGURE 9.5. Differential Diagnosis of Overelevation in Adduction

Inferior oblique overreaction
Dissociated vertical deviation
Aberrant regeneration of cranial nerve III
Rectus rotation in patients with craniosynostosis
Tether effect in patients with Duane syndrome

positive forced duction testing. Head tilts and turns to avoid diplopia are common in this group.

Therapy is indicated not only for esthetic reasons and to increase the range of comfortable single binocular vision but also to obviate the need for head posturing to avoid visual confusion and diplopia. Some patients respond to vertical prisms, but many require surgery. Older patients should be warned of the possibility of temporary postoperative diplopia.

INFERIOR OBLIQUE UNDERACTION

Many patients with limitation of elevation in adduction have Brown syndrome, associated with V-pattern exotropia in upgaze, similar duction and version limitation of elevation (worse in adduction than in abduction), and tight forced duction testing. A few have true inferior oblique palsy, a difficult entity to reconcile neuroanatomically but one that is analogous to superior oblique palsy. These patients may have a hypodeviation in primary position if fixing with the nonparetic eye (Fig. 9.6), secondary overaction of the antagonist superior oblique, and an A-pattern exotropia with better elevation in abduction than in adduction. Elevation is better on duction than on version testing, and forced duction testing is unrestricted unless the superior oblique is contracted. Some patients may respond to vertical prisms, but many require surgery; recession of the contralateral superior rectus or weakening of the ipsilateral superior oblique are the usual procedures.

Secondary inferior oblique underaction caused by inhibitional palsy of the yoke of the antagonist to a paretic inferior rectus is occasionally seen. If the patient chooses to fixate with the paretic eye, a hypodeviation in the other eye in primary position will be present.

PRIMARY SUPERIOR OBLIQUE OVERACTION

Superior oblique overactions (overdepression in adduction) without known cause are similar to primary inferior oblique overactions, in that they are usually asymptomatic, and exhibit objective evidence of torsion (here incyclotorsion) of the fundus, positive forced duction testing, and a negative Parks–Bielschowsky three-step test. However, some patients with primary superior oblique overaction have a vertical strabismus in primary position. Because of the tertiary abducting effect of the superior oblique in downgaze,

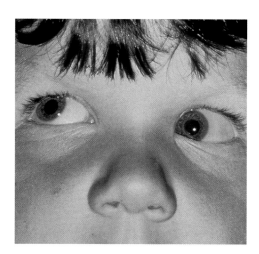

9.6 | This child has inferior oblique underaction in the left eye and underelevation in adduction. This must be distinguished from the more common Brown syndrome. (From Cheng KP, Biglan AW, Hiles DA: Pediatric ophthalmology, in Zitelli BJ, Davis HW (eds): *Atlas of Pediatric Physical Diagnosis*, ed 2. New York: Gower Medical Publishing, 1992, 19.11.)

some have an A-pattern strabismus as well (Fig. 9.7). Superior oblique overactions can be seen in esotropia and exotropia, and occasionally without any horizontal strabismus. Antagonist inferior oblique function is often normal, but occasional underactions can be demonstrated.

Prism therapy for a vertical strabismus will benefit some patients. If the condition is esthetically significant, the superior oblique can be weakened by tenotomy, tenectomy, graded recession, or lengthening. If the tenotomy spares the intermuscular septum, contractile force will be transmitted around the tenotomy to the distal tendon, thus preventing superior oblique palsy; some advocate simultaneous inferior oblique weakening to delay or prevent the onset of superior oblique palsy. Tenectomy seems to be more associated with palsy than does tenotomy. Measured recessions, although more technically challenging, offer reproducibility and less likelihood of palsy. Lengthening by interposition of Silastic material appears a promising method for superior oblique weakening. Many are cautious of weakening overacting superior obliques in patients fusing in primary position, choosing to treat A-pattern strabismus with horizontal or vertical rectus translations. Recent reports describe little, if any, eso shift in primary position after bilateral superior oblique weakening procedures.[6]

9.7 | Child with bilateral superior oblique overaction, overdepression in adduction, and an A-pattern exotropia.

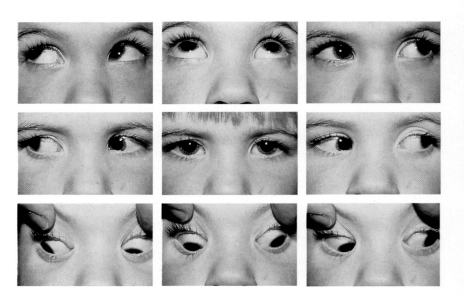

Secondary superior oblique overactions are usually caused by ipsilateral inferior oblique palsy or contralateral inferior rectus palsy (if the patient fixes with the paretic eye). In the latter case, the patient may exhibit a hypodeviation in the nonparetic eye. Patients with secondary superior oblique overaction may have a vertical deviation in primary position, a head posture, and can be expected to show a positive Parks–Bielschowsky three-step test. They also have objective evidence of globe torsion, as mentioned above. Some patients can be treated with vertical prisms, but many require strabismus surgery.

Superior oblique palsy is the most common form of cyclovertical muscle weakness. Its diagnosis and treatment are described in Chapter 11. Before spread of comitance to other cyclovertical muscles, the patient will have underdepression in adduction (Fig. 9.8), excyclotorsion of the fundus of the paretic eye, and a head posture. The Parks–Bielschowsky three-step test will be positive. Adults with recent onset superior oblique palsy will admit to torsion on Maddox rod, Bagolini lens, or Lancaster red–green testing; children or adults with chronic palsy often will not. Some patients respond to vertical prisms but many require surgery.

Occasionally, a patient with superior rectus palsy in the contralateral eye will present with a secondary superior oblique underaction if the patient chooses to fix with the paretic eye.

SECONDARY SUPERIOR OBLIQUE OVERACTION

SUPERIOR OBLIQUE UNDERACTION

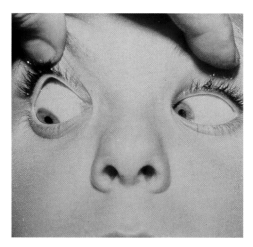

9.8 | Child with left superior oblique underaction and underdepression in adduction. (From Cheng KP, Biglan AW, Hiles DA: Pediatric Ophthalmology, in Zitelli BJ, Davis HW (eds): *Atlas of Pediatric Physical Diagnosis*, ed 2. New York: Gower Medical Publishing, 1992, 19.11)

10 | ALPHABET PATTERN STRABISMUS

Gary R. Diamond

This diverse group of ocular misalignments has incomitance from upgaze to downgaze as its unifying theme. It should be suspected in any patient with a history or presentation of chin-up or chin-down posture, and can be associated with eso, exo, or no deviation in primary position. Every patient should be evaluated for alphabet pattern strabismus by prism and alternate cover test measurements at distance fixation with the chin elevated 30°, depressed 30°, and in primary position. Figure 10.1 gives the relative incidence of alphabet pattern strabismus.

Every muscle group (obliques, horizontal recti, vertical recti) has been incriminated as causative in these patients. Those without oblique overaction have been postulated to have anatomic alterations in the rectus position on the globe. Patients with A-pattern esotropia tend to have lateral canthi higher than medial ("mongoloid" facies), and those with V-pattern esotropia tend to have lateral canthi lower than medial ("antimongoloid" facies), but no predilection can be determined for exotropes.[1,2]

Figure 10.1. Relative Incidence of Alphabet Pattern Strabismus

	V	A	TOTAL
ESOTROPIA			
	41%	25%	66%
EXOTROPIA			
	23%	11%	34%
TOTAL			
	64%	36%	100%

(From Costenbader FD: Introduction, in Symposium: The "A" and "V" pattern in strabismus. Published courtesy of *Trans Am Acad Ophthalmol Otolaryngol 1964;68:354.*)

V-PATTERN ESOTROPIA

This very common pattern presents with esotropia greatest in downgaze, and often with a chin-down posture to maintain comfortable single binocular vision. The cause of the V pattern in some patients is inferior oblique overaction, as the abductive effect of the inferior obliques in upgaze produces an exo shift in horizontal alignment. The ultimate deviation in upgaze represents a sum of the underlying eso deviation and the abductive pull of the inferior obliques in upgaze (Fig. 10.2).

The cause of the V pattern is obscure in patients with normally functioning oblique muscles. Some authorities have postulated anatomic variations in the horizontal recti that permit greater effect of the lateral recti in upgaze and the medial recti in downgaze.[3] Others have incriminated the vertical recti, claiming the superior recti to be temporally translated and the inferior recti nasally translated, thus permitting the former to act as abductors in upgaze and the latter as adductors in downgaze.

Mild amounts of incomitance (less than 15 prism diopters difference from upgaze to downgaze) can be ignored unless they cause a chin posture. Antiaccommodative measures (plus lenses or miotics) are effective for some patients, but the progressively increasing esotropia in downgaze will confound the use of bifocals in most of those with V-pattern esotropia and a high AC/A ratio. If surgery is indicated, inferior oblique overaction should be reduced together with the horizontal misalignment. If the obliques function normally, the lateral recti can be translated upward and the medial recti downward for a variable degree, up to perhaps one half of tendon width. Likewise, the superior recti can be translated nasally and the inferior recti

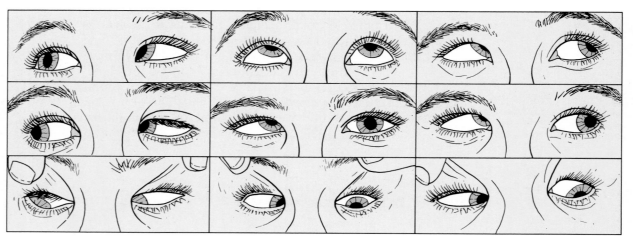

10.2 | Child with V-pattern esotropia has bilateral inferior oblique overaction, with increasing esotropia from upgaze to downgaze. A chin-down head posture is common.

temporally to a similar degree. Translations larger than one half of tendon width tend to be unpredictable. In children, the resultant globe torsion is well tolerated; adults, however, may complain postoperatively of torsional diplopia. To avoid overcorrection in patients with large incomitant strabismus, horizontal surgery for the least eso deviation (upgaze) should be performed when combined with horizontal tendon translations.

A three-step head tilt test should be performed in all patients with V-pattern esotropia to investigate the presence of bilateral superior oblique palsy, which can accompany this picture. A left hyperdeviation greater on left head tilt and right hyperdeviation greater on right head tilt will confirm the diagnosis.

V-PATTERN EXOTROPIA

Patients with V-pattern exotropia commonly present with a chin-up head posture to place the eyes in a position of least horizontal strabismus (Fig. 10.3). Evidence of overaction of the inferior obliques should be sought, and if surgery is undertaken the inferior obliques should be weakened. If the obliques function normally, the lateral recti can be translated upward and the medial recti downward, as discussed above.

An occasional patient with a Y-pattern strabismus consisting only of exotropia in upgaze can be treated with oblique weakening alone if the obliques are overacting, or with a pure upward translation of the lateral recti if the obliques are not overacting.

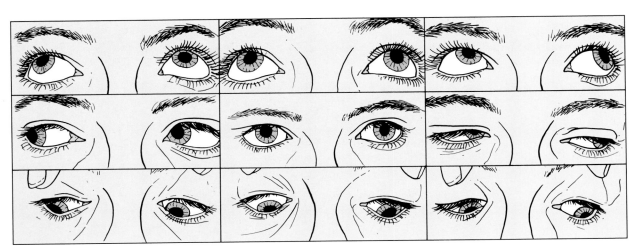

10.3 | Child with V-pattern exotropia has bilateral inferior oblique overaction, with increasing exotropia from downgaze to upgaze. A chin-up head posture is common.

A-PATTERN ESOTROPIA

This common pattern should be suspected in patients who maintain a chin-up posture and have esotropia in upgaze. Some have overaction of the superior oblique muscles and will harness the abducting effect of the superior obliques in downgaze to overcome the esotropia. Others have normally acting obliques and a less clear cause for the A pattern (Fig. 10.4).

Traditionally, caution has been recommended when considering superior oblique weakening procedures in patients fusing in primary position, because postoperative primary position hyperdeviations were feared. Modern graded superior oblique recession procedures are available to provide symmetric superior oblique weakening in such patients without as large a risk.[4] Those with normally acting superior obliques will benefit from downward translation of the lateral recti, upward translation of the medial recti, or both, combined with necessary surgery to reduce the horizontal strabismus. Another approach in patients with little horizontal misalignment is temporal translation of the superior recti and/or nasal translation of the inferior recti.

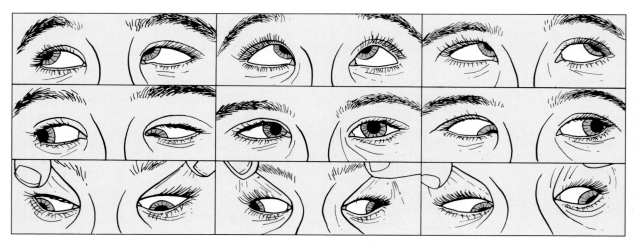

10.4 | Child with A-pattern esotropia has bilateral superior oblique overaction, with increasing esotropia from downgaze to upgaze. A chin-up head posture is common.

A-PATTERN EXOTROPIA

Patients with this pattern have a chin-down posture to move the eyes away from the position of maximum exotropia (Fig. 10.5). Those without superior oblique overaction should undergo translation of the lateral recti upward, the medial recti downward, or both, together with surgery for the exotropia. Graded recessions of the superior oblique, if the muscles are overactive, should prevent asymmetric weakening by tenotomy or tenectomy and the creation of a vertical strabismus in primary position. Patients with little exodeviation in primary position (λ, or λ pattern) can benefit from pure translation of the lateral recti downward or the inferior recti nasally.

X-PATTERN STRABISMUS

Patients with longstanding exotropia may develop secondary contracture of all four oblique muscles and an X-pattern strabismus. Alternatively, the lateral recti may contract, yielding a "tether" effect on upgaze and downgaze and providing an X pattern. Because these are approached by different surgical techniques, evidence of true oblique overaction should be sought by forced duction testing, observation of fundus torsion, and consideration of staged surgery. Lateral rectus recessions alone will alleviate the X pattern if it is caused only by tether effect.

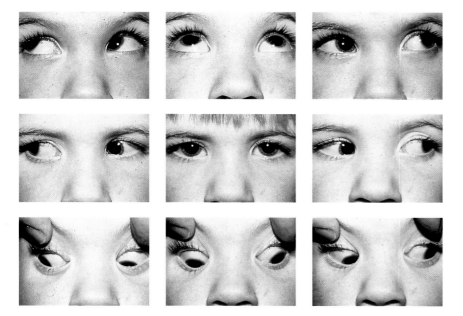

10.5 | Child with A-pattern exotropia has bilateral superior oblique overaction, with increasing exotropia from upgaze to downgaze. A chin-down head posture is common.

CONGENITAL, COMITANT, AND PARETIC VERTICAL STRABISMUS

Howard M. Eggers

CONGENITAL ANOMALIES

The most common congenital anomaly is an abnormal muscle insertion.[1] The insertion may be too far anterior or posterior or in an altogether anomalous location. Fascial bands may restrict rotations. Muscles may be absent or hypoplastic, fused with adjacent muscles, and bifurcated or reduplicated. The resulting deviation depends on the nature and location of the anomaly.

VERTICAL RETRACTION SYNDROME

A vertical retraction syndrome, analogous to the horizontal involvement in Duane syndrome, is rare.[2] Elevation or depression may be limited, and there is retraction of the globe with narrowing of the lid fissure on attempted upgaze or downgaze. The etiology is presumably a peripheral aberrant innervation pattern to the extraocular muscles, in analogy with Duane syndrome.

COMITANT VERTICAL DEVIATIONS

Most vertical deviations are incomitant, and therefore can be shown to represent a weakness or overaction of one of the vertically acting muscles. Small comitant vertical deviations do occur but are rare.[3] Most cases prove on repeated, careful examination to be incomitant. The etiology of these small comitant deviations is obscure. The principal differential diagnosis is skew deviation, a small, usually but not necessarily incomitant vertical divergence of the eyes associated with brainstem or cerebellar lesions.[4] Skew deviation does not invariably carry a serious prognosis. Depending on the location of the lesion there may be other neurologic signs or symptoms. Because a skew deviation, which can be the result of a central nervous system lesion, may not be identifiably different from the benign, comitant small vertical deviations of unknown cause, the latter require evaluation of possible cause, including neurologic.

Because of the comitance of the deviation, these patients are ideally suited for treatment with prisms. Electromyographically guided injection of botulinum toxin into a vertical muscle may also be helpful.

PARETIC VERTICAL DEVIATIONS
FOURTH NERVE PARALYSIS

Superior oblique paresis is usually divided into congenital and acquired forms[5,6] (Fig. 11.1). The term "congenital" here means early life and with the absence of a specific cause located at a later point in time. Supporting evidence for a diagnosis of congenital superior oblique paresis are a history of diplopia or abnormal eye position (i.e., hypertropia observed by parents), photographs of a childhood head tilt, and no history of head trauma. A history of some head trauma, at some time in life, is common. The role of relatively minor head trauma in producing superior oblique paresis is unknown, but it appears in some cases that relatively minor trauma is responsible. In cases of superior oblique paresis presenting later in life without any apparent cause, sometimes childhood photographs are found that show a head tilt. The presumption is that the deviation was controlled for many years, but with time the same fusional effort could no longer be exerted and the deviation presented. This situation is interpreted as a decompensated congenital paresis.

Acquired superior oblique paresis is most commonly due to trochlear palsy. Causes of trochlear palsy are trauma (closed-head or neurosurgical), diabetes (in the older age group), vascular disease, decompensated congenital paresis, superior orbital fissure and cavernous sinus syndromes, *Herpes zoster*, and posterior fossa tumors.[7,8] The differential diagnosis includes other causes of superior oblique paresis or underaction: Graves' ophthalmopathy, orbital pseudotumor, injury to trochlea, and myasthenia. The susceptibility of the IV nerve to injury during closed-head trauma is probably due to its location adjacent to the edge of the tentorium. In acquired IV nerve paresis and in the absence of a history of significant head trauma, clinical evaluation

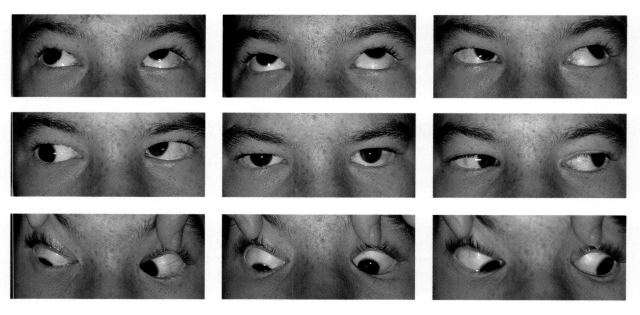

11.1 | Eye rotations, left superior oblique paresis. In primary position (center) the band of sclera visible above the lower lid shows the left eye to be higher than the right. The left hypertropia is greater in right gaze and less in left gaze. On rotations up and to the right the left inferior oblique is seen to overact relative to the right superior rectus, and down to the right the left superior oblique is underacting relative to the inferior rectus.

should include a traction test, Tensilon testing, and a glucose tolerance test. Radiologic tests are of minimal value when the only clinical finding is superior oblique paresis. In the Mayo clinic series, acquired IV nerve palsies were due in approximately equal numbers to unknown factors, head trauma, and everything else.

All forms of superior oblique paresis can produce a head tilt, which is functional and serves to minimize the vertical deviation. The chief symptom of acquired superior oblique paresis is diplopia, vertical or torsional. In addition to diplopia, more longstanding paresis can have symptoms of neck strain or muscle spasms from efforts to tilt the head, and the neck muscles may be hypertrophied on one side. Sometimes the presenting symptom is asthenopia. Whereas image tilting as a symptom occurs only in recently acquired superior oblique paresis, vertical diplopia can occur in congenital pareses.

In unilateral superior oblique paresis, as the muscle becomes incrementally weaker the hypertropia first occurs in the field of action of the muscle (downgaze to the side). The deviation depends on the direction of gaze, i.e., it is incomitant. With further weakness, the alignment in lateral gaze and in primary position also is affected. There is typically a spread of the deviation to other fields of gaze, which can occur as early as 3 weeks after the onset of the paresis, regardless of whether binocular vision is maintained or which eye is used for fixation. Congenital and acquired superior oblique pareses show the same variety of patterns of spread of deviation. A large intermittent deviation in primary position (up to 35 or 40 prism diopters) implies a high degree of fusional control and is taken as a sign of a longstanding deviation.

Knapp introduced a useful classification scheme for superior oblique paresis.[9] The classes are distinguished by the direction of gaze in which the maximal deviation occurs, corresponding to the field of action of particular muscles: Class I, field of the direct antagonist (inferior oblique) (Fig. 11.2);

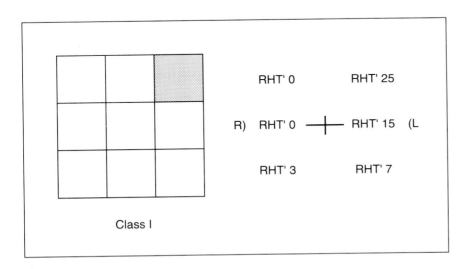

11.2 | Class I superior oblique paresis. The maximal deviation is in the field of action of the direct antagonist to the paretic muscle. RHT = right hypertropia.

Class II, field of the agonist (paretic superior oblique) (Fig. 11.3); Class III, both agonist and direct antagonist (Fig. 11.4); Class IV, agonist, direct antagonist and yoke (contralateral inferior rectus) (Fig. 11.5); Class V, agonist and ipsilateral depressor ("double depressor") (Fig. 11.6); Class VI, bilateral supe-

11.3 | Class II superior oblique paresis. The maximal deviation is in the field of action of the paretic superior oblique.

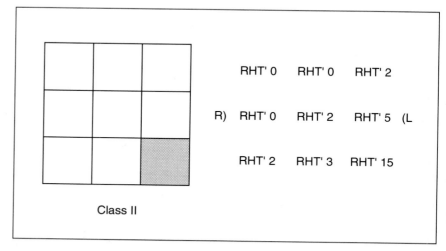

RHT' 0   RHT' 0   RHT' 2

R)   RHT' 0   RHT' 2   RHT' 5   (L

RHT' 2   RHT' 3   RHT' 15

Class II

11.4 | Class III superior oblique paresis. The maximal deviation is in the field of both the paretic agonist and the direct antagonist.

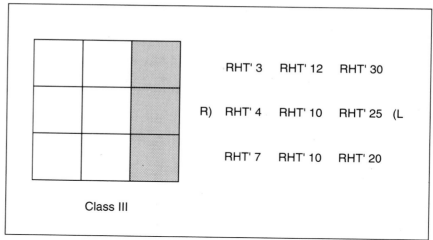

RHT' 3   RHT' 12   RHT' 30

R)   RHT' 4   RHT' 10   RHT' 25   (L

RHT' 7   RHT' 10   RHT' 20

Class III

11.5 | Class IV superior oblique paresis. The maximal deviation is in the field of action of the paretic agonist, the direct antagonist, and the yoke (the contralateral inferior rectus).

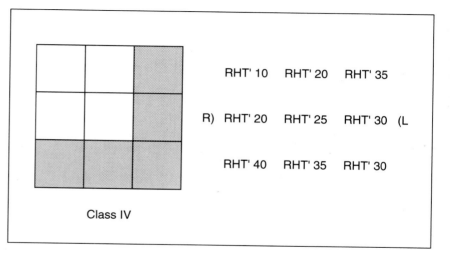

RHT' 10   RHT' 20   RHT' 35

R)   RHT' 20   RHT' 25   RHT' 30   (L

RHT' 40   RHT' 35   RHT' 30

Class IV

rior oblique (Fig. 11.7); and Class VII, superior oblique paresis from trauma in trochlear region with restricted elevation in adduction (Fig. 11.8).

The patterns of spread of the deviation are found regardless of which eye is used for fixation. The importance of the patterns of spread of deviation is to show that the direction of maximal deviation is not always in the field of action of the paretic superior oblique. More consistent is the direction of

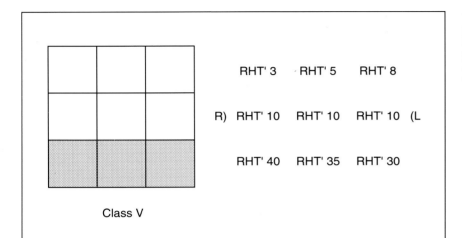

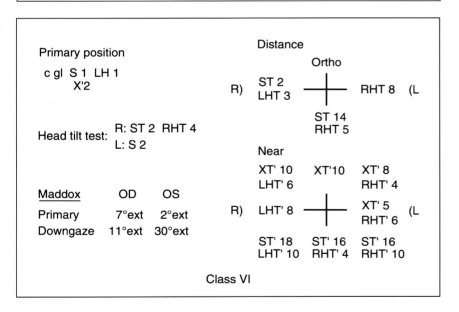

11.6 | Class V superior oblique paresis. The maximal deviation is in the field of action of the paretic agonist and the ipsilateral depressor ("double depressor weakness").

11.7 | Class VI superior oblique paresis (bilateral). S = esophoria; ST = esotropia; XT = exotropia; RHT = right hypertropia; LHT = left hypertropia; X(T), RH(T), LH(T) = intermittent deviations; c gl = wearing distance spectacle correction; ext = extorsion; R) = rightward gaze; (L = leftward gaze; ' = measurement at near. Note that in primary position there is a torsional strabismus and diplopia. Near primary position the vertical elements of the two superior oblique pareses nearly cancel each other out, and right and left hypertropias show up only in lateral gaze. The torsional components of the pareses summate, frequently producing an excyclotropia. The weakness of the secondary actions of the superior oblique (abduction in downgaze and incycloduction) leads to an esotropia in downgaze and an incomitant excyclotropia, worse in downgaze. The torsional misalignment of the images prevents fusion even if the horizontal and vertical deviations were controlled. The head-tilt test shows little difference on the two sides. A chin-down head position is common. It avoids the esotropia and cyclotropia of downgaze.

the least deviation, diagonally across from the field of action of the paretic muscle.[10] The patterns of cyclotropia have not been systematically studied, but the cyclotropia can also be incomitant, increasing in downgaze.

Bilateral superior oblique paresis is characterized by less vertical deviation in primary position than the usual unilateral case, because the vertical deviations cancel each other out. A right hypertropia may be found in left gaze and a left hypertropia in right gaze. With asymmetry of the bilateral involvement, the opposite vertical deviation is sometimes observed only in the upper diagonal field. The torsion produced by a unilateral superior oblique paresis averages about 8° and ranges up to 15°. Owing to the wide range of possible torsion there is no specific amount of torsion that is diagnostic for bilateral paresis, although larger amounts of torsion should make one suspect a bilateral paresis. A V pattern is typically present, and horizontal diplopia in downgaze is a frequent symptom.

The development of a superior oblique paresis on the opposite side after surgery for unilateral superior oblique paresis is called a masked bilateral paresis.[11,12] There is no characteristic of the history, cause, or strabismus exam that allows distinguishing a masked bilateral paresis in advance of surgery. In one series the incidence was 8% and the average presentation was 10 weeks postoperatively. Presentation after several months is possible.

HEAD TILT TEST

The most useful application of the head tilt test is to confirm the diagnosis of superior oblique paresis (Fig. 11.9). In theory it can distinguish pareses of other vertical muscles, but in practice its results are most clear-cut for the obliques. The head-tilt test is based on the fact that the two intorters or extorters of each eye (both superior or inferior to the eye) have opposite vertical actions, one an elevator and the other a depressor. Torsional synergists are vertical antagonists. When the head is tilted, both intorters are activated on the low side of the head and both extorters on the high side. The torsional actions add and the vertical actions cancel, but in the presence of a paresis the vertical actions do not cancel and the hypertropia is worse with tilt to one side. Biomechanical modeling of the extraocular muscles on a computer confirms the role of the superior rectus in producing the hypertropia elicited by the head-tilt test.[13] With time the hypertropia increases, implying a greater superior rectus force, consistent with some element of contracture of that muscle from the chronic hypertropia.[14] Contracture of the superior rectus may play a role in spread of the deviation across the lower fields of gaze.

11.8 | Class VII superior oblique paresis, resulting from trauma in the region of the trochlea. The superior oblique is paretic from restriction of the tendon sliding through the trochlea. Scarring also prevents lengthening of the tendon as the muscle is inhibited, creating the functional equivalent of a Brown syndrome.

	R)				(L
		X(T)' 10 RH(T)' 8	X(T)' 10 RH(T)' 3	X(T)' 10	
		XT 10 LHT 10	X' 6 LH' 3	X(T)' 10	
		XT' 14 LHT' 30	XT' 12 LHT' 30	XT' 12 LHT' 30	

Class VII

Parks introduced a three-step test to determine the paretic vertical muscle.[15] The first step determines the deviation in primary position. For example, a right hypertropia implies a weak depressor in the right eye or a weak elevator in the left. In the second step, the side of maximal vertical deviation is noted. A right hypertropia greater in right gaze implies involvement of the muscles with their field of action to the right. The muscle at fault is either the right inferior rectus or the left inferior oblique. These are both extorters and will be activated on *contralateral* head tilt. The third step is the head-tilt test. The direction of tilt for which the vertical actions do not cancel and the hypertropia becomes maximum is contralateral to the paretic side. Thus, in this example, the left inferior oblique would be implicated by a greater hypertropia on tilt to the right. To complete the listing of possibilities, a right hypertropia greater in left gaze implies a weak right superior oblique or left superior rectus (both intorters). Head tilt to the *ipsilateral* side will activate both intorters, but the vertical actions will not cancel out for the pair of intorters containing the paretic muscle and the vertical deviation will be maximum to that side. Thus, the vertical deviation from a superior oblique paresis is greater on ipsilateral head tilt.

Helveston devised a similar test with two steps.[16] The first step is to consider the position of the adducted eye in the lateroversion of greatest vertical tropia. A hypertropic adducted eye implies a paretic superior muscle (ipsilateral superior oblique or contralateral superior rectus). A hypotropic

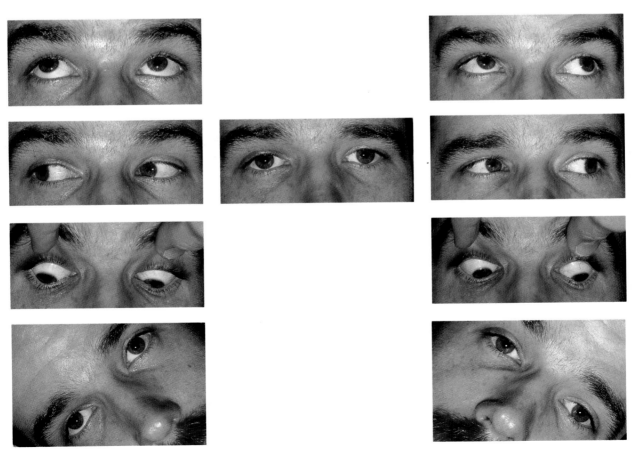

11.9 | Right superior oblique paresis. A mild elevation in adduction, overaction of the right inferior oblique, and underaction of the right superior oblique can be seen. The head tilt test confirms the diagnosis by showing a right hypertropia greater with head tilt right.

adducted eye implies a paretic inferior muscle (ipsilateral inferior oblique or contralateral inferior rectus). The second step is the head-tilt test. If the greatest vertical tropia results from tilting the head to the side of the higher eye, an oblique muscle is paretic. If the greatest vertical tropia results from tilting the head to the side of the lower eye, a rectus muscle is paretic.

The interpretation of the head tilt test requires that there be normal function of the vestibular apparatus, that there be only a single muscle palsy, and that there be no mechanical restrictions to eye movements. Paretic obliques show a greater increase in vertical deviation during head tilt than do the vertical rectus muscles because of the strong vertical actions of their torsional synergists (the vertical recti). The obliques have a weaker vertical effect and therefore their vertical action, when unopposed by a paretic rectus muscle, will produce a less marked hypertropia.

TREATMENT

The treatment of superior oblique paresis is based on the symptoms. Prisms may provide relief of diplopia in mild cases, although incomitance and torsion may provide insuperable barriers to fusion. A good surgical result is considered to be relief of symptoms and correction of the head tilt; however, a deviation frequently persists in extreme positions of gaze. Surgery is done according to the nature of the deviation, and no standard, stereotypical procedure is possi-

Figure 11.10. Surgical Treatment of Superior Oblique Paresis

CLASS	PROCEDURE
I	Weaken inferior oblique
II	Tuck superior oblique, recess yoke inferior rectus (adjustable)
III	Weaken inferior oblique, weaken yoke inferior rectus (adjustable), tuck superior oblique if >25 PD hypertropia
IV	Same as Class III and recess ipsilateral superior conjunctiva, wait for improvement in ipsilateral lower field
V	Tuck superior oblique, weaken yoke inferior rectus (adjustable), recess ipsilateral superior conjunctiva, wait for improvement in ipslateral lower field
VI	Depends on amount of cyclotropia, V pattern, and pattern of hypertropia
VII	Free restriction near trochlea. Treat remaining superior oblique paresis according to measurements of deviation

ble.[17] The classification scheme of Knapp is useful in planning surgery (Fig. 11.10). The muscles to be operated are those having their field of action in the direction of gaze where the deviation is maximum. Thus, a deviation that is maximum in the upper corner will benefit from having the inferior oblique weakened. Correction of the hypertropia should lead to correction of the head tilt. In bilateral superior oblique paresis, if the vertical deviations cancel out it may be sufficient to correct only the torsion and the V pattern.[18] Class VII is difficult to treat. At least two stages must be planned. In the first, the restriction of elevation due to scarring should be freed. The second procedure is aimed at correcting the superior oblique paresis.

THIRD NERVE PALSY

The muscles innervated by the III nerve may become palsied individually or in groups, according to the divisions of the nerve. Third nerve palsies are due to vascular lesions (diabetes, arteriosclerosis, and hypertension) or to undetermined causes in 20%–25% of cases each. The remaining cases are distributed in approximately equal numbers in groups resulting from head trauma, neoplasm, aneurysm, and miscellaneous. In children, most III nerve palsies are congenital. Unilateral, congenital III nerve palsies are usually not associated with other neurologic disease, but neoplasms are present in approximately 10%.[19,20] These patients frequently have amblyopia and aberrant regeneration. Acquired III nerve paralysis in children is most commonly caused by blunt trauma or infectious processes, either local or systemic.

Complete III nerve palsy causes the eyes to be in a position of abduction, mild depression, and intorsion, a position determined by the pull of the remaining, functioning muscles: the lateral rectus and the superior oblique. The pupil is dilated, unreactive to light, and there is a paralysis of accommodation. During the recovery process, nerve axons may reinnervate the wrong distal structure, a phenomenon called aberrant regeneration. Typically, nerve fibers to the medial or inferior rectus innervate the levator, resulting in upper lid retraction when the eye attempts adduction or downgaze. The lid retraction on downgaze is called a pseudo-Graefe sign.

The rare entity of oculomotor paresis with cyclic spasms occurs after early life injuries to the oculomotor nerve.[21] Typically, every second minute the ptosis, exotropia, and impairments of the pupil and accommodation resolve for 10–30 sec. It has been speculated that the oculomotor axons undergo retrograde degeneration from the injury and that there is then a failure of supranuclear connections to form properly.

Partial oculomotor paralysis that involves only one muscle is rare. Common presentations are congenital or the result of trauma. Head trauma can damage the III nerve intracranially by way of contusion necrosis of the proximal nerve or avulsion of the rootlets. Perineural hemorrhage can also be found at the superior orbital fissure. In the orbit, primary hemorrhages can occur in individual muscles, usually associated with fractures of the orbital bones.[22]

Isolated paralysis of the superior, inferior (Fig. 11.11), or medial rectus, or inferior oblique (Fig. 11.12) is rare. More commonly, it is part of a superior or inferior division paralysis or represents the most obviously weak muscle when several are involved. Weakness of the vertically acting muscles leads to a deviation that is maximal in the field of action of that muscle. There may be a chin-up or down head position or a face turn to allow fusion. Weakness of the inferior, extorting muscles will lead to incyclotropia, mild for the inferior rectus and greater for the inferior oblique. Weakness of the superior rectus will lead to mild excyclotropia. In inferior oblique paresis, there is usually a head tilt towards the paretic side and the head-tilt test is positive on tilting the head towards the normal side. The superior oblique may be overacting. Weakness of the medial rectus will give an incomitant exotropia and possibly poor convergence as well. There may be a head turn to favor the field with the smaller deviation.

The differential diagnosis of isolated vertical muscle paresis includes mechanical restriction to rotation. For superior rectus paresis this means restrictive lesions that limit elevation: inferior rectus fibrosis or entrapment in a floor fracture. For inferior oblique paresis, a Brown syndrome must be excluded. A traction test must be done to demonstrate whether the eye fails to move because of mechanical restriction or muscle paresis.

The therapy of vertical deviations from III nerve palsy depends on the severity of the strabismus. Small deviations can be functionally cured with prisms. For the rectus muscles, if there is any function in the paretic muscle a resection of the paretic muscle and recession of its direct antagonist is appropriate. Recession of the superior or inferior rectus in the other eye may also be indicated, depending on the incomitance. Any oblique weakening should

11.11 | Right inferior rectus paresis; 67-year-old man with abrupt onset of diplopia in downgaze. Negative history and work-up.

Primary position   sc   XT 3 RHT 7
                      X(T)' 25 RH(T)' 16

```
              X 3                          X(T)' 20              X(T)' 16
                                           RH(T) 2
        R | L    X 3
RHT 5   -----    RH 2                      XT' 20    R | L    XT' 14
          |                                RHT' 5    -----    RHT' 2
                                                       |
        RHT 16

                                           XT' 16              XT' 12
Head    R: RHT 3                           RHT' 18             RHT' 14
tilt test: L: RHT 3
```

Rotations: mild limitation depression OD, greater in abduction be done cautiously to avoid creating problems with torsion. If there is complete paresis of a superior or inferior rectus, a reasonable result can be obtained by a full-tendon transposition of the medial and lateral recti to the ends of the muscle insertion.

A paresis of the medial rectus is treated with resection of the paretic muscle and recession of the direct antagonist. Depending on the deviation, the yoke and the antagonist of the yoke can also be recessed. Alternatively, botulinum toxin can be injected into the antagonist, the ipsilateral lateral rectus under electromyographic control. This is most effective when done soon after the onset of the deviation, before the formation of any contracture.[23]

A complete III nerve palsy is difficult to treat. The vertical deviation may well be minimal because of equal paresis of the superior and inferior recti. The lateral rectus must be given a large recession along with the lateral conjunctiva and Tenon's capsule. If there is any function in the medial rectus at all, a large resection will help. If the muscle is completely paralyzed, the trochlea can be fractured and the superior oblique tendon swung down and attached near the medial rectus tendon to provide an anchoring muscle force. Prisms may be needed postoperatively to adjust any remaining small vertical deviation.

An inferior division III nerve palsy is treated by a full tendon transfer of the functioning superior rectus to the medial rectus and of the lateral rectus to the inferior rectus, and a tenectomy of the superior oblique.

An inferior oblique paresis is treated by weakening of the ipsilateral superior oblique. A tenotomy, tenectomy, or tendon lengthening may be performed. The contralateral superior rectus may need to be recessed as well.

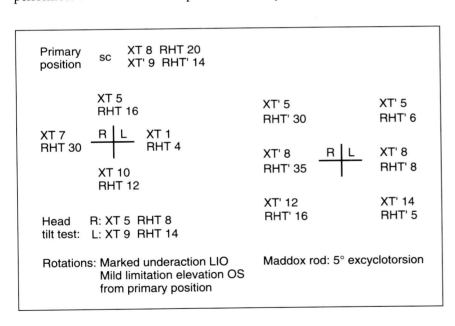

11.12 | Inferior oblique paresis; 16-year-old girl with abrupt onset of vertical diplopia. Negative history and work-up.

OCULAR MYASTHENIA GRAVIS

Myasthenia gravis may produce weakness of any of the extraocular muscles and thus can mimic any ocular muscle paresis. It must always be considered in the differential diagnosis (Fig. 11.13). It can occur at any age. The ocular symptoms are diplopia and ptosis. The extraocular muscle paresis can be of any degree and can affect any combination of muscles. The ptosis may be unilateral or bilateral and of any severity. A muscle weakness that does not fit into a pattern consistent with a neurogenic cause should indicate the possibility of myasthenia. However, a paresis that shows a neurogenic pattern may also be due to myasthenia. In this case a variability in the deviation would point to myasthenia.

The diagnosis is made by the improvement of the deviation produced by intravenous administration of edrophonium chloride (Tensilon®). Electromyography shows improved neuromuscular conduction immediately after Tensilon injection in myasthenia. However, the potential cholinergic side-effects of Tensilon include cardiopulmonary arrest. A sleep test is safer, moderately sensitive, and specific.[24] The procedure is to measure the deviation or ptosis in the office after a 30-min nap. Myasthenics show a substantial improvement immediately after this short period of sleep.

Treatment is aimed at symptomatic relief and functional rehabilitation, if possible. Anticholinesterase agents may be helpful but frequently do not alleviate all the ocular symptoms. Lid crutches fitted to spectacles may help. Fresnel prisms can be used for diplopia, or one eye can be occluded. The deviation can change spontaneously, even after long periods of time. This potential for change, combined with the weakness of the muscles, makes it usually best to avoid muscle surgery. Because of the muscle weakness the results of surgery are unreliable and unpredictable. Small adhesions and the spring forces provided by the passive tissues surrounding the eyes become more prominent in determining the eye position, and in the presence of weak muscles postoperative adhesions that usually would not be noticed may spoil a surgical result. Similarly, lid surgery is best avoided owing to the risk of corneal exposure.

11.13 | Ocular myasthenia; 66-year-old woman. In this case the left hypertropia occurs in a pattern not characteristic of any single muscle or nerve weakness, although myasthenia can masquerade as a muscle or nerve paresis.

Primary position	sc	LHT 20 XT' 10 LHT' 20	
	LH(T) 12	XT' 14 LHT' 18	XT' 12 LHT' 8
LHT 30 R | L LHT 10		XT' 10 R | L XT' 8 LHT' 30 LHT' 16	
	LH(T) 12	XT' 10 LHT' 10	XT' 8 LHT' 10
Head tilt test:	R: XT 6 LHT 12 L: LHT 25		

Rotations: Mild limitation elevation OU
Mild limitation depression OS in abduction

12

OTHER VERTICAL STRABISMUS

Howard M. Eggers

SUPRANUCLEAR DISORDERS
DISSOCIATED VERTICAL DIVERGENCE (DVD)

Dissociated vertical divergence is characterized by a spontaneous upward deviation of one eye or the other (if there is bilateral involvement)[1] (Fig. 12.1). After a period usually of no more than a few tens of seconds, or on a shift of gaze, the eye returns down and may even become mildly hypotropic. The deviation may occur with or without daydreaming or fatigue, although these states will make the deviation worse or the spontaneous dissociation more common. The deviated eye is suppressed, so there are rarely visual symptoms.[2] Rarely, the suppression is not deep enough and vertical diplopia occurs. Occasionally a patient may find it physically uncomfortable for the eye to turn up. In cover testing, updrift occurs behind the occluder, the eye returning downwards when the occluder is removed. Because each eye drifts upward under cover and moves downward on removal of the cover, it is not possible to accurately measure a

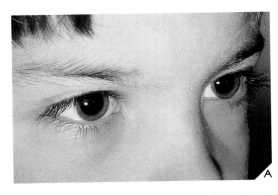

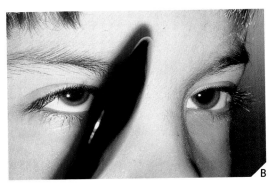

12.1 | Dissociated vertical divergence (DVD). The eyes are approximately straight in primary position (A). Occlusion of an eye leads to an upward drift of the covered eye (B). DVD is usually bilateral, although it may show asymmetrical amounts of drift. On cover testing each eye drifts up under cover. A measure of a simultaneous vertical deviation is the prism power that equalizes the amplitude of the vertical drift in the two eyes.

vertical deviation in the presence of DVD. The best that can be done is to find the prism the makes the vertical drift symmetrical.

Further characteristics are that the amplitude of the updrift is usually not equal in the two eyes. The upward movement is typically accompanied by extorsion of the eye and sometimes a movement in the exo direction. DVD can occur with any strabismus that develops early in life, although it is most common with congenital esotropia. While usually associated with a strabismus, DVD can occur as an isolated defect. Elevation in adduction, producing an apparent inferior oblique overaction, is a common initial presentation. Latent or manifest nystagmus and poor binocular sensory fusion are also common in congenital esotropia. Frequently present at birth, DVD is seldom a new finding after the age of 2 or 3 years. In isolated cases of DVD that appear to develop later in life, DVD has seldom been positively and totally ruled out as a preexisting condition.

The cause of DVD has been a subject of much speculation. In summary, it is unknown. Because versions and ductions are normal, it must be a defect in supranuclear control of eye position. The Bielschowsky phenomenon is another curious characteristic of DVD that must be related to the abnormal supranuclear control of vertical eye position. It is demonstrated by occluding one eye to make it deviate upwards. Then, a neutral density wedge is placed before the opposite, unoccluded eye. The eye behind the cover will make a gradual downward movement in proportion to the attenuation of light reaching the open eye.

Therapy for DVD is aimed at strengthening the patient's fusional mechanisms. This is done by eliminating any concurrent strabismus and optimizing vision through accurate refractive prescription and treatment of amblyopia. Indications for surgery are visual symptoms or the disfigurement produced by the updrift. A variety of surgical procedures have been advocated for DVD, which indicates that none of them is entirely satisfactory. Advocated procedures have included resection of the inferior recti, tuck of the superior obliques, large recession of the superior recti, and recession of the superior rectus with Faden procedure. Good results can be obtained with superior rectus recession combined with Faden procedure[3,4] or with large superior rectus recessions.[5]

OVERACTION OF THE INFERIOR OBLIQUE (STRABISMUS SURSOADDUCTORIUS)

Strabismus sursoadductorius refers to a marked elevation of an eye when in the adducted position, and is commonly ascribed to overaction of the inferior oblique (Fig. 12.2). The elevation in adduction may be bilaterally symmetric or asymmetric. There is no vertical deviation in primary position, a right hypertropia in left gaze, and a left hypertropia in right gaze. The head-tilt test result is negative. The patient may have esotropia, exotropia, or a V pattern. Strabismus sursoadductorius may be due to primary overaction of the inferior obliques (i.e., the cause for the overaction is unknown). The differential diagnosis includes secondary inferior oblique overaction (from a paretic superior oblique or superior rectus), Duane syndrome, and dissociated vertical divergence. Overaction secondary to superior oblique paresis will show a positive head-tilt test.

Strabismus sursoadductorius commonly occurs in congenital esotropia, in which it is frequently confused with DVD. Genuine inferior oblique overaction should produce a V pattern and show measurable vertical deviations in lateral gaze. A DVD undergoes dissociation of the eyes by occlusion of much of the visual field of the adducted eye by the nose and eyebrow, resulting in elevation of the occluded eye. The deviation in lateral gaze is not measurable by prism and cover because each eye moves downward on removal of the occluder.

The distinction of DVD from inferior oblique overaction is important because different surgical procedures are used, depending on the diagnosis. In DVD the adducted eye may be elevated, but when the cover is switched to the abducted eye, that eye becomes elevated. In inferior oblique overaction the abducted eye will become lower as the high, adducted eye takes up fixation. The deviation in inferior oblique overaction is the same, regardless of which eye is fixating. In DVD, if the adducting eye is the fixating eye there will be much less or no elevation in adduction, and occlusion of the abducted eye can make that eye elevate, thus reversing the hypertropia findings. The vertical fixation shift with alternation of the cover is faster in inferior oblique overaction, occurring at saccadic velocities. In DVD the updrift and recovery movements are slower and accompanied by extorsion as the eye rises and intorts during recovery.

When elevation in adduction is genuinely due to inferior oblique overaction, a weakening procedure should be done on these muscles.[6] If, in fact, a DVD was responsible for the elevation in adduction, this weakening will have little effect. A procedure for DVD must then be done. Unilateral inferior oblique weakening can lead to overaction of the opposite inferior oblique following surgery. Assuming no mechanical restriction to have resulted from the inferior oblique surgery, this indicates that a DVD was probably initially at fault. Apparent overaction of the inferior obliques may also dissappear after surgery for esotropia.

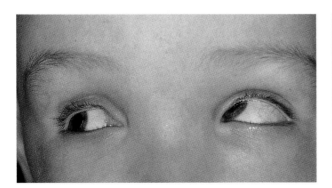

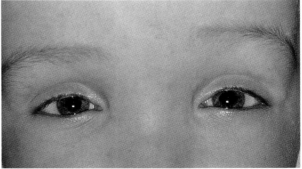

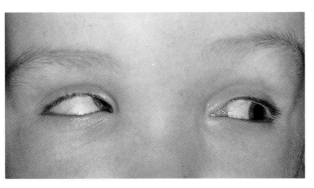

12.2 | Elevation in adduction. The apparent overaction of the inferior oblique must be confirmed with cover testing. A DVD frequently gives the same appearance on testing versions. True inferior oblique overaction will give a measurable deviation in lateral gaze and may produce a V pattern. In DVD, the abducted eye may sursumduct under occlusion.

DOUBLE ELEVATOR PALSY

Paralysis of both elevators (superior rectus and inferior oblique) of one eye results in a rather large hypotropia on the affected side (Fig. 12.3). It may be congenital or acquired. The levator palpebrae may or may not be involved, and Bell's phenomenon may be present or absent. If the latter is present, a supranuclear lesion is implied. The pupil is normal, as are horizontal rotations. The etiology of the congenital forms is not known. The acquired cases have all been adults with small lesions in the pretectum.[7] The differential diagnosis includes mechanical restriction of elevation: orbital floor fracture, Graves' disease, congenital fibrosis of the inferior rectus, and Brown syndrome (which can sometimes affect primary position). A traction test will determine whether or not there is restriction.

If there is no mechanical restriction of movement, surgical treatment is to transfer the entire tendon of both the medial and lateral rectus muscles to the ends of the superior rectus insertion.[8] Horizontal rotations are only slightly impaired, and vertical rotations are remarkably improved. If the lid height does not improve with the raising of eye position, lid surgery may also be required.

A similar entity of double depressor paralysis occurs only in congenital form. The inverse surgical procedure is effective.

RESTRICTION OF EYE MOVEMENT
SUPERIOR OBLIQUE TENDON SHEATH SYNDROME (BROWN SYNDROME)

The motility features of the superior oblique tendon sheath syndrome are due to a short anterior sheath of the superior oblique tendon[9] (Fig. 12.4). Brown distinguished true from simulated sheath syndrome by whether the causative defect was actually a short anterior sheath or some other anomaly. This differentiation cannot be made on clinical features, but only at the time of surgery.

The most striking clinical feature is restriction of elevation in adduction, which is limited to the horizontal plane. The lid fissure may widen when the eye is adducted. The limitation, being due to mechanical factors, is the same on versions, ductions, and traction test. The maximal possible elevation increases as the eye moves from adduction to abduction, where it should be normal. There is divergence in gaze up from primary position but normal elevation into the ipsilateral upper corner field (normal superior rectus function). The ipsilateral superior oblique usually does not overact. In Brown's original series there was a 3:2 predominance of females to males and nearly twice as many cases involving the right eye as the left. Ten percent

12.3 | Congenital double elevator palsy in a 27-year-old woman.

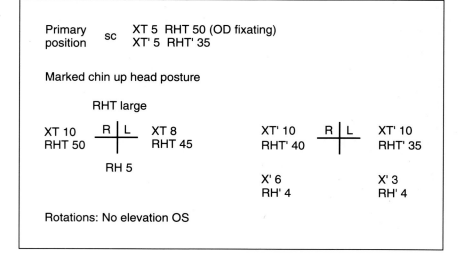

were bilateral. Variable features are head tilt and tropia in all fields. Familial occurrence of Brown syndrome has been reported.[10]

The simulated sheath syndrome can be congenital or acquired. Acquired cases are due to orbital trauma,[11] direct trochlear trauma, orbit or muscle surgery, scleral buckling, frontal sinusitis or sinus surgery, and inflammation of the superior oblique tendon or sheath. A Brown syndrome is easily produced during surgery to tuck the superior oblique if the tendon sheath is not adequately stripped away or if the surgery is done too close to the trochlea. Inflammation of the superior oblique tendon has occurred in rheumatoid arthritis and juvenile rheumatoid arthritis.[12-14] Intermittent forms of Brown syndrome have been associated with a click, upon which the restriction is released (superior oblique click syndrome).[15]

The congenital simulated sheath syndrome is due to structural anomalies other than a short sheath. Other fibrous adhesions may be present around the trochlear area. Orbital floor fractures can trap the orbital tissue in such a way as to simulate a Brown syndrome. Adhesions around the inferior oblique have also been reported.

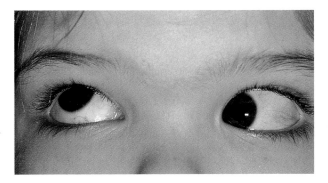
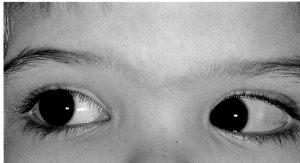
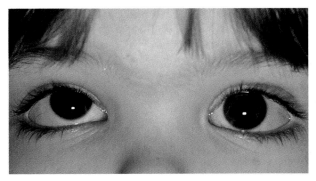
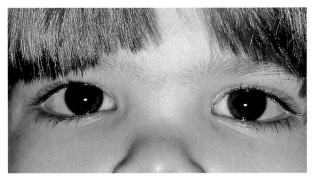
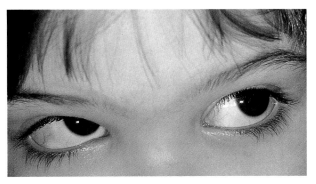

12.4 | Brown syndrome. Elevation of the left eye is impaired most in right gaze. The differential diagnosis is inferior rectus paresis. Brown syndrome has a positive traction test for elevation in adduction and the muscle paresis does not.

If binocular vision is present and there is no head position no treatment is necessary. Treatment is required for visual symptoms, strabismus, or head position. Acquired cases with active inflammation of the tendon may benefit from local steroid injections in the region of the trochlea.[12] Prisms may provide some relief from diplopia in acquired forms.

Surgery aims to restore free ocular rotations. Brown advocated stripping the superior oblique tendon. The results of such a procedure are frequently unsatisfactory due to re-formation of scar tissue. Tenotomy of the superior oblique tendon has also been advocated.[16] This has the disadvantage of frequently producing a superior oblique paresis.[17] Furthermore, if the tendon was not tight the tenotomy may not improve the restricted movement. This author favors surgery without any preconception as to the site of restriction. During surgery a traction test must be frequently repeated until the globe rotations are free. Recession of conjunctiva in the inferotemporal quadrant can provide additional freeing of rotations. If the restrictive adhesions are not found near the trochlea, they must be searched for elsewhere around the globe. After the rotations are as free as possible the eye should be anchored in an elevated, adducted position for up to 2 weeks. This maneuver is intended to prevent the reformation of scar tissue in the same places. In healing, the eye position will shift for several months after surgery. A second procedure is frequently required.

CONGENITAL FIBROSIS

A rare and usually familial form of vertical strabismus is congenital fibrosis.[18–20] The inheritance pattern is often autosomal dominant. The eyes are typically tethered in a downward position by a fibrotic inferior rectus. There is blepharoptosis and a compensatory elevated chin position. Attempts at upward eye movements may result in convergence. Many of the extraocular muscles are fibrotic, not just the inferior recti. Histology shows replacement of muscle fibers with fibrotic tissue. The differential diagnosis includes Graves' disease, Brown syndrome, orbital floor fracture, double elevator palsy, and chronic progressive external ophthalmoplegia.

Surgical treatment can only relieve the extreme downward tethering of the eyes. The head position will improve as a result. The lids may need to be raised but caution is necessary because the upward rotation of the eyes is limited and the normal Bell's phenomenon does not occur with blinking. It is therefore easy to produce corneal exposure.

FRACTURES OF THE ORBITAL FLOOR

Ocular motility may be impaired in orbital floor fractures owing to proptosis and edema from the original trauma, intraorbital hemorrhage, herniation of the orbital fascia, and muscle entrapment.[21] Eye movements in general, but particularly elevation and depression, may be limited (Fig. 12.5). The inferior rectus is the muscle most commonly affected. The pathophysiology of any resulting strabismus is the herniation of the orbital contents—fat, connective tissue septa, and muscle—into the fracture and a consequent tethering of the eye.

The presence of a floor fracture does not require repair if there is no disturbance of motility.[22] The initial treatment is to wait up to 2 weeks for regression of edema. This can result in significantly improved motility. The diagnosis of inferior rectus entrapment is made by the presence of limited elevation on the affected side, resulting in hypotropia, and by a positive traction test. Depression may also be limited by the entrapment or by damage to the nerve to the inferior rectus.

Diplopia may persist after the inferior rectus has been freed. If the entrapment is old, the muscle can become permanently fibrotic and inelastic. There may also be a paresis of the inferior rectus, presumably resulting from trauma to the nerve to the inferior rectus. On occasion, the inferior rectus can be devitalized by compromise of its blood supply. The muscle is then found at time of surgery to be quite friable.

GRAVES' DISEASE

Graves' ophthalmopathy is an autoimmune inflammatory condition that involves the orbital tissues, primarily the muscles and fat.[23] The muscles are affected by a myositis, showing histologic features of interstitial edema and round cell infiltration. The muscles enlarge and become fibrotic and inelastic. Other findings are lid edema, proptosis, lid retraction, and optic neuropathy (Fig. 12.6).

The usual motility findings are caused by the inelasticity of the muscles. Most commonly the inferior rectus is affected, producing a limitation of elevation. When more severe, the eye may be tethered down by the inferior rectus, producing a hypotropia in primary position. The medial rectus is the next most commonly involved, followed by the superior and lateral recti.

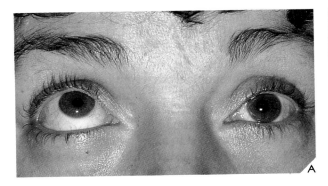
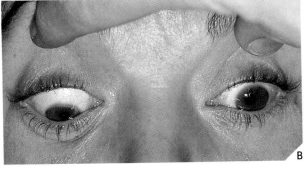

12.5 | Orbital floor fracture with entrapment and paresis of the left inferior rectus. *A:* Upgaze. *B:* Downgaze. The muscle and the orbital connective tissue are caught in the floor fracture. Because of insufficient elasticity of the short, anterior free portion of the muscle, the left eye elevates just to primary position. The left eye also has limited depression. This is due in part to the entrapment of the orbital connective tissue. After surgical freeing, a residual paresis is commonly present, implying damage to the nerve to the inferior rectus. Note the enophthalmos and deep upper lid sulcus resulting from atrophy of the orbital fat.

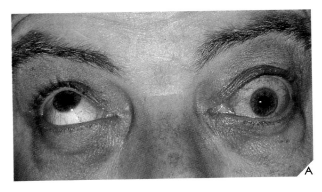
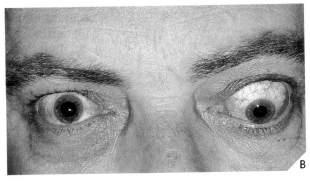

12.6 | Graves' disease. *A:* Upgaze. *B:* Primary position. The left eye is markedly proptotic and the inferior rectus is inelastic. The left inferior rectus has become fibrotic and inelastic from the inflammation of Graves' disease. On attempted upgaze, the left eye barely reaches primary position.

13

Howard M. Eggers

Amblyopia is a developmental defect of spatial visual processing that occurs in the central visual pathways in the brain. It is defined as a reduction of best-corrected visual acuity in an eye that is otherwise normal to clinical examination. The conventional definition assumes that the measure of visual acuity is a Snellen chart. However, other aspects of spatial visual performance also are compromised, such as position acuity, reflected in vernier acuity and visual bisection tasks, and pure resolution, such as grating acuity. In addition, there is an exaggeration of spatial interference effects (crowding).

The stimulus to vision is the contrast and resolution of the retinal image. To diagnose amblyopia, when a refractive error is present it must be corrected so that each eye has a visual stimulus of the same contrast, containing the same resolution of detail. The clarity and imaging quality of the refractive media, beginning with the corneal tear film, also must be normal. Scars and other opacities or irregularitites can reduce the image resolution or scatter light, reducing contrast. Finally, no retinal or optic nerve disease should be present to explain the lack of acuity. When all these criteria are met, the neural signal sent to the brain along the optic nerve will be the same in the two eyes. If amblyopia exists, the central visual pathways will be able to perform better with the signal provided by one eye than that from the other.

Amblyopia occurs in two forms: when the image in one eye is reduced in contrast or resolution, or with strabismus. The amblyopic eye in either form is said to have experienced a deprivation in its visual experience. In strabismus it is not obvious what the deprivation of visual experience is. The amblyopia is said to be caused by an abnormal binocular interaction. The clinical psychophysical findings in the two forms of amblyopia have many features in common; in addition, the anatomic and physiologic findings are similar.

Some terms in the older clinical literature—suppression amblyopia, amblyopia of arrest, amblyopia ex anopsia—all assume particular theories of causation and should be avoided.

NEUROPHYSIOLOGIC BACKGROUND

Amblyopia is best understood in a conceptual framework based on neurophysiologic and anatomic results of animal experiments. The two animals used preeminently in this work are the cat and the monkey, and various forms of amblyopia have been studied in these animal models. The defects in visual performance that are produced mimic very closely those seen in human subjects.

Vision occurs through the analysis of the changing two-dimensional pattern of light on the retina (Fig 13.1). It is generally accepted that this analysis in the human adult is mediated by parallel processing at each retinal locus by a number of different mechanisms, each tuned in spatial frequency, orientation, and temporal frequency. The mechanisms can be studied by various psychophysical testing techniques, visual evoked potentials (VEPs), or neurophysiologic recordings in animals. These mechanisms are present in the infant but become modified with growth and development and become both more sensitive and more finely tuned, i.e., selective for a specific stimulus.

Compared with that of adults, the infant visual system has a reduced grating resolution and reduced contrast sensitivity at all spatial frequencies. With growth, anatomic changes occur in the eye relevant to visual acuity: migration of cones into the fovea, whereby the intercone spacing is reduced; enlargement and elongation of the eye; and lengthening of the cone outer segments.[1] The axial elongation of the eye and the change in spacing of cones lead to a change in scale for spatial information processing at all subsequent levels in the visual system and thus results in better visual acuity. The increased length of the cone outer segments enables a greater number of photons to be captured and allows greater sensitivity to small increments of illumination. These changes are probably sufficient to account for most of the increase in resolution and contrast sensitivity that occurs with maturation. These developmental processes are undisturbed by amblyopia.

A period of synaptogenesis occurs in the striate cortex extending from 3 to 8 months of age, followed by a decline to adult levels by the age of 10 years.[2] During this period visual information processing tasks that depend on inhibition develop: the reduction of contrast sensitivity at low spatial fre-

13.1 | The neural processes serving visual perception are decentralized in the brain. A two-dimensional pattern of light is created on each retina by the dioptric apparatus of the eye. The information contained in these images is sampled and filtered by the response of the rods and cones and the retinal neural circuitry. The resulting neural representations of the world are sent to the primary visual cortex and are available for further stages of analysis by other visual areas of the brain. Analysis for features such as color, motion, and stereopsis is carried out in different locations.

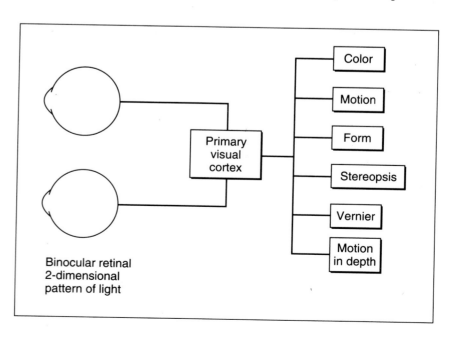

quencies; improved selectivity of tuning to the orientation of gratings; phase discrimination (vernier acuity); stereopsis; binocular rivalry; and the oblique effect (the reduced contrast sensitivity to gratings that are diagonal, i.e., not vertical or horizontal).

The visual cortex contains neurons that respond to patterns of light (bars or sine-wave-modulated gratings) in a restricted area of the visual field (the receptive field of that cell) (Fig. 13.2). The response of individual cells is studied by recording with an electrode the action potentials elicited in that neuron by a particular visual stimulus. In the visually normal animal, most cells respond to some extent to visual stimulation of the receptive field through either eye, a feature known as binocularity. Cortical cells can be characterized by the degree to which they are driven by the input through one eye compared to that through the other eye, and the results can be displayed as a histogram of the ocular dominance distribution. The areas of the cortex dominated by either eye are arranged in irregular bands or stripes, in a pattern reminiscent of a fingerprint.[3]

Neurophysiologic recordings of single neurons in the visual cortex of neonatal cats[4] and monkeys show the presence of selectivity for spatial frequency and orientation;[5] however, the responses are characterized by low sensitivity and broad selectivity (tuning). With aging a rapid improvement occurs in responsiveness and selectivity to grating spatial frequency and orientation, regardless of the quality of visual experience up to a certain age (3 weeks in the kitten). Beyond this age, in the absence of visual experience the proportion of unresponsive cells increases again.[6-8] It appears that the func-

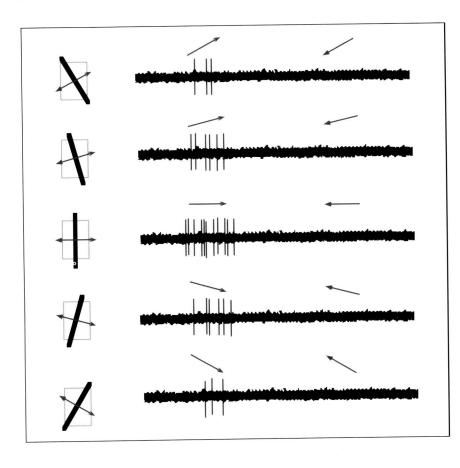

13.2 | The receptive field of a neuron is the portion of the visual field in which it responds to stimulation by light (dotted rectangle in left column). A bar, light or dark with respect to the background, is an adequate stimulus for most neurons in the primary visual cortex. As the bar moves across the receptive field the neuron fires action potentials (tracing at right). Many neurons are selective for stimuli moving in a particular direction, with a particular orientation of the bar.

tion of these cells must be validated by experience if they are to continue to function. If the quality of the visual experience is asymmetric between the two eyes, the eye with the stronger input (from a better contrast in its retinal image) will take over the cortical cells that were once binocular. This leads to an ocular dominance shift through a mechanism of competition between the two eyes for cells in the visual cortex[3,9] (Fig. 13.3). (This dominance is not necessarily the same as the dominance in a fixation or siting task.) Therefore, amblyopia is not merely the result of disuse, because competition between the eyes is also present. More cells in the visual cortex will respond to stimulation through the eye that has had the more normal visual experience; a reduced number will respond to visual stimulation through the eye that has had the lower-quality visual experience.[10] Because contrast of the retinal image is the stimulus that drives the neural responses, the eye with the better contrast in its retinal image will come to be dominant in terms of the number of cortical cells that respond to its input.

The period of time in which the functional capability of the visual cortex can deteriorate is known as the critical period (approximately 3 weeks to 3 months in the cat).[11] The capacity of the functional properties of the cortical neurons to be modified by visual experience during this period is known as plasticity. It is thought that this period of plasticity functions to allow the development of visual capabilities that cannot be anatomically or physiologically predetermined with sufficient accuracy at the genetic level.

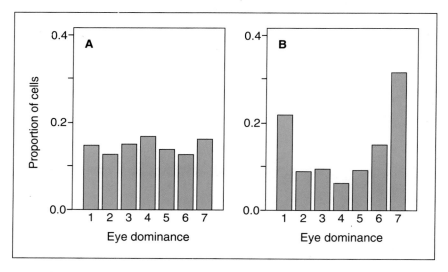

13.3 | Ocular dominance histograms. *A:* Pooled data from four normal control monkeys (384 cells). *B:* Similar data from a monkey reared with chronic atropinization of the right eye as a model of anisometropic amblyopia (316 cells). Cells dominated by atropinized eye are in groups 1–3, cells dominated by the untreated eye are in groups 5–7. Group 4 responds equally well to receptive field stimulation in either eye. Adjacent groups are progressively unequal in responses until groups 1 and 7 respond to only one eye. The atropinized monkey shows a mild loss of binocular cells and more cells responding to the untreated eye. The reduction in number of cells responding through the amblyopic eye is not amblyopia per se but a corollary finding. The quality of cell function is not addressed by the ocular dominance histogram. (Data from Movshon JA, Eggers HM, Gizzi MS, et al: Effects of early unilateral blur on the macaque's visual system. Physiological observations. *J Neurosci* 1987;7:1340–1351.)

Beyond asymmetrical retinal image contrast, more severe forms of visual deprivation occur. Lid suture of one or both eyes has been used as the standard way to remove all pattern visual input. This simulates the clinical condition of a lid tumor that prevents the eye from opening and results in occlusion amblyopia. In anisometropia the level of accommodation can be accurate only for one eye (Fig. 13.4). A defocus is produced in the other eye, resulting in a reduction of image contrast and resolution in the more ametropic eye.

Strabismus leads to a loss of binocular cells.[12,13] In strabismus without concurrent anisometropia, amblyopia is present only when a preferred use of one eye (for whatever reason) exists. This brings out another feature about cortical development, i.e., the role played by attentional mechanisms in visual development. If the image quality is equal, the exercise of attention when viewing with only one eye is enough to unbalance cortical development and lead to amblyopia. It is said that sometimes an abnormal binocular interaction occurs, but the nature of the abnormal interaction is not known. Amblyopia occurs when a selection exists of which eye to use, and even though vision occurs in the nonpreferred eye, which may be of equivalent optical quality, that eye becomes amblyopic.[14]

Visual deprivation can also be selective, only certain features of visual experience being absent. For example, kittens reared with only vertical visual contours in their environment have a reduced number of cortical neurons that respond to horizontal contours.[15] Similarly, the presence of an uncorrected astigmatic refractive error results in a blurring and loss of contrast for contours at a particular orientation.[16] Clinical testing shows reduced contrast sensitivity for gratings in this orientation (meridional amblyopia), reflecting the reduced responsiveness of the neurons having this orientation in their receptive fields. Anisometropia, through the mechanism of defocus, pro-

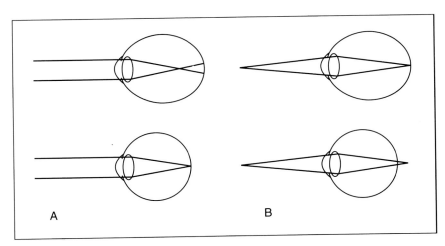

13.4 | Anisometropia. The upper eye in each drawing is myopic, the lower emmetropic. A: Distant target. The image is in focus only for the emmetropic eye. B: Near target. Only the myopic eye is in focus. With anisometropia only one eye is in focus at a time. If both eyes are hyperopic, the more ametropic eye may never be in focus because accomodation is exerted only until one eye is clear. The eye having a chronically unclear image will become amblyopic owing to deprivation of high spatial frequencies. Anisomyopia may have no amblyopia if objects fall within the far point of each eye. In unilateral high myopia the highly myopic eye is too myopic to have much experience of clear images.

duces selective deprivation of high spatial frequency experience in the more ametropic eye. The high spatial frequencies in this eye have a reduced contrast. This leads to a reduction in the number of cortical cells that respond to this eye at high spatial frequencies. At low spatial frequencies, however, much less shift occurs in the ocular dominance. The amount of ocular dominance shift thus is spatial frequency dependent[17] (Fig. 13.5). In anisometropic myopia it may be possible to fixate near objects with either eye. In such a case amblyopia may not result because the visual experience is not sufficiently asymmetric. One would expect a mild reduction in binocularity in the cells that respond to the high spatial frequencies which are blurred by the anisometropia.

Monocular visual deprivation (lid suture in the experimental animal or lid tumor in the child) affects both the anatomic and the functional connections of the central visual pathways. In most animal studies the retina has

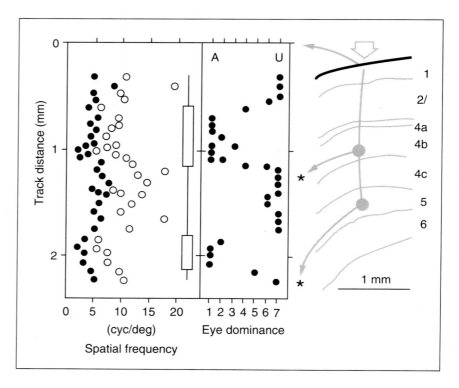

13.5 | Summary of a single microelectrode penetration in area 17 of the visual cortex of the same monkey reared with chronic atropinization as shown in Fig. 13.3. *Right:* Sketch of the penetration with electrode track (open arrow) and electrolytic lesions (filled circles). The asterisks mark the location of landmarks in the track. *Left* and *center* panels: Neuronal properties encountered. The closed circles indicate the spatial frequency showing the highest contrast sensitivity on the left (optimal spatial frequency), and the ocular dominance class in the center. *A* and *U* indicate the atropinized and untreated eyes, respectively. The open circles indicate the highest spatial frequency reponding to a high contrast grating (spatial resolution). Thick sections of the vertical bar indicate regions of the penetration dominated by the atropinized eye. Note that both optimal spatial frequency and spatial resolution increase in cells driven by the untreated eye. These differences in spatial frequency responses are the neural substrate for poor vision in amblyopia, because the cells driven by the blurred (atropinized) eye on average have poorer responses. (Data from Movshon JA, Eggers HM, Gizzi MS, et al: Effects of early unilateral blur on the macaque's visual system. Physiological observations. *J Neurosci 1987;7:1340–1351.*)

remained anatomically normal.[18] The most obvious anatomic change is in the lateral geniculate nucleus (LGN), where cell size and basophilia are reduced in layers driven by the amblyopic eye. The cell size reduction ranges up to 30%. Milder forms of amblyopia (esotropia, exotropia, late eyelid suture, and atropinization to simulate anisometropia) predominantly affect the parvocellular geniculate layers.[19] In the more severe forms of amblyopia produced by neonatal eyelid suture or aphakia, the magnocellular geniculate layers also are affected. Although cell size may be reduced, the function of LGN cells is entirely normal. A study of the physiologic responses of neurons in the monkey LGN after 5 years of monocular deprivation showed no qualitative or quantitative abnormalities.[20]

One human lateral geniculate nucleus has been studied from a patient who had anisometropic amblyopia.[21] It exhibited the expected cell size changes, predominantly in the parvocellular layers. The change in cell size is believed to reflect the size of the axonal tree that the cell has to support. A smaller area of cortical tissue is occupied by afferents from the amblyopic eye, and therefore a smaller axonal arbor would be expected. The cell size change says nothing about the functional quality of the synapses made by the smaller cells and by itself does not indicate amblyopia, which can be defined only behaviorally or physiologically. Physiologic recordings of cells in the LGN show completely normal responses in amblyopia produced by anisometropia or by lid suture. Physiologically, the first cell to show abnormal functional responses is in the visual cortex.

In the visual cortex the more severe forms of amblyopia cause a reduction in the cortical area driven by afferents from the deprived eye. The ocular dominance stripes become uneven in size on the basis of competition of afferents in layer 4c of the visual cortex, the amblyopic eye having less territory. Lid suture and other severe reductions in the input from one eye lead to a decrease in the cytochrome oxidase staining of the areas of cortex previously driven by that eye. Cytochrome oxidase is present in nerve terminals, axons, dendrites, and cell bodies. However, in the atropinization model of anisometropic amblyopia the cytochrome oxidase activity increases in area 4Cb, where the parvocellular layer afferents synapse; therefore, the exact pattern of staining seems to depend on the magnitude of the amblyopia.[19,22]

Physiologic recordings in the cortices of lid-sutured animals show very few, poorly responding units driven by the severely amblyopic eye and very few binocular units. In anisometropic amblyopia a much more modest loss of binocularity occurs. Units driven by the amblyopic eye show a shift in the population means of maximum spatial resolution, spatial frequency of maximum contrast sensitivity, and maximum contrast sensitivity to lower values. In esotropic amblyopia similar but more marked changes are found.

Human amblyopes have been examined with positron emission tomography[23] (Fig. 13.6). Deprivation, anisometropic, and strabismic amblyopes all showed similar findings. A significant reduction occurs in visual cortical blood flow and glucose metabolism during visual stimulation of the amblyopic eye compared with periods of stimulation of the normal eye. This implies a lower level of activity, or fewer cells responding, or both.

CLINICAL FEATURES

It is estimated that amblyopia occurs in 2% of the population, the exact number depending on the population studied and the definition criteria used. It occurs in several clinical contexts: occlusion of vision of an eye by an eyelid (Fig. 13.7) or an opacity in the refractive media; anisometropia; strabismus; and bilateral marked blurring of the images in both eyes by refractive error (ametropic amblyopia). Amblyopia can be acquired and treated

13.6 | Positron emission tomogram of the brain, horizontal section, in strabismic amblyopia. *Right:* Active glucose metabolism while viewing through the sound eye (arrow). *Left:* Greatly reduced glucose metabolism while viewing through the amblyopic eye. The greater activity is from the high spatial frequency responding neurons that are not driven by the amblyopic eye. Amblyopia is a disease of the visual areas of the brain.[23]

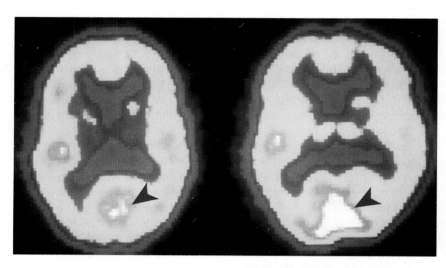

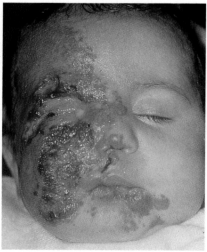

13.7 | Facial hemangioma. Occlusion of the eye by lid tumor results in a very profound amblyopia. There is little to no activation of the visual sensory neural pathways originating in the occluded eye. (Courtesy of Dr. M. Lieb.)

only during the period of plasticity of the visual cortex (the sensitive period). This sensitive period begins at or shortly after birth for humans. The visual system loses its ability to acquire amblyopia or, conversely, to improve with treatment usually somewhere between ages 7 and 8 years, depending on the individual.

Amblyopia is considered to be a functional defect that can be reversed with treatment. Any anatomic defect is only at a microscopic level, in terms of synaptic morphology and dendritic branching patterns in the cortex. Clinically, such microscopic anatomic defects are completely undetectable. During treatment these defects presumably reverse with the recovery of function. An occasional patient does not respond to adequate treatment. The clinical presumption is that an undetected organic defect that prevents improvement must exist in this patient. The term "organic amblyopia" is then sometimes applied. Typically, most patients who do not fully recover visual acuity are those whose treatment was instituted at an older age or who comply poorly with treatment. In general, the prognosis for treatment depends on the age at onset, duration since onset, age at treatment, and compliance with treatment. Use of the term "organic amblyopia" to refer to optic atrophy reflects an archaic and different use of terminology.

Amblyopia may be superimposed on organic disease. Therefore, structural anomalies of the refractive media or retina may limit the best visual acuity that can be achieved. Nevertheless, a superimposed amblyopia may be present simultaneously. Treatment of this amblyopia will lead to some improvement in vision even though the best acuity possible is limited.[24]

The performance of an eye with anisometropic or strabismic amblyopia depends on the acuity test used. Detection of a sine- or square-wave-modulated grating of a particular contrast, spatial frequency, velocity, and orientation is considered to be a *resolution acuity* because the grating can be detected by resolving the bars (Fig. 13.8). Performance is limited by the size of the smallest foveal cones (about 30 sec arc) and the point spread function of the eye, which spreads the image of a point over several cones.

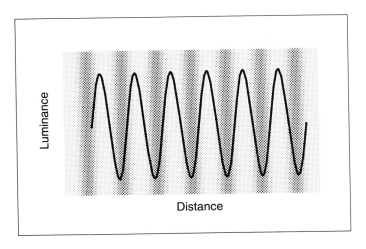

Distance

13.8 | Sine-wave, luminance-modulated grating. Such gratings contain one spatial frequency. The grating is characterized by its spatial frequency, orientation, contrast, drift velocity and temporal frequency. The contrast is defined as

$$\frac{L_{max} - L_{min}}{L_{max} + L_{min}}$$

where L_{max} is the maximum luminance and L_{min} the minimum. The tracing shows the luminance of the corresponding location in the background grating.

Performance on a grating resolution task is frequently characterized by the contrast sensitivity function, which records for each spatial frequency tested the reciprocal of the contrast required for threshold detection of a sine-wave-modulated grating (sensitivity = 1/threshold contrast). Contrast sensitivity is reduced in the amblyopic eye in rough proportion to the severity of the amblyopia. Higher spatial frequencies show greater elevations in threshold contrast. For a particular range of Snellen acuity no difference exists in contrast sensitivity between anisometropic and strabismic amblyopia. An amblyopic eye may have a nearly normal contrast sensitivity at 0.25 cycles/degree but with a Snellen acuity of 20/200 typically shows a tenfold reduction in contrast sensitivity at 4 cycles/degree.

A second class of acuity tests requires detecting the spatial offset of a line or point relative to a reference (Fig. 13.9). The most studied task in this group is *vernier acuity*. The general name for these tasks is hyperacuity or position acuity. The visual system is remarkably good at these tasks and spatial thresholds are five to ten times finer than the best grating resolution or intercone spacing—3 to 6 arc sec or better. Resolution therefore exceeds the size of the smallest pixel (foveal cone). It is thought that hyperacuity results from cortical processing and plays a role in the analysis of form and shape. Snellen acuity requires the analysis of shape and form, and Snellen acuity and hyperacuity are degraded similar amounts in amblyopia.

The normal eye has a vernier threshold (0.1 min arc) about eight times better than its Snellen threshold (0.8 min arc). In both strabismic and anisometropic amblyopia these two acuities are reduced proportionately. For example, a twofold rise in Snellen threshold will be accompanied by a twofold rise in vernier threshold. It seems that whatever process reduces one acuity also reduces the other. It is of interest that the severest form of amblyopia—complete deprivation of vision—shows a supernormal vernier acuity in the sound eye.[25]

Strabismic and anisometropic amblyopia differ in their performance to grating acuity in proportion to Snellen acuity.[26] Snellen acuity is reduced to a greater degree than grating acuity in strabismus. In anisometropia the reduc-

13.9 | Tests of vernier acuity. The vernier resolution task is to detect the offset in the grating (left) or line (right). The smallest detectable offset (threshold) is expressed as an angle at the viewing distance used. Under optimal conditions vernier acuity can be as good as 3–6 sec arc.

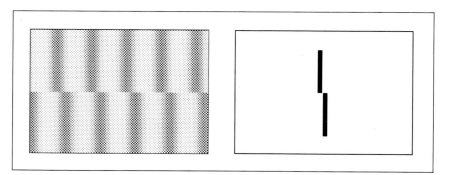

tion is proportional. Therefore, in strabismus a measurement of grating acuity will overestimate Snellen acuity[27] (Fig. 13.10).

Spatial interference effects refer to the interference to seeing a visual contour that is produced by a nearby, adjacent contour (crowding effect). Such effects occur for stereoacuity, vernier acuity, Snellen acuity, and orientation discrimination. Flanking, interference lines produce a maximum elevation of threshold at a spacing 30 times the threshold acuity for normal foveal and peripheral vision and for both eyes of amblyopes of any type. Therefore, the maximum effect on normal foveal vernier acuity (threshold of 0.1 min arc) is at a spacing of 2 to 4 min arc away from the target.[28] The eye with strabismic amblyopia has a vernier acuity much more degraded than grating acuity, so that resolved targets are subject to spatial interference effects. Clinically, this effect is seen as better performance on Snellen acuity when isolated letters are shown compared with rows of letters. For the eye with strabismic amblyopia the performance on a row of letters depends on the spacing between the letters. Amblyopes who have anisometropia and strabismus show results on these various acuity tests appropriate for strabismus.

The accommodative response is subnormal in amblyopic eyes.[29] The slope of the stimulus/response function is reduced, and larger errors of accommodation are required to produce a response.[30] Optical correction of mild hyperopic refractive errors therefore may help in the treatment of amblyopia.

Severe degrees of amblyopia are associated with the phenomenon of *eccentric fixation*.[31,32] The diagnosis of eccentric fixation is made by observing the fundus through an ophthalmoscope that projects a fixation target onto

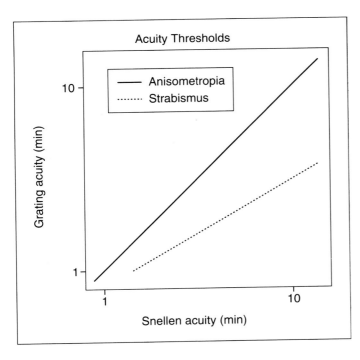

13.10 | Grating acuity thresholds vs. crowded Snellen acuity thresholds. Schematic representation of data, showing that Snellen acuity is much more affected than grating acuity in strabismic amblyopia.[61]

the retina[33] (Fig. 13.11). The portion of retina used to fixate this target then can be directly observed. The normal eye uses the fovea to fixate such a target. The deeply amblyopic eye may fixate anywhere within a broad non-foveal location which is fairly consistent for the individual. A loose association exists between the depth of amblyopia and the degree of eccentricity. Esotropes and exotropes do not necessarily eccentrically fixate on the nasal and temporal retina, respectively,[32] nor does eccentric fixation correlate well with anomalous retinal correspondence. The best use of eccentric fixation is as a sign of depth of amblyopia and resulting poor prognosis for treatment.

The retinal sensitivity to light is mildly abnormal in amblyopia. The threshold to increments of light presented as a small spot on a background is elevated on average about a half log unit over the central 5° of the visual field, both the depth and extent of the relative scotoma depending on the depth of the amblyopia.[34,35]

Neutral-density filters reduce the Snellen visual acuity of an eye with an organic lesion.[36] In amblyopia the visual acuity is minimally reduced by the reduction in light level produced by the filter. This difference can serve as a useful clinical test.

The control and execution of eye movements is impaired in amblyopia, and both eyes may be affected.[37–40] The sound eye shows unsteady fixation (nasal drifts alternating with temporal saccades) and asymmetries of pursuit tracking. In the amblyopic eye there is a reduction of position and velocity sensitivity. Saccades in response to 3° 0.5 Hz square-wave target displacements are small and variable. Saccades in a temporalward direction are smaller and more frequent than saccades in a nasalward direction. Pursuit movements are impaired for nasalward-moving retinal images (temporalward moving target in space). The pursuit velocity is slower than the target velocity, and saccades correct the position error resulting from the mis-

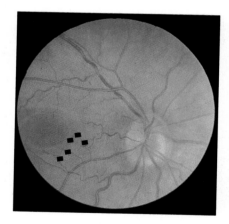

13.11 | To diagnose eccentric fixation a target is projected onto the retina with a special ophthalmoscope and the observer examines where the fixation target falls on the retina relative to the fovea. The marks indicate the locations of successive fixations in a case of eccentric fixation. In general, the poorer the vision the greater the scatter and the greater the distance from the fovea.

matched velocity. The ratio of nasalward to temporalward pursuit velocities, reflecting the pursuit asymmetry, is correlated with the depth of amblyopia.

TYPES OF AMBLYOPIA
PATTERN DEPRIVATION

Occlusion or pattern deprivation amblyopia shows profoundly poor performance on all visual acuity tests but is probably analogous to anisometropic amblyopia in pathophysiology. The essential feature responsible for producing this form of amblyopia is the deprivation of any contrast in the light pattern on the retina. It arises most commonly from severe media opacity (such as cataract or corneal scar), uncorrected aphakia, the use of patching for therapeutic reasons,[41] or blepharoptosis. It may be unilateral or bilateral. A secondary exotropia or esotropia may result from the poor vision. It is the most difficult form of amblyopia to treat. The contrast sensitivity function is profoundly depressed.[42]

A review of a large number of cases of simple congenital ptosis showed that 17% developed amblyopia and 19% developed strabismus. The types of amblyopia were divided as follows: stimulus deprivation 14%, anisometropic 21%, and strabismic 51%.[43]

STRABISMIC

Strabismic amblyopia occurs uniocularly and is present equally under monocular and binocular viewing conditions (Fig. 13.12). Under binocular

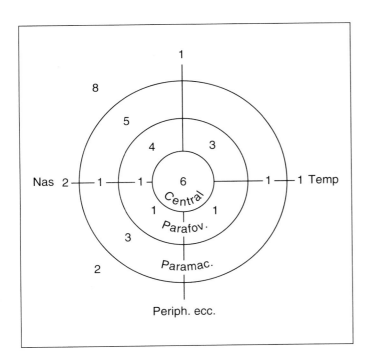

13.12 | The location of the fixation area in 40 esotropic amblyopes. The largest number use an area superonasal to the fovea, but temporal fixation is possible. The scatter of fixation areas makes it difficult to arrive at a simple explanation of why a particular area is used.[32]

conditions a fixation preference exists for the sound eye. If the sound eye is covered, fixation of necessity will be with the amblyopic eye. After the cover is removed, fixation will return to the sound eye after a period of time that is roughly correlated with the extent of amblyopia[44] (Fig. 13.13). No correlation exists between the severity of the amblyopia and the angle of deviation.[45] Exotropes tend to alternate fixation and not develop amblyopia. The reason for such common alternation is not understood. Amblyopia in an exotrope is usually associated with anisometropia. The development of ambyopia in esotropes depends on the fixation preference. Usually the less hyperopic eye is used for both distance and near fixation tasks and the more hyperopic eye becomes amblyopic. If the second eye is myopic, one eye can be used at distance and the other at near, resulting in no amblyopia. Hypertropes tend to either fuse or alternate. Amblyopia develops less frequently when intermittent sensory fusion exists. Amblyopia may be present with or without suppression; no necessary relationship occurs between the two.

ANISOMETROPIC

Amblyopia due to poor retinal image quality results in unilateral amblyopia in the context of anisometropia. Only a rough correlation exists between the degree of anisometropia and the depth of amblyopia.[46] If the image quality is poor in both eyes, it is possible to have amblyopia present in both eyes. This form of amblyopia is uncommon. Possibly owing to the balance of retinal inputs, competitive mechanisms in the cortex are not triggered. Both eyes have equally degraded performance as the high spatial frequency mechanisms are not validated through the visual experience of either eye.

TREATMENT

The standard treatment for amblyopia has been patching of the sound eye, which forces use of the amblyopic eye (Fig. 13.14). Simultaneous with this, any defect in image quality in the amblyopic eye should be rectified. This could be removal of whatever is occluding vision (e.g., lid tumor, cataract) as soon as possible, or merely the prescription of spectacles based on a cycloplegic refraction. Keeping in mind the subnormal accommodation of the amblyopic eye, it is probably best to prescribe most or all of the hyperopia

13.13 | *A:* Fixation preference in esotropia with amblyopia. The patient habitually fixates with the sound right eye. *B:* Occlusion forces fixation to be taken up by the amblyopic left eye. *C:* After removal of the occluder, fixation switches back to the sound eye. A scale of depth of amblyopia can be constructed by observing how long it takes to refixate with the sound eye. An immediate refixation is called a fix. Refixation after a momentary delay is called a strong prefer. Holding fixation with the amblyopic eye to, but not through, a blink is called a moderate prefer. Holding through a blink and then refixating with the sound eye at some time later is called a prefer.

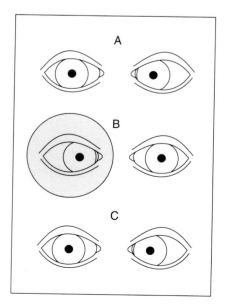

that is found. This will minimize the risk of developing a strabismus from the occlusion, which disrupts peripheral fusion. When esotropia exists the full cycloplegic refraction must be given. In either case, the full cylindrical correction should be given to establish the best possible quality of the retinal image.

Occlusion can be done in many ways. The strictest way is to wear an opaque patch on the face around the clock. More practical is to use it for the waking hours. Partial occlusion is given by doing less than full-time, opaque occlusion or with translucent occlusion, usually full time but possibly part time as well. If significant refractive error occurs in the sound eye, that eye can be blurred with cycloplegia. With cycloplegia or translucent occlusion it must be verified that the occlusion is sufficient to switch fixation to the amblyopic eye under binocular viewing conditions. Bangerter introduced a convenient graded series of plastic occluding films that adhere to the back surface of the spectacle lens. Translucent occlusion has the advantage that large forms still can be visible to the occluded eye and peripheral fusion is not so disrupted.

The practical implementation of patching may by rather difficult, depending on the depth of amblyopia and the age and personality of the child. Psychologic methods, from ordering to pleading, threatening, or bribery, may have to be used by the parents. In very young children arm restraints can be used to make removal of the patch more difficult. Tincture of benzoin can be applied under the adhesive rim of the patch to increase its adhesiveness and to help protect the skin. Children frequently peek around an opaque patch on spectacles, but the frequency of peeking may be sufficiently low so that the amblyopia does improve. Conversely, the peeking may be enough to prevent further improvement. An improvement in vision that stops short of equality with the sound eye can be caused by peeking; treatment should never be discontinued as ineffective if peeking has been a possibility. Regardless of the occlusion method, once the child has gotten a little used to it and the vision has started to improve the patch is much better accepted.

In some patients latent nystagmus is elicited by occlusion. Initially, this might be expected to reduce visual acuity. Nevertheless, it is not a contraindication to occlusion therapy, and visual acuity does respond to treatment in the presence of the nystagmus.[47]

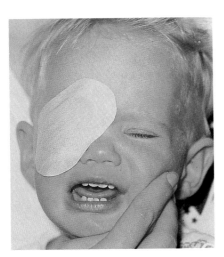

13.14 | Application of a patch to the sound eye of a child reduces vision in proportion to the degree of amblyopia, frequently resulting in crying or efforts to remove the patch. This response can be used to diagnose poor vision in one eye. The child cries with the patch on one eye but not with it on the other eye.

Once occlusion therapy has been started, the vision or fixation pattern of the child must be monitored at frequent intervals. The previously sound eye may experience a loss in vision due to the occlusion.[48] This most likely will occur before age 2, and seldom to any serious extent after age 5. On examination the patched eye should be given a few minutes to adjust to seeing without the patch before vision is measured. A rule of thumb frequently used is that occlusion can safely be done for 1 week for each year of age. Younger children respond more rapidly to treatment. Total failure of response to treatment should be concluded only after 6 months of full-time occlusion with full compliance and no improvement in the vision. Once the vision has started to improve, treatment should be continued until no further improvement occurs. Along with the improvement in vision the contrast sensitivity and the near point of accommodation also improve.

Until 2 years of age, the extreme responsiveness of infants and children to occlusion therapy sometimes leads one to use inefficient methods of occlusion. This takes the form of omitting occlusion every other, second, or third day or of alternating the patch to occlude the amblyopic eye itself, also every other, second, or third day.

After the initial treatment, once vision has been equalized or made as good as possible, maintenance treatment should be continued until the child is at least 8 years old. This can take the form of part-time occlusion at home, the wearing of a thin Bangerter film, or spectacles that correct one eye for distance and the other for near. Sometimes as little as +0.50 overcorrection for distance in one eye can lead that eye to be used for near while the eye that is not overplussed is used for distance. When maintenance therapy is finally discontinued, minimal decline should occur in vision in the formerly amblyopic eye. The reason for keeping vision under treatment so long is that it is not known for how long vision can be kept optimal and then allowed to decline and yet retain the ability to recover in later life should the sound eye be damaged. Recovery of function in the formerly amblyopic eye is known to occur when the sound eye is lost or injured later in life,[49] but in many cases vision improves only partially. A history of the visual acuity at various times is seldom available and one usually does not know what the best treated vision was. The safest procedure, therefore, is to keep the acuity optimal as long as possible.

Alternatives do exist to occlusion therapy. One alternative called penalization, involves optically correcting one eye to distance and the other to near.[50] The sound eye may be atropinized and corrected for distance and the amblyopic eye corrected for near. Thus, alternation between the eyes is forced as gaze shifts from distance to near. Alternatively, the sound eye is atropinized and corrected for near and the amblyopic eye corrected for distance. Atropinization may not sufficiently decrease visual acuity in the sound eye to ensure use of the amblyopic eye, and the pupil dilation may lead to difficulties with dazzle from sunlight.

Bangerter[31] and Cüppers[33] devised special, intensive treatment methods for patients with eccentric fixation, known as pleoptics. The peripheral retina, including the eccentrically fixating area, was bleached with bright light administered through an ophthalmoscope-like device. The therapist could visualize the fundus and shade the anatomic macula with an occluding disc. The macula would then function for a brief period better than the peripheral eccentric fixation location. Repeated application of this treatment led to improved visual acuity under all viewing conditions. Although initially promising, a randomized study showed pleoptics to have no superiority over conventional occlusion treatment.[51]

In 1978, Campbell et al[52] proposed a new form of amblyopia treatment, the Cam vision stimulator, which involved the use of brief periods of occlusion during which visual attention is given to viewing a slowly rotating disc with any of a range of spatial frequencies of bar grating on it. While the disc was viewed, games or pictures were drawn on a piece of clear plastic just above the rotating disc. Remarkable improvements were obtained by giving weekly treatments of 7 min each. Subsequent results in the hands of others were much less successful, and the best the treatment achieved in controlled clinical tests was to equal the efficacy of patching, but only when used daily.[53-55] The device has gradually dropped out of use. This episode demonstrated the importance of visual attention with the amblyopic eye when the better eye is occluded. A similar strategy has been used in the past with visual tasks involving small pictures or drawings.[56]

Video games have also been used, with brief periods of occlusion while the game is being played. They have the advantage of capturing the subject's attention. The are somewhat limited in that very small objects cannot be presented. Improvement in vision has been variable.[57]

Occasionally, later in life, the vision of the sound eye is damaged. The amblyopic eye is sometimes able to recover some vision beyond its level of performance at the time of the injury. The recovery rate is not well known, but appears to be in the 30–50% range.[58] The best prognostic factors for improvement are foveal fixation in the amblyopic eye and loss of the good eye. The improvement occurs over several weeks and can be five Snellen lines or more.[59] Improvement only after loss of the good eye implies release from an inhibitional influence from the good eye.

Amblyopia also can be a risk factor for loss of vision in the good eye. Trauma is involved in more than half of such cases. A study in Finland showed a threefold greater risk of loss of the healthy eye when the companion eye has amblyopia.[60]

14 | OTHER FORMS OF NONSURGICAL STRABISMUS MANAGEMENT

Gary R. Diamond

SECTOR OCCLUSION

A popular form of strabismus management in Europe, not well known in the United States, involves the use of partial lens occlusion, termed "sector occlusion." A sector is a piece of translucent adhesive paper applied to the posterior surface of a lens or lenses to obstruct vision of an eye in a particular direction (Fig. 14.1). This method, unlike prisms or optical penalization, does not alter the shape, size, or localization of a viewed object.

Sector occluders are devised to obstruct the areas responsible for diplopia and visual confusion. A large frame is provided so that exact placement of the sector occluders can be performed.

In one study, of 384 children with constant horizontal strabismus, orthophoria was obtained in 169 (44%), in 85% of those with a deviation less than 30 prism diopters, in 25% of those with a deviation between 30 and 50 prism diopters, and in only 3% of those with a deviation over 50 prism diopters. An additional 57 (15%) achieved final deviation of less than 15 prism diopters. The remaining 157 children (41%) required surgery.[1]

Sector occluders of a different shape are used for treatment of amblyopia (Fig. 14.2).

ORTHOPTICS

The treatment of strabismus by means of orthoptics (literally "straight eyes") has a long history, although today this technique is used more extensively in Europe than in the United States. Its basic principle is the gradual expansion of fusional version amplitudes by exercises, either in open space or by viewing targets through devices intended to isolate the eyes (haploscopic devices, such as the major amblyoscope). Fusional vergence amplitudes are expanded through the use of gradually stronger prisms held in the appropriate direction before one or both eyes, or by the use of spherical lenses to utilize the accommodation–convergence relationship to change ocular alignment.

Historically, the success of orthoptic training has been greatest in cooperative patients with phorias or intermittent strabismus of comitant nature. Patients with alphabet pattern strabismus, torsional symptoms, highly incomitant strabismus, and little cooperation fared less well. Patients with longstanding constant tropias were less likely to regain fusional vergence amplitudes despite orthoptic training.

Today, the most common indications for orthoptic expansion of fusional vergences include convergence insufficiency, intermittent exotropia of relatively small amplitude, and decompensating accommodative esotropia. Published series of successfully treated patients followed for long periods are difficult to find, and it is uncertain whether orthoptic training must be continued throughout life to be effective. It is also uncertain whether preoperative fusional expansion improves long-term surgical results.

Diplopia recognition training for patients with anomalous retinal correspondence and suppression is rarely performed today because of the risk of intractable diplopia.

PRISMS

Prisms can be very useful in the treatment of certain patients with a small degree of horizontal and vertical strabismus.

Patients who have superior oblique palsy and a vertical deviation in primary position may benefit from a vertical prism before the paretic eye. Confounding the usefulness of this technique is the simultaneous excyclotorsion associated with this palsy; some patients, however, will cyclofuse successfully if the vertical deviation is collapsed with a prism. The minimal

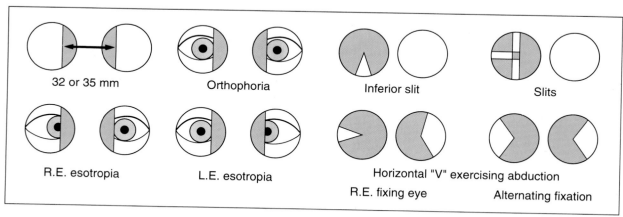

14.1 | Various forms of sector occlusion for treatment of strabismus, diplopia, and visual confusion.

14.2 | Various forms of sector occlusion for treatment of amblyopia.

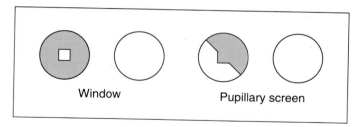

amount of prismatic correction necessary to provide comfortable single binocular vision should be prescribed after an office and home trial with Fresnel membrane prisms, as described below. Because many patients with this palsy have incomitant deviations when viewing from right to left, the field of single binocular vision is likely to be limited. In addition, vertical fusional vergence amplitudes are likely to wither under prism correction, and the patient becomes more strabismic when the prism is removed.

Some patients with VI nerve palsies and esotropia in primary position can benefit from a base-out prism over the paretic eye; this may obviate the need for a face turn to view in forward position. Some patients with congenital nystagmus and a face posture may benefit from prisms before one or both eyes to position the null point of least nystagmus and best acuity in the forward position with the head straight. In the case of a horizontal face position, the bases of the prisms should be placed in the direction of the face turn. Because the amount of prismatic correction is quite large, this approach usually is impractical.

The use of prisms for treatment of patients with typical intermittent horizontal and vertical strabismus is often contraindicated, because they place fusional vergence amplitudes at rest and consign the patient to permanent, often increasing, prismatic correction. However, certain elderly or debilitated patients may benefit from prismatic correction when surgery is not indicated or when the deviation is small and symptomatic.

The prism adaptation test involves the preoperative use of prisms to neutralize a deviation with prisms for a given period of time, followed by performance of surgery for the amount of strabismus fully neutralized by the prisms. Thus, the prism neutralization may predict the outcome of surgery for a given deviation, may determine the maximal deviation, and may estimate fusion potential at that deviation (Fig. 14.3). In addition, some patients exhibit a different deviation with the prism adaptation test than with cover testing. It remains to be shown whether the former provides better surgical results than the latter. In a controlled, randomized study of patients with acquired esotropia, 60% underwent prism adaptation and 40% did not; of those who responded to prisms with motor stability and sensory fusion, half underwent conventional surgery and half underwent augmented surgery based on the prism-adapted deviation.[2] Success rates were highest (89%) in prism adaptation responders who underwent augmented surgery, 79% in those who underwent traditional surgery, and lowest (72%) in those who did not undergo prism adaptation.

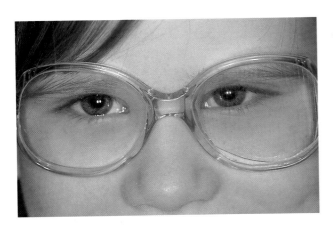

14.3 | Prism adaptation test: a child with esotropia is wearing a Fresnel membrane prism over the left eye of sufficient strength to neutralize the esotropia.

The amount of prism to be provided a patient for comfortable single binocular vision can be arbitrarily assumed to be one third to one half of the maximal phoria obtained on cover testing or can be titrated to the subjective response of the patient.[3] Fresnel membrane prisms are easily obtained, relatively inexpensive, and can be readily adjusted in strength. They are somewhat dysesthetic, yellow, peel after about 3 months in place, and do degrade acuity (about one line per 5 prism diopters). Available from 1 to 30 prism diopters, they can be confined to one or both lenses (plano carriers in the case of patients not wearing a correction), trimmed to fit a bifocal segment, distance correction, or part of the field of a lens, or prescribed to an oblique axis orientation for those who have both horizontal and vertical deviations (Fig. 14.4). Patients should be given a trial of Fresnel prism wear. If agreeable and the deviation is relatively small (under about 10 prism diopters), the prism can be permanently ground into glasses. Some patients prefer to continue wearing the Fresnel membrane, simply changing it after 3 months or so.

BOTULINUM TOXIN

The use of type A *Clostridium botulinum* toxin (Oculinum®) to paralyze temporarily human extraocular muscles by chemodenervation, thus permitting the antagonist to contract and effect a permanent alignment change, is credited to Alan B. Scott and colleagues at the Smith–Kettlewell Eye Research Foundation.[4] The toxin interferes with acetylcholine release from nerve endings by antagonizing serotonin-mediated calcium ion release. The toxin is usually injected in the conscious patient, with the syringe needle connected to an auditory EMG device that amplifies the muscle action potentials; on successful injection, the muscle immediately becomes silent as the action potential disappears. Within 3 days the injected muscle becomes paralyzed and an overcorrection is noted. Alternatively, the muscle can be injected under direct visualization during general anesthesia.

Oculinum is provided to investigators as a freeze-dried lyophilate in vials containing 50 ng of toxin prepared under FDA supervision. The toxin is stable for up to 4 years at freezer temperature but degrades in an hour when thawed to room temperature. Immediately before use it is reconstituted with normal saline. Each vial contains less than 1/40 of the lethal dose for 50% of

14.4 | A Fresnel membrane prism as received from the manufacturer (3M Health Care Specialties Division, St. Paul, MN 55144-1000). The prisms are pre-punched in circular format and the base is clearly marked.

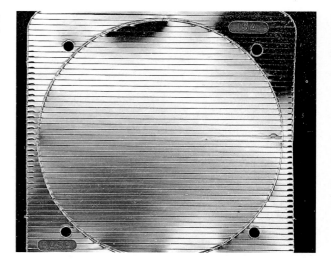

humans; the nanogram dose injected is too small to stimulate antibody formation.

Oculinum would be predicted to be most useful in cooperative adults but has been injected successfully in children as young as 9 years. Younger children can be sedated in the operating room with ketamine and then injected. The protocol suggests titrated dosages proportional to the deviation, with children's dosages also proportional to body weight. Injections are preceded by administration of topical anesthetic drops.

Many patient series have been reported. A recent series by Biglan et al found best results in patients with surgical overcorrections (87.5% controlled with Oculinum) and mild VI nerve palsy (43.7% controlled), and worst results in patients with comitant exotropia (13.3% controlled) and infantile esotropia (33.3% controlled).[5] Significant complications included blepharoptosis, hypertropia, globe perforation, and subconjunctival hemorrhage. Complications reported by others include transient pupillary dilatation, retrobulbar hemorrhage, spread of paralysis to noninjected muscles, missed injection site, patient disorientation, diplopia, and corneal irritation.[6]

Oculinum appears to be most useful in patients who are not medically fit for surgery (because of illness or history of malignant hyperthermia), who refuse surgery, who have had multiple strabismus operations, or who have acute VI nerve palsies and mild esotropia in primary position. Oculinum is contraindicated in patients with a history of myasthenia gravis and is unlikely to be effective in patients who have mechanical restriction of eye movement caused by scar tissue or entrapment of tissue.

15 | TECHNIQUES IN STRABISMUS SURGERY

Robert W. Lingua

Preoperatively, one may consider a variety of factors that can assist the surgeon in performing the optimal procedure for the strabismus patient.

The potential of the anticipated surgery to compromise further the blood supply to the anterior segment is to be evaluated in light of previously operated muscles, prior cryotherapy in the vicinity of the long posterior ciliary arteries, the presence or absence of encircling elements, chronic intraocular inflammation, and previous trauma.

Selection of the type and location of the conjunctival incision is based on the number and location of muscles on which to be operated, the anticipated presence or absence of scarring, and the status of the conjunctiva and Tenon's capsule in light of the patient's age and health. Tenon's capsule is typically sparse in the elderly, and the conjunctiva is often friable. In this case, one may select a conjunctival incision that will not require stretching and therefore avoid irregular conjunctival tears. I prefer the cul-de-sac approach in eyes that have not been previously operated on, and especially in the young, where the tissues are more elastic. In patients undergoing reoperation, those with extremely thin conjunctiva, and those intended to undergo an adjustable suture procedure, I employ an incision over the insertion of the tendon (after Swan). When conjunctival recession is planned or in cases involving exploration for the tendon, the exploration begins from the cornea with a limbus-based peritomy. In resections, especially of the medial recti, where one anticipates redundant conjunctiva, I prefer the Swan approach, entering the conjunctiva at the base of the semilunar fold, or employ the limbus-based incision with recession or resection of the conjunctiva in order to minimize chemosis at the nasal limbus postoperatively. Prolonged chemosis may lead to dellen formation and ulceration, especially in the elderly or in the medically compromised patient. When horizontal and oblique or vertical rectus muscles are to be operated on simultaneously, fornix incisions between the muscles will often provide adequate exposure for the entirety of the case, e.g., in A-pattern esotropia with superior oblique overaction or V-pattern exotropia with inferior oblique overaction. Similar planning is necessary when horizontal or vertical transpositions of the recti are to be performed.

Especially in cases of reoperation, at the conclusion of the conjunctival incision, fastidious hemostasis of all conjunctival vessels will minimize the occurrence of hemorrhage in Tenon's capsule, which can obscure tissue planes. A constant awareness of your position relative to the vortex veins and periocular fat will minimize trauma to these structures. Hemorrhage from a torn vortex vein will cease with the direct pressure of a cotton tip applicator over its transverse scleral canal, and cautery of its distal aspect in the periocular fascia. Violation of the fat pad can be managed by primary closure with plain gut sutures, and is advised, especially in the presence of any bleeding. Realizing that the horizontal and vertical recti insert between 4 and 8 mm from the limbus, introduction of the muscle hook more posteriorly than the anticipated location of the tendon is to be avoided, since it may draw the posterior Tenon's capsule forward, along with the fat pad, and complicate the dissection. Additional caution is exercised in engaging the lateral rectus, where introduction of the hook along its inferior border more than 8 mm posterior to its insertion is likely to engage the inferior oblique muscle. Likewise, in surgery of the superior rectus, the superior oblique should be visualized prior to cutting the intermuscular fascia and thus assure its integrity.

As in patients with high myopia, those with a long exposure to alcohol have a rubberlike texture to the sclera which in the former case may also be very thin. In such cases, the "microtip" spatula needles will pass more easily through the sclera with less tissue drag, but may present a greater risk of perforation. When perforation occurs in the elderly, liquified vitreous may spontaneously drain through the site. In any case of suspected perforation, the pupil is dilated and the area visualized with indirect ophthalmoscopy. When penetration of the retina has occurred, a single small application of cryotherapy over the perforation site is indicated, as well as retinal consultation in the postoperative course.

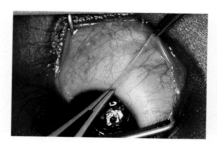 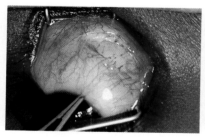 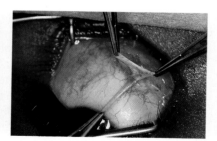

15.1 | This and subsequent figures display a recession of the left medial rectus as viewed from the surgeon's twelve o'clock position. The 0.3-mm forceps are placed at the seven-thirty position and grasp the conjunctiva and Tenon's capsule at the limbus. The eye is elevated and abducted. A second 0.3-mm forceps elevates the conjunctiva approximately 8 mm posterior to the limbus.

15.2 | Westcott scissors are used to incise the conjunctiva.

15.3 | Both surgeon and assistant elevate Tenon's capsule out of the plane of the conjunctival incision.

In general, absorbable suture material can be used when the tendon is secured to the globe at the point of intended attachment. In other situations, e.g., where one might anticipate difficulty in the localization of the tendon if reoperation is necessary (superior oblique tenectomy or large adjustable recessions of the medial or superior rectus), or suspension in the vicinity of a silicone element, or in posterior fixation cases, a nonabsorbable suture may be preferred. When a tendinous insertion is particularly vascularized, as in thyroid eye disease, or as is routinely noted in the vertical recti, light applications of cautery prior to the passage of the spatula needle will minimize hemorrhage in the distal tendon. A hematoma at the insertion can obscure the anatomy and lead to an insecure passage and/or lock of the tendon. Improper locking of the suture to the Tenon's capsule rather than tendon may lead to muscle slippage. Closure of the conjunctiva can be accomplished with plain gut suture. Passing the needles close to the edge of the conjunctival incision will minimize the risk of inclusion cyst formation.

Recessions alone tend to widen the palpebral fissures, while recess/resect procedures tend to narrow them. The possible consequences of the intended procedure on eyelid position should be discussed with the patient preoperatively and may often be employed to one's advantage when an asymmetry exists preoperatively.

Retrobulbar anesthesia is satisfactory for most adult strabismus surgery. However, caution must be exercised in those with thyroid eye disease, where the necessary volume of anesthetic for anesthesia and akinesia may compromise blood supply to the eye. The longer-acting anesthetics (e.g., bupivacaine) are avoided when one is planning to adjust sutures the following morning. If one intends to perform a passive "spring-back balance" test under general anesthesia, then the use of a long-acting paralytic agent such as Pavulon may be discussed with the anesthetist. If, however, one chooses to elicit a contraction of the extraocular muscle during the procedure, as in certain paralytic, adjustable suture, transposition, or slipped muscle cases, then inhalation anesthesia alone will allow the introduction of succinylcholine as necessary during the case. The skeletal muscle paralysis from succinylcholine will resolve within three minutes of injection, but the increased tension effect in the extraocular muscle typically peaks by 60 seconds after injection and then gradually declines over a period of 10 to 20 minutes. Therefore, when succinylcholine has been used to facilitate general anesthesia, preoperative forced ductions will be influenced by this induced muscular tension.

The assistant grasps the eye at the conjunctiva–Tenon's junction with a 0.3-mm forceps and rotates the eye into elevation and abduction (Fig. 15.1). The surgeon then elevates the conjunctiva at the base of the fornix, and incises the conjunctiva the desired distance from the limbus (Fig. 15.2). At this point, all visible conjunctival vessels are lightly cauterized to ensure good visibility through the localization of the tendon. The assistant and the surgeon grasp the fascia within the conjunctival incision with gentle pressure against the sclera, and elevate it from the globe (Fig. 15.3). The scissors are

RECESSION OF A RECTUS MUSCLE

then used to incise Tenon's capsule at this point, exposing bare sclera (Fig. 15.4). Visualization is maintained with the posterior forceps.

The large muscle hook can then be passed behind the medial rectus muscle without any further posterior movement of the hook than the site of the incision itself (Fig. 15.5). When the medial rectus is on the hook, one should confirm that the entire tendon has been engaged. The posterior arm of the 0.3-mm forceps can be used as a probe to locate the superior pole of the muscle (Fig. 15.6). Securing it with the forceps, the muscle hook is withdrawn to the inferior aspect of the tendon (Fig. 15.7), being sure to release the hook from entrapment in the insertion. Then, it is passed beyond the superior pole held by the forceps (Fig. 15.8). In this way, one can be certain of having completely secured the full length of the tendon. A large Jameson muscle hook, or the Greene hook, will assist in the following dissection.

The small tenotomy hook is introduced between the insertion of the tendon and Tenon's capsule anterior to it (Fig. 15.9) and used to dissect bluntly the fascia from the surface of the tendon, moving posteriorly along its long axis (Fig. 15.10). Overcoming some resistance to blunt dissection at this point is important in order to visualize adequately the tendon during the remainder of the case. When the conjunctiva and Tenon's capsule have been satisfactorily reflected over the tip of the large muscle hook (Fig. 15.11), the scissors are used to incise the superior aspect of Tenon's fascia (Fig. 15.12). Visualization of bare sclera superiorly is accomplished by the introduction of the closed scissor blades into the fascial incision and rotation of them over the tip of the hook (Figs. 15.13 and 15.14). Two small tenotomy hooks are then passed posteriorly along the tendon, against bare sclera, and elevated to expose the intermuscular fascia (Figs. 15.15 and 15.16) for dissec-

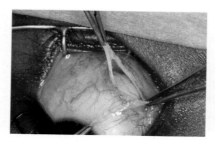

15.4 | Tenon's capsule is incised, exposing sclera.

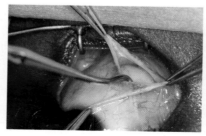

15.5 | The Greene or Jameson muscle hook is inserted under the tendon of the medial rectus muscle, keeping the toe of the hook flat against the sclera at all times.

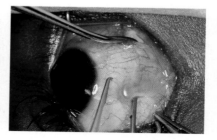

15.6 | The surgeon can grasp the superior pole of the muscle through the conjunctiva to ensure that the entire tendon is on the muscle hook.

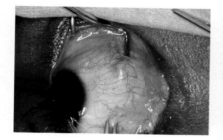

15.7 | The superior pole of the rectus muscle is held by the forceps and the muscle hook is partially withdrawn.

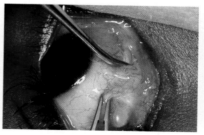

15.8 | The muscle hook has been replaced, clearing the forceps and thus capturing the entire tendon.

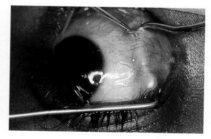

15.9 | A small Stevens muscle hook is placed under the conjunctiva on the limbal side of the rectus muscle tendon.

tion. The 0.5-mm Castroviejo locking forceps are then applied to the distal aspect of the tendon superiorly (Fig. 15.17) and inferiorly. These forceps serve as globe handles throughout the case, obviating the need for traction sutures at the limbus. Also, the superior forceps maintains full exposure of the insertion, keeping the distracted conjunctiva and fascia securely above the superior pole when the inferonasal fornix incision is used.

Gentle traction by the assistant, away from the operated muscle, allows the surgeon to control the hook beneath the tendon and accomplish suture passage at the insertion (Fig. 15.18). The surgeon may then control the for-

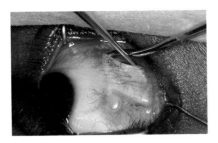

15.10 | The small Stevens hook is manipulated forward and backward over the tendon and under the conjunctiva to separate the conjunctiva from the underlying Tenon's capsule and tendon.

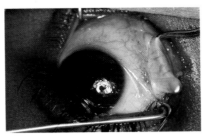

15.11 | The small muscle hook is placed perpendicular to the globe at the superior tendon border to expose intermuscular septum and Tenon's capsule.

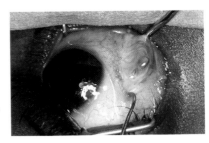

15.12 | A small opening is created at the tip of the muscle hook through intermuscular septum and Tenon's capsule.

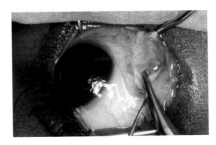

15.13 | The closed scissors can be used to dissect bluntly the superior pole of the tendon.

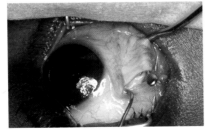

15.14 | A Stevens muscle hook is placed perpendicular to the sclera through the incision and swept around the superior pole of the tendon to ensure that the entire tendon is captured on the muscle hook.

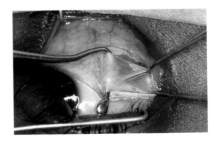

15.15 | Two Stevens muscle hooks retract the conjunctiva and Tenon's capsule to expose the length of muscle.

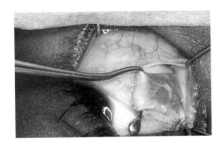

15.16 | The muscle is exposed as far posteriorly as desired.

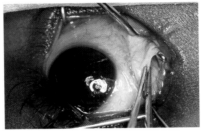

15.17 | The locking forceps are applied to both the superior and inferior poles of the tendon insertion to control the exposure as well as the position of the globe.

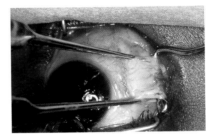

15.18 | The surgeon holds the muscle hook and the assistant the locking forceps.

ceps during the scleral passes to position optimally and control the globe. The needle is passed from the middle to the superior edge of the tendon, where it is positioned for regrasping. A second "through-and-through" lock to the edge of the tendon (Figs. 15.19 to 15.21) is performed. The Westcott scissors suffices for removing the tendon (Fig. 15.22). Visualization of the tendon may be preserved by passing a dry cotton pledget between the tendon and the globe (Fig. 15.23). The anterior pole of the caliper is positioned at the crotch of the original insertion (Fig. 15.24). The ideal scleral pass imparts an opaque translucency to the needle (Fig. 15.25).

Because the spatula needle is a "side-cutting" needle, it is important to avoid the tract of the previously passed suture and not inadvertently cut it. Likewise, it is important to have the exits of the sutures not so far apart as to

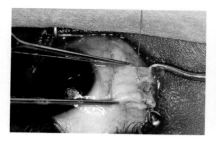

15.19 | While controlling the position of the eye with the muscle hook, the surgeon places the suture from the middle of the tendon to the margin, parallel to the insertion.

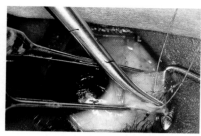

15.20 | A lock bite is performed at the margin of the muscle.

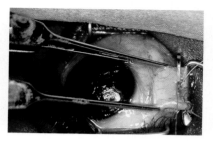

15.21 | A similar maneuver is performed using the second arm of the double-armed suture, through the remaining half of the tendon.

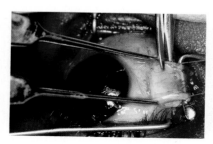

15.22 | The tendon is disinserted from the globe.

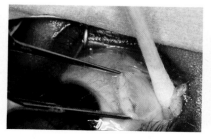

15.23 | Note the thin sclera posterior to the muscle insertion. Any hemorrhage from the cut tendon can be controlled with cotton swabs.

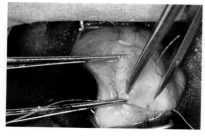

15.24 | The appropriate position for muscle reattachment is measured from the original insertion.

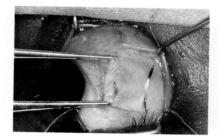

15.25 | The first arm of the double-armed suture is placed through the sclera, parallel to the original insertion.

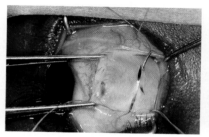

15.26 | The second needle of the double-armed suture is placed in similar fashion, with slight overlapping of exit sites.

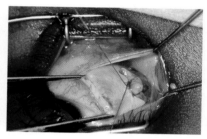

15.27 | The muscle is pulled fully to the desired recession site.

create a buckling effect when the knot is tied (Fig. 15.26). The sutures are then drawn in the direction they were passed (Fig. 15.27) to avoid pulling the sutures through their scleral paths. The recessed muscle is demonstrated where one has attempted to preserve the original orientation of the tendon to the globe at its normal width (Fig. 15.28). After securing the tendon to the globe, the tenotomy hook is then introduced above the superior pole of the old insertion and the fascia is rotated inferiorly (Figs. 15.29 and 15.30) over the operative site. The incision is then closed with a single 6-0 plain suture in a "bury-the-knot" fashion, to minimize a foreign body sensation (Fig. 15.31). In the young, the conjunctiva is routinely closed, since the complication of Tenon's capsule prolapse can require additional anesthesia for management.

Elevating the semilunar fold (Fig. 15.32), its junction with the bulbar conjunctiva can be visualized and incised (Fig. 15.33). The conjunctival vessels are cauterized and Tenon's fascia entered. The large muscle hook is passed beneath the tendon, going no further posteriorly than the insertion itself (Figs. 15.34 and 15.35). The Tenon's capsule beneath the olive tip of the large

RESECTION OF A RECTUS MUSCLE

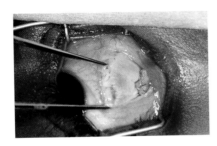

15.28 | The sutures are tightened, tied, and cut.

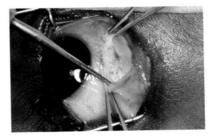

15.29 | Tenon's capsule is repositioned over the incision site.

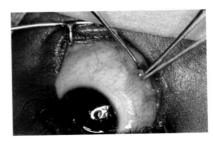

15.30 | The conjunctiva is smoothed over the incision site.

15.32 | This series demonstrates the resection of the left medial rectus as viewed from the twelve o'clock surgeon's position. The surgeon has chosen a superonasal incision site so the eye is grasped with 0.3-mm forceps at the ten-thirty o'clock limbus and held inferotemporally.

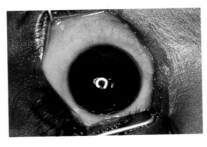

15.31 | The incision may be closed with a single buried knot suture.

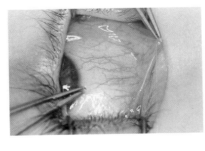

15.34 | A large muscle hook is placed under the insertion of the rectus muscle.

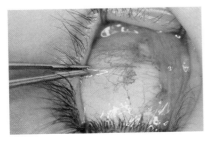

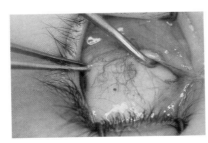

15.33 | The conjunctiva and Tenon's capsule are incised in layers.

muscle hook is incised (Fig. 15.36) in order to visualize bare sclera at both poles of the tendon. Two small tenotomy hooks are passed along the long axis of the tendon in order to expose the perimuscular fascia for incision (Fig. 15.37). A second large muscle hook is passed beneath the tendon and traction is applied between the two, keeping the insertion and both hook tips parallel. The anterior arm of the caliper is placed on the midportion of the anterior hook, and the posterior portion delineates the site for needle passage (Fig. 15.38). A marking pen or the cautery may be used if remeasuring during suture passage is not desired.

The same technique of suture passage is employed as was used for recession. The needle is passed tangentially to the tendon and globe and woven through the tendon from its midportion to the superior pole and then locked upon itself. The needle at the opposite end of the suture is then passed from the midportion to the inferior pole and once again locked, securing the tendon at the point of desired resection (Fig. 15.39). A "mosquito" hemostat is placed across the tendon just ahead of the suture (Fig. 15.40). The tendon is then cut ahead of the clamp (Fig. 15.41), and the resection of tendon then completed at the original insertion (Fig. 15.42). The hemostat can remain on the tendon until all scleral passes have been performed, permitting a clean operating field.

Passage of the needles through the original insertion takes advantage of the differential scleral width at this location. Since the scleral thickness is at its minimum just posterior to the insertion, there is a differential step of 0.5 to 0.7 mm from just behind to just in front of the insertion. Orienting each needle tangentially to the globe just posterior to the insertion will allow a forward movement of the needle through the step of sclera, accomplishing

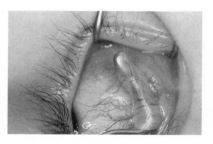

15.35 | Appearance of the tendon after the conjunctiva has been displaced from the muscle belly.

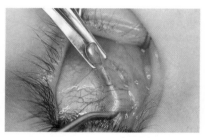

15.36 | A small incision is made in the inferior pole of the tendon through Tenon's capsule and intermuscular septum.

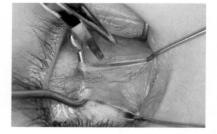

15.37 | Two small Stevens muscle hooks are used to lift Tenon's capsule and intermuscular septum from the muscle belly for incision.

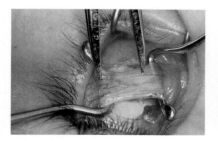

15.38 | A second large muscle hook is placed underneath the muscle belly. The amount of muscle to be resected is measured with a caliper.

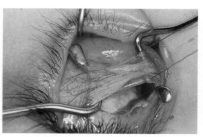

15.39 | A double-armed suture is placed in the measured position for the resection procedure.

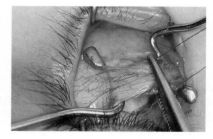

15.40 | A small hemostat is placed just anterior to the suture in the muscle belly.

a secure attachment, without ever having to direct the tip of the needle toward the globe (Fig. 15.43). The passage of the needles through the insertion can be in a diagonal fashion in order to maintain the normal width of the tendon at the posterior insertion, and yet have their exit points approximate one another to facilitate tying (Fig. 15.44). Once one is satisfied with the location and depth of the scleral pass, the first suture throw is placed before the muscle is pulled forward. The hemostat is removed from the distal tendon and the muscle drawn forward and knotted (Figs. 15.45 and 15.46). The assistant may slightly adduct the globe at this time to minimize the suture tension required to complete the knot. The conjunctiva can be closed with two interrupted 6-0 plain sutures in a bury-the-knot fashion (Fig. 15.47). The conjunctiva from the limbus to the insertion is left undisturbed.

Resections of the lateral recti and superior recti should include visualization and preservation of the neighboring oblique muscles prior to per-

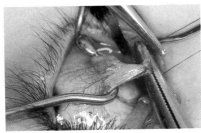

15.41 | The tendon is cut just anterior to the hemostat.

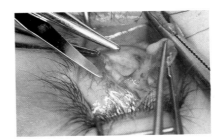

15.42 | The resected tissue is removed from the muscle insertion.

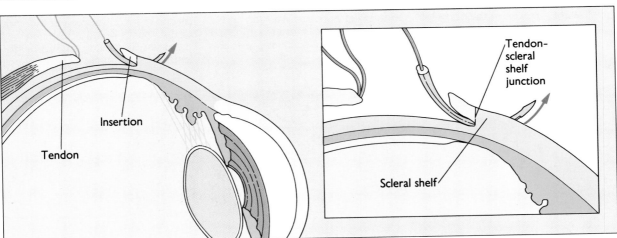

15.43 | The needle is returned through the insertional step of sclera.

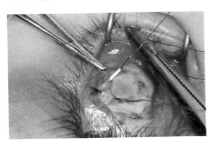

15.44 | The needles can be returned in diagonal fashion to maintain normal tendon width.

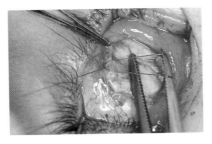

15.45 | The hemostat is released and the distal muscle is brought to the original insertion.

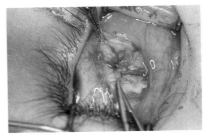

15.46 | The resected muscle has been returned to the original insertion.

forming the procedure. The frenulum between the superior rectus and superior oblique should be visualized and incised, and the common fascial attachments between the lateral rectus and inferior oblique likewise removed to avoid undesired effects on oblique muscle functions.

LEAVING THE RECESSED OR RESECTED MUSCLE FOR ADJUSTMENT

In this case of dysthyroid ophthalmopathy, the inferior rectus has been exposed through a modified Swan incision and placed on a large muscle hook (Fig. 15.48). After placing the locking forceps at the nasal and temporal aspects of the insertion and securing the 6-0 Vicryl suture to the distal aspect of the tendon, the muscle is removed from the globe (Fig. 15.49). In order to facilitate engagement of the sclera during the subsequent needle pass, 1 to 2 mm of tendon is left at the insertion (Fig. 15.50). As in the resection procedure, the tip of the spatula needle is oriented tangentially to the globe at the posterior aspect of

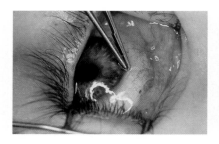

15.47 | Tenon's capsule and conjunctiva are replaced in their original position and the incision is closed.

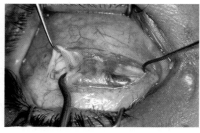

15.48 | An incision is made anterior to the inferior rectus insertion and the inferior rectus muscle is engaged on a large muscle hook as previously described.

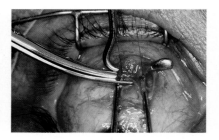

15.49 | A double-armed suture is placed in the insertion and the ends of the inferior rectus tendon are grasped with locking forceps by the assistant. The muscle is then detached from the globe.

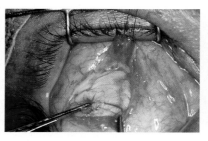

15.50 | One to 2 mm of tendon are left attached to the sclera.

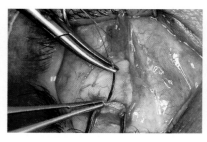

15.51 | The needles are placed in the tendon stump, approximately 3 mm apart.

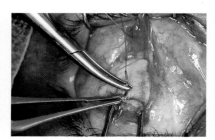

15.52 | Gently lifting the needle should prove the solidity of the suture in the tendon stump.

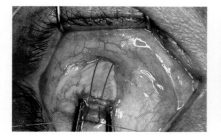

15.53 | A double throw surgeon's knot is performed.

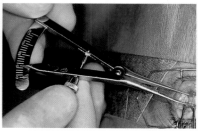

15.54 | The suspected amount of appropriate recession is measured with a caliper.

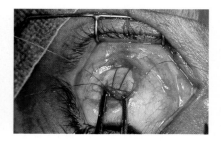

15.55 | A single bow knot is now placed as the second throw of the suture.

the insertion. While the assistant maintains the eye in an elevated position with the use of the locking forceps, the surgeon may gently elevate the residual tendon (Fig. 15.51). The needle is advanced forward through the "shelf" of sclera ahead of the insertion (Fig. 15.52). A gentle elevation effort, prior to releasing the needle, should reveal a satisfactory engagement of the sclera. If a pass is too superficial, involving only the tendon, the needle will easily pull through. Two such passes are performed in parallel, approximately 3 mm apart.

Once both passes have been accomplished, the first double throw of a surgeon's knot is performed (Fig. 15.53). The tendon is then suspended from the insertion by the suspected amount of appropriate recession (Fig. 15.54), or drawn forward to the insertion in the case of resection. The second throw of the suture should accomplish a single bow knot (Figs. 15.55 and 15.56). The bow and both ends of the suture are left 4 to 5 inches long. In vertical muscle cases where exposure of the tendon can be difficult postoperatively, an additional globe handle can be placed consisting of a 5-0 Prolene suture knotted as a loop (Fig. 15.57). The conjunctiva may be closed (Fig. 15.58), and both the loop *and* two ends of the suture are taped to the lateral (or nasal) canthal area to avoid any disturbance of the knot until the time of adjustment (Fig. 15.59). An antibiotic–steroid ointment is placed between

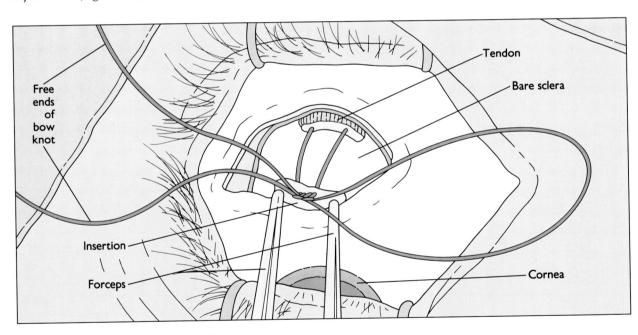

Free ends of bow knot

Tendon

Bare sclera

Insertion

Forceps

Cornea

15.56 | Drawing of the bow knot in place.

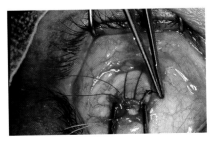

15.57 | If desired, a globe handle consisting of 5-0 Prolene suture knotted as a loop can be placed at one end of the insertion.

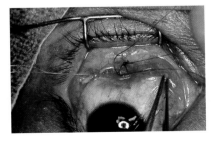

15.58 | The conjunctiva may be closed.

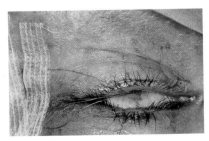

15.59 | Both suture ends and the globe loop are taped to the canthal skin.

the lids, the eye is securely patched, and the area of the sutures protected until the folIowing morning.

   If, on the following morning, the patient has had a satisfactory amount of surgery performed, then one may expand the loop of the knot, pulling the free end through, and thereby complete the fist square knot without disturbing the position of the muscle (Fig. 15.60). If, however, the position of the muscle needs to be adjusted, the free end of the suture may be pulled to reduce the size of the loop until the second throw has been pulled through (Fig. 15.61). In the latter case, a single double throw exists that can be loosened or drawn forward to adjust the position of the tendon before the square knot is completed.

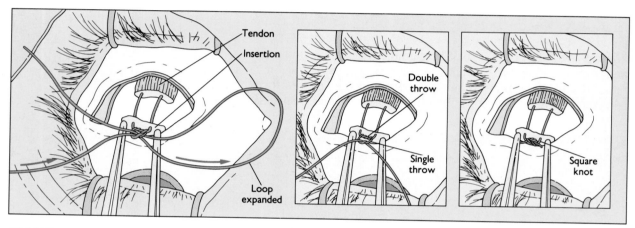

15.60 | If no adjustment of muscle position is necessary, the loop is expanded and the free end pulled through, tightened, and tied, thereby not disturbing the muscle position.

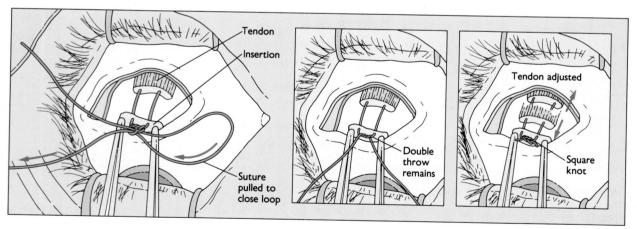

15.61 | If muscle position adjustment is necessary, the loop is closed and the position of the muscle is adjusted as necessary before the square knot is completed.

The medial rectus muscle has been exposed through a conjunctival incision over the distal tendon (Fig. 15.62). The fascia is dissected posteriorly for at least 1 cm from the insertion (Fig. 15.63). After the application of the locking forceps at the insertion, a double-armed 6-0 Vicryl suture is woven and locked at the distal tendon (Fig. 15.64). The tendon is removed from the globe and the Desmarres retractor placed beneath the medial rectus to accomplish exposure of the globe 10–12 mm posterior to the original insertion (Fig. 15.65). If resistance is encountered, a larger conjunctival incision is performed.

A double-armed 5-0 Mersilene suture is passed through the superficial sclera at the desired point of posterior fixation, leaving equal amounts of suture to either side of the scleral canal (Figs. 15.66 and 15.67). The Desmarres retractor is removed, and, visualizing the global aspect of the medial rectus, the inferior half of the Mersilene suture is then introduced into the junc-

POSTERIOR FIXATION SUTURE

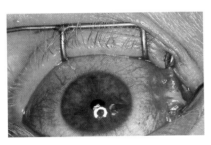

15.62 | The medial rectus muscle is isolated on a large muscle hook through a conjunctival incision.

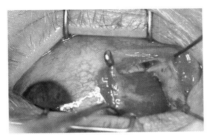

15.63 | The intermuscular septum and Tenon's capsule are cleared from the muscle belly for at least 10 mm posterior to the insertion.

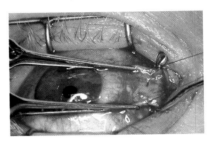

15.64 | The ends of the muscle insertion are grasped with locking forceps.

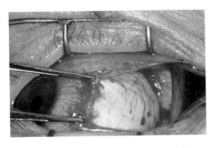

15.65 | Disinsertion of the muscle is performed.

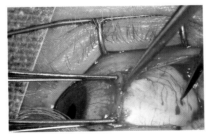

15.66 | The position of the posterior fixation suture is measured from the insertion site.

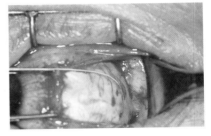

15.67 | A 5-0 Mersilene suture is passed through the sclera at the desired point of posterior fixation, leaving equal amounts of suture to either side of the scleral canal. A Desmarres retractor provides excellent exposure.

tion of the middle with the inferior third of the medial rectus tendon (Fig. 15.68). The point of introduction through the medial rectus is determined by the desired amount of accompanying recession that will minimize muscle slack between the anterior and posterior fixation. If the posterior fixation distance is intended to be 12 mm posterior to the original insertion, and the accompanying recession of the anterior insertion 5 mm posterior to the original insertion, then the sutures are passed through the muscle at a point 7 mm from the distal aspect of the tendon.

The tendon is brought against the globe, allowing penetration at the desired distance (Fig. 15.69). The superior half of the suture is similarly passed at the junction of the middle third with the superior third of the medial rectus (Fig. 15.70). The suture is then securely tied on top of the middle third of the muscle, realizing that any laxity in the knot will defeat the

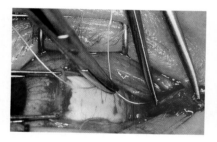

15.68 | The needles of the Mersilene suture are brought through the muscle at the appropriate point.

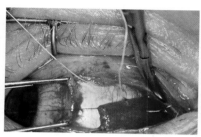

15.69 | The inferior needle is brought through the muscle 1/3 of the way from the inferior border.

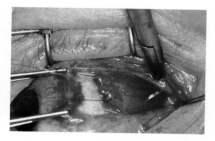

15.70 | The superior needle is brought through the muscle 1/3 of the way from the superior border.

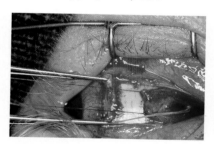

15.71 | The suture is tightly tied on top of the muscle.

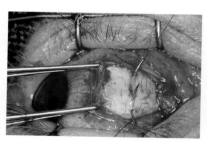

15.72 | The rectus muscle is reinserted to the globe.

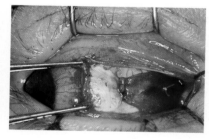

15.73 | The suture ends are tightened, tied, and cut. Notice the knot of the Mersilene suture on the muscle belly.

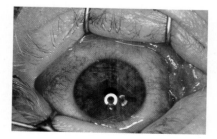

15.74 | Closure of the incision can be accomplished with a single suture.

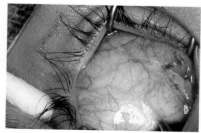

15.75 | Surgeon's twelve o'clock view of the inferotemporal quadrant of the left eye. The globe is held superonasally by forceps at the four-thirty limbus.

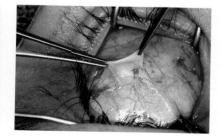

15.76 | To elevate Tenon's capsule through a conjunctival incision, 0.3-mm forceps are used.

effect of the posterior fixation by allowing slippage of the tendon along the globe at that point (Fig. 15.71). The anterior recession is then completed with passage of the Vicryl sutures (Figs. 15.72 and 15.73) and, after hemostasis, closure of the conjunctival incision can be accomplished with running or interrupted 6-0 plain sutures in a bury-the-knot fashion (Fig. 15.74).

With the eye maximally rotated superonasally (Fig. 15.75), Tenon's fascia is elevated between two forceps (Fig. 15.76) and incised to expose bare sclera (Fig. 15.77). With two large muscle hooks placed beneath the lateral rectus muscle, a single-armed 4-0 black silk suture is passed beneath the tendon (Fig. 15.78). The hooks are removed, and by drawing nasally on the inferior aspect of the suture, the eye will rotate into a superonasal position (Fig. 15.79). The eye is then secured in this position with a clamp to the drapes. Since this may elevate intraocular pressure, one should periodically release the suture, especially with elderly patients. Using a large and a small muscle hook, the inferotemporal fornix is exposed (Fig. 15.80), and the inferior oblique muscle may be seen as a purple discoloration, running in close approximation to the periorbital fat. The small tenotomy hook is introduced against the globe and moved posterior to the inferior oblique. The hook is rotated up to engage the muscle, allowing the point of the hook to penetrate the fascia between the muscle and the fat (Fig. 15.81). At this point, a myectomy or recession may proceed.

For a myectomy, the large muscle hook supports the inferior oblique muscle and two small tenotomy hooks will expose the intermuscular fascia between it and the lateral rectus (Fig. 15.82). These are then incised and the

APPROACH TO THE INFERIOR OBLIQUE MUSCLE

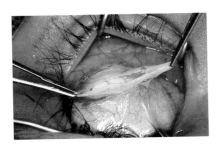

15.77 | After incision of Tenon's capsule, the sclera can be viewed.

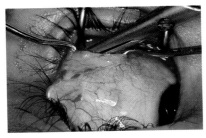

15.78 | The lateral rectus muscle is hooked and the eye is held fully in adduction. A 4-0 black silk suture is passed under the lateral rectus tendon and through the conjunctiva.

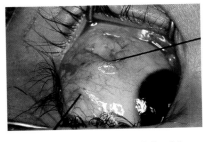

15.79 | The eye is held in full adduction by the black silk suture, which can be clamped to the drape.

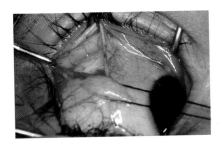

15.80 | Using two muscle hooks, the inferotemporal fornix is exposed and the inferior oblique muscle is seen as purple tissue under Tenon's capsule.

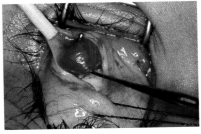

15.81 | A small muscle hook is used to trap the muscle against the orbital bone; the muscle is brought into the surgical field.

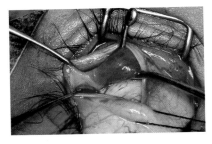

15.82 | The small muscle hook has been replaced with a large muscle hook and the inferior oblique muscle cleaned of fascial connections to its insertion on sclera.

inferior oblique is removed, flush with the globe (Fig. 15.83). The desired portion of the muscle is then resected, and the stump of the muscle is lightly cauterized (Fig. 15.84) before removal of the clamp, allowing it to retreat beneath the inferior rectus (Fig. 15.85).

In the case of recession, the inferior oblique is placed on a large muscle hook, and distracted inferotemporally. In this way, one may see that no residual muscle remains in the periorbital fat (Fig. 15.86). With nasal traction on the muscle, two small tenotomy hooks elevate the intermuscular connections, which are then incised (Fig. 15.87). The muscle is then removed flush with the globe (Fig. 15.88) and placed on a double-armed 6-0 Vicryl suture (Fig. 15.89). With a large muscle hook beneath the inferior rectus for maximal supraduction, the temporal border of the inferior rectus

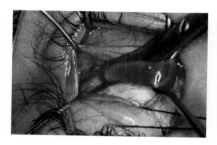

15.83 | Under direct visualization, the inferior oblique muscle is detached from the sclera.

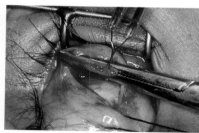

15.84 | After myectomy, the stump of muscle in the clamp is cauterized.

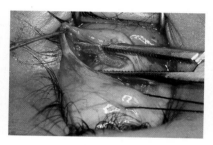

15.85 | The cauterized stump is freed from the clamp and permitted to retract into the orbit.

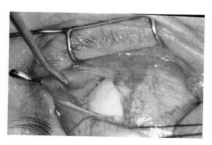

15.86 | If a measured recession is planned, the muscle is hooked as before and cleaned to its insertion.

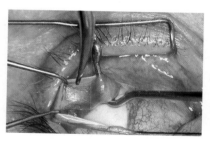

15.87 | Small muscle hooks expose the insertion of the inferior oblique muscle.

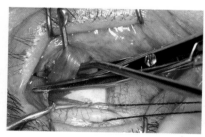

15.88 | The muscle is cut flush with the sclera to disinsert.

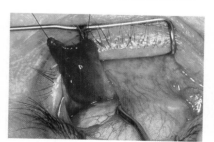

15.89 | A double-armed 6-0 Vicryl suture is placed at the insertion of the inferior oblique muscle.

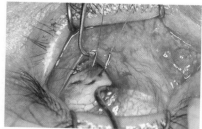

15.90 | The desired replacement position of the muscle is marked, and each suture placed in sclera along the course of the inferior oblique muscle.

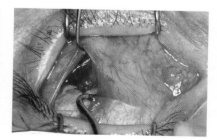

15.91 | The muscle is pulled up, the sutures are tightened and tied.

muscle is exposed and the desired amount of recession performed by two scleral passes (Fig. 15.90). The muscle is thus secured to the globe along its original direction of passage (Fig. 15.91), and the conjunctiva then closed with a gut suture (Fig. 15.92).

With the eye rotated inferotemporally, a conjunctival incision is made in the superonasal fornix (Fig. 15.93). A large hook is placed beneath the superior rectus muscle and the eye is maximally infraducted (Fig. 15.94). Gently distracting the overlying conjunctiva and Tenon's capsule, the nasal border of the superior rectus is visualized (Fig. 15.95). With the muscle hook maximally distracting the eye inferotemporally, a Desmarres retractor is placed in the incision and used to expose the superonasal quadrant. The oblique tendon is first visualized, and engaged on a tenotomy hook (Figs. 15.96 and 15.97). One can see how the large muscle hook, when passed deeply behind the superior rectus, may engage the posterior fascia and drag the superior oblique tendon into the hook along with the rectus tendon. Furthermore, trauma to the superior oblique tendon can occur if not visualized and preserved prior to a dissection of the intermuscular fascia. The intermuscular fascia ("sheath") may be dissected from the superior oblique

APPROACH TO THE SUPERIOR OBLIQUE TENDON

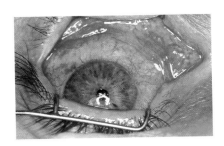

15.92 | The conjunctival incision site may be closed with a suture, if necessary.

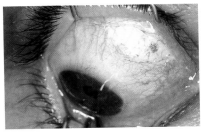

15.93 | Approach to the right superior oblique tendon with surgeon sitting at six o'clock. The eye is drawn inferotemporally and a superonasal fornix incision through the conjunctiva and Tenon's capsule is performed.

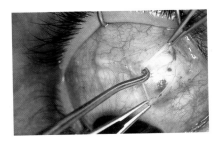

15.94 | The superior rectus muscle is isolated on a large hook.

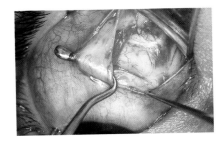

15.95 | The nasal border of the superior rectus muscle is visualized.

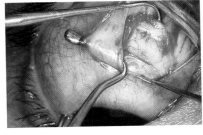

15.96 | The superior oblique tendon is isolated on a small muscle hook.

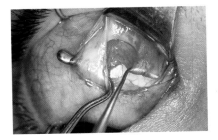

15.97 | The superior oblique tendon is brought out of the surgical field on the small muscle hook.

tendon (Fig. 15.98) and, at this point, one may perform a tuck, tenotomy, or tenectomy. A tenotomy may proceed by incising the tendon after protecting the nasal border of the superior rectus with the Desmarres retractor (Figs. 15.99 and 15.100). A tenectomy is performed after grasping the tendon with a hemostat, and sectioned on both sides, removing approximately 4 mm of tendon (Figs. 15.101 and 15.102). The conjunctival incision may then be closed with a running or interrupted 6-0 plain gut suture.

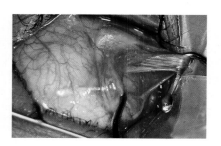

15.98 | The intermuscular septum may be dissected from the superior oblique tendon.

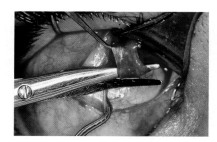

15.99 | Tenotomy of the superior oblique tendon.

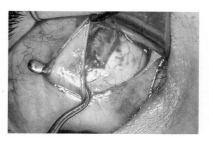

15.100 | The cut tendon is returned to its position on the sclera.

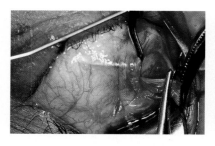

15.101 | If tenectomy is desired, two hemostats grasp the tendon roughly 4 mm apart, and the interposing tendon is removed.

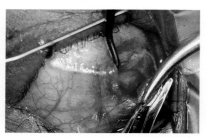

15.102 | Completing the superior oblique tenectomy.

This chapter previously was published in Lingua RW: Techniques in Strabismus Surgery, in Jaffe NS (ed): *Atlas of Ophthalmic Surgery*. New York: Gower Medical Publishing, 1990.

INTRODUCTION TO GENETICS

Gary R. Diamond

HUMAN CHROMOSOME STRUCTURE AND NUMBER

Although the easily stainable material in the nuclei of human cells was recognized and named "chromatin" by Walther Flemming in 1889, it was not until 1902 that W. B. Sutton suggested that the transmission of Mendel's factors of inheritance (genes) was associated with chromatin. By 1952 it was certain that genes consisted primarily of deoxyribonucleic acid (DNA). Until 1956 it was believed that the human genetic material was contained in 48 chromosomes, as in other primates; in that year, Tijo recognized the true human chromosome complement as 46 chromosomes (23 pairs).

Unwound, the DNA contained in each human cell would be 2 meters in length. Given one hundred million base pairs (one of two purine-pyrimidine base combinations, either adenine-thymine or cytosine-guanine) per chromosome, each cell contains three billion total base pairs. By chemical analysis, each chromosome consists mostly of DNA, but small amounts of ribonucleic acid (RNA) and two classes of proteins are also found. One protein class, the histones, can be further divided into five types: H1, H2A, H2B, H3, and H4. In addition, small amounts of nonhistone protein are present.

The typical chromatin fiber is 1,000 nanometers in diameter and is structured as a repeating array of ellipsoidal discs. Each disc is a combination of wedge-shaped octamer histone protein (two each of H2A, H2B, H3, and H4) wrapped left-handed 1.8 times around 146 base pairs of DNA. The ultrastructure of a chromosome is shown in Figure 16.1. H1 is positioned outside the ellipsoidal disc (called a nucleosome) and connects one nucleosome to the next with the "linker" DNA. These connecting regions of linker DNA and H1 histone protein are often areas at which initiation of transcription of DNA to messenger RNA (mRNA) takes place. Each chromosome consists of a number of smaller segments called genes, each of which codes for a single trait, often for a single polypeptide chain. The average gene is 20,000 to 50,000 base pairs in length, but 90% of the

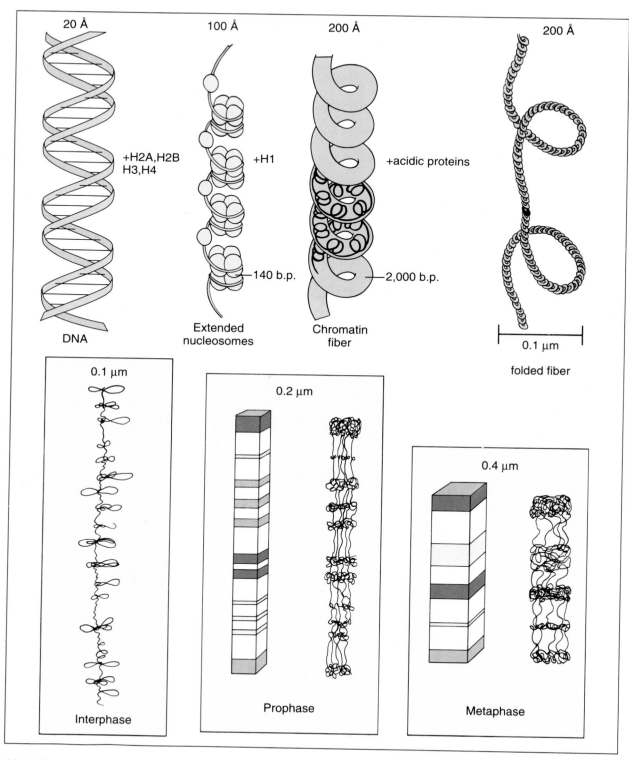

20 Å

100 Å

200 Å

200 Å

+H2A,H2B
H3,H4

+H1

+acidic proteins

140 b.p.

2,000 b.p.

0.1 μm

DNA

Extended
nucleosomes

Chromatin
fiber

folded fiber

0.1 μm

0.2 μm

0.4 μm

Interphase

Prophase

Metaphase

16.1 | Chromosomal DNA is coiled into nucleosomes, and each nucleosome is "supercoiled" into chromatin. Note the large number of base pairs in each chromatin super-coil. Between cell divisions (interphase) the chromatin is loosely folded, but then it compresses as mitosis begins (prophase). By the mitotic metaphase the chromatin is maximally compressed for ease of segregation into daughter cells. The box-like structures next to the chromatin in the lower drawings represent the appearance under banding techniques of the prophase and metaphase chromatin. (Courtesy of Dr. Jorge Yunis, Hahnemann University, Philadelphia.)

bases in each gene do not form protein and are termed *noncoding (intron)* DNA. In addition, more than one copy of each gene may exist on a chromosome; human DNA is about 20% highly repetitious, 20% moderately repetitious, and 60% single sequence.[1]

Each chromosome has ultrastructural features recognizable with conventional and special staining. Giemsa or Feulgen techniques stain all chromosomes dark, enabling them to be distinguished on the basis of relative size, length, and location of centromeres, satellites, and secondary constrictions (Fig. 16.2). The constricted part of the chromosome (centromere) divides it into two portions or arms. Depending on the relative size of the arms, chromosomes are considered metacentric (equal-sized arms), submetacentric (unequal-sized arms), or acrocentric (centromere near one end of the chromosome) (Fig. 16.3). Some chromosomes occasionally exhibit unique morphology (1, 2, 3, 16), but conventional staining techniques permit separation only into roughly similarly appearing groups, consisting of chromosomes 1–3, 4–5, 6–12, 13–15, 16–18, 19–20, 21–22, X, and Y.

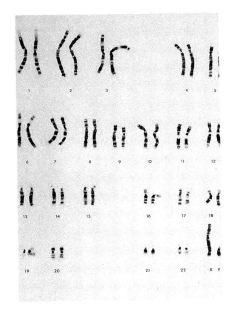

16.2 | Giemsa-banding pattern of normal male chromosomes stained with Wright's stain. (Courtesy of Dr. Jorge Yunis, Hahnemann University, Philadelphia.)

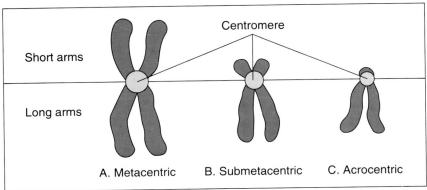

16.3 | *A:* Metacentric chromosome. *B:* Submetacentric chromosome. *C:* Acrocentric chromosome. (Courtesy of Dr. Myron Yanoff.)

Other special staining techniques also permit refined identification of subtle chromosome abnormalities and allow more exact identification of a given chromosome. These "banding" techniques permit identification of inversions, duplications, translocations, and deletions of chromosomal material; each band represents about 34 genes (Fig. 16.4). Q, or quinidine, banding provides fluorescence under ultraviolet light and discloses about 320

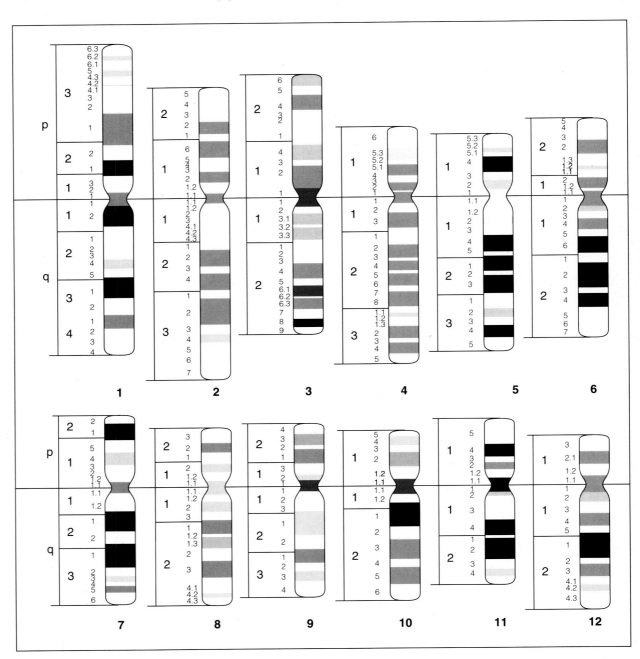

16.4 | Refined chromosomal banding possible with modern techniques. By convention, p ("petite") represents the short arm, q the long arm of a chromosome. Numbering of bands proceeds from the centromere (constriction in the drawing) in both directions. Large bands are divided into sub-bands, using decimals if necessary. (Courtesy of Dr. Jorge Yunis, Hahnemann University, Philadelphia.)

bands per cell. The popular and routine G banding consists of Giemsa staining after trypsin digestion; the genetically active euchromatin stains light and the inactive heterochromatin stains dark. R, or reverse Giemsa, banding consists of phosphate buffer treatment of the chromosomes followed by Giemsa stain; euchromatin stains dark and heterochromatin light. C banding stains centromeres and the long arm of the Y chromosome.

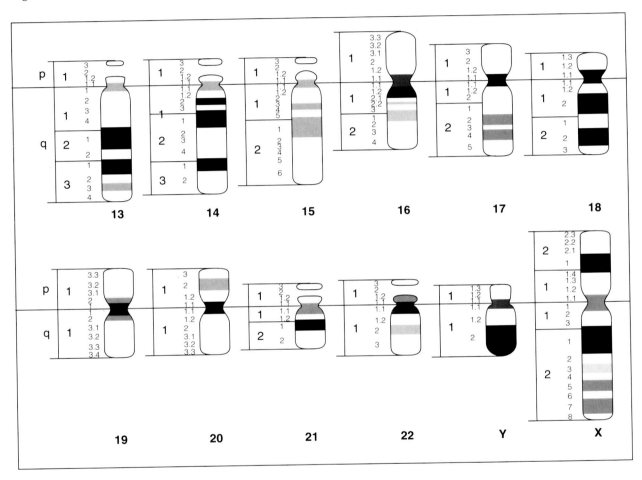

16.4 | (Continued)

Chromosome analysis, or *karyotyping,* was formally established at four international conferences held between 1960 and 1971. The human chromosome complement was arranged in seven autosomal groups (A–G) on the basis of size and centromere location. Standards of terminology also were established (Fig. 16.5).

Sex determination is dependent on the presence or absence of the Y chromosome; if present, a male develops under normal circumstances and if absent, a female. A second X chromosome is essential for normal ovarian function. In 1949, Barr and Bertram described a wedge-shaped mass of heterochromatin *(Barr body)* against the nuclear envelope in 65% of buccal smear cells from females only; this has been determined to be inactivated X chromosome material. Mary Lyon, in 1961, hypothesized that only one X chromosome is active in protein synthesis in any given cell, preventing a double-dosage effect in females. Both X chromosomes are active early in embryogenesis until relatively random inactivation occurs. In the adult, prior to meiosis in gamete formation the inactive X becomes reactivated. The Y chromosome is small, about 70,000 base pairs in length, and is believed to contain few genes (Fig. 16.6). There are homologous areas on the X and Y chromosomes, and rare transfer of genetic material *(crossing-over)* between these chromosomes can lead to the puzzling phenomenon of an XX male with the male-determining piece of the Y chromosome surreptitiously attached to one X chromosome. Also described is the rare occurrence of an XY female whose Y chromosome is missing the essential male-determining piece.[2]

Indications for karyotyping include: clinical diagnosis in the newborn with multiple malformations, especially those involving more than one organ system; diagnosis of mental retardation without clear cause; investigation of multiple miscarriages in the first or second trimester without clear cause; studies of juvenile malignancies such as retinoblastoma, Wilms tumor (associated with aniridia), and leukemia; and prenatal diagnosis in the setting of advanced parental age, known translocation or X-linked carrier state, or a previous child with a chromosome abnormality.

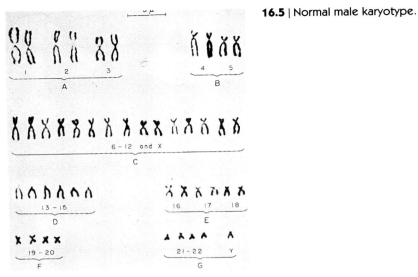

16.5 | Normal male karyotype.

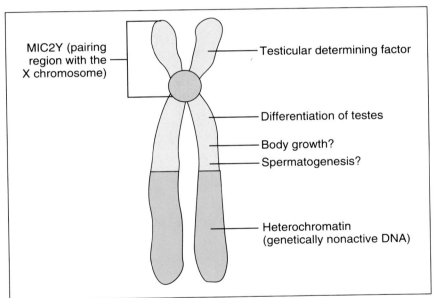

16.6 | Schematic structure of human Y chromosome.

DNA REPLICATION

The function of mitosis is to ensure equal distribution of chromosomal DNA into each of two descendant cells (*diploid* complement) (Fig. 16.7). At the beginning of mitosis, two pairs of homologous chromosomes (chromatids) are present in each nucleus. This phase of the cell cycle takes roughly 1 hour and consists of the following stages. In interphase, homologous chromosomes form centromere attachments. During prophase, the chromatids shorten, thicken, and spindle fibers appear. Metaphase is characterized by dissolution of the nuclear envelope and movement of chromatids towards the equatorial plane of the cell. Finally, in anaphase, chromatids and centromeres move to opposite ends of the cells. The maximum number of cell divisions varies among species; cells from a mouse are capable of 20 divisions and cells from a Galapagos tortoise are capable of 100.

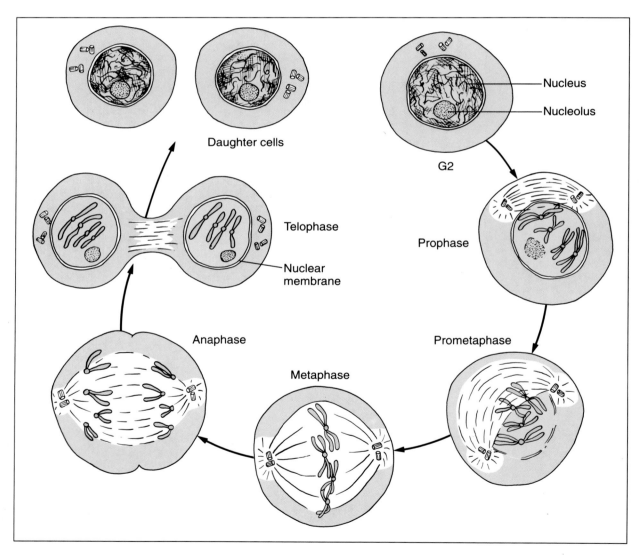

16.7 | Characteristics of mitotic cell division. *G2:* second phase of DNA synthesis. *Prophase:* sister chromosomes (chromatids) become more compact. *Prometaphase:* spindle fibers appear, attached to each chromatid at the centromere. *Metaphase:* chromatids move to equator of cell. The nuclear membrane melts. *Anaphase:* the chromatids separate to opposite cell ends. *Telophase:* the cell membrane divides, forming two identical sister cells. The nuclear membranes reform.

The function of meiosis (Fig. 16.8) is to produce four gametes from each cell, each with one half the normal number of chromosomes (*haploid* complement). Through the mechanism of crossing-over, with its resultant exchange of genetic information among sister chromatids, genetic variation can take place. Meiosis consists of two nuclear divisions, termed meiosis I and meiosis II. Three essential differences exist between mitosis and meiosis. In meiosis, homologous chromosomes pair along their entire length, not just at the centromeres, the number of chromosomes per cell is reduced by half, and variability is ensured by crossing-over. Meiosis I consists of a complicated prophase in which homologous pairing of sister chromosomes occurs, associated with crossing-over. At the end of the first anaphase, homologous chromosomes migrate to opposite poles of the spindle and the cell divides,

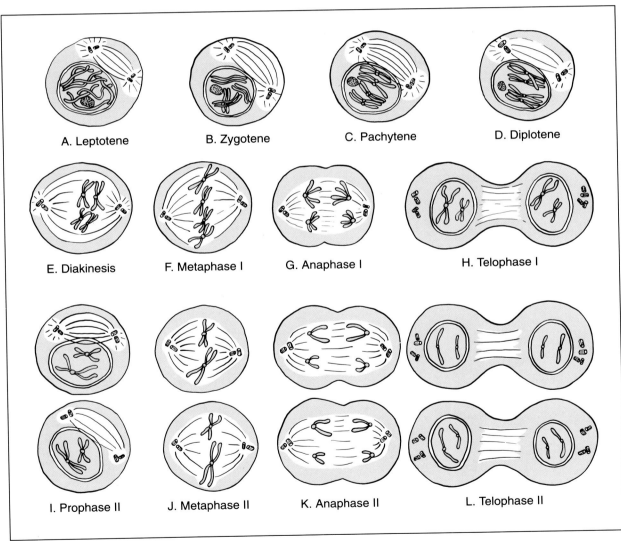

A. Leptotene   B. Zygotene   C. Pachytene   D. Diplotene

E. Diakinesis   F. Metaphase I   G. Anaphase I   H. Telophase I

I. Prophase II   J. Metaphase II   K. Anaphase II   L. Telophase II

16.8 | Characteristics of meiotic cell division. During *Prophase,* the following sub-stages are present. *Leptotene:* diploid number of chromosomes in nucleus. *Zygotene:* sister chromatids pair along entire length. *Pachytene:* crossing-over may occur between sister chromosomes. *Diplotene:* sister chromosomes sep- arate. *Diakinesis:* chromosomes coil tightly. The remaining stages (*Metaphase I* through *Telophase I* and *Prophase II* through *Telophase II*) are similar to those seen in mitotic cell division.

each daughter cell possessing a haploid chromosomal complement (23 chromosomes). Meiosis II is similar to mitosis, as the number of chromosomes per daughter cell is the same as that of the parent; four haploid gametes result.[3]

PEDIGREE ANALYSIS

Useful information can be concisely depicted in a genetic pedigree drawing using universal symbols as depicted in Figure 16.9. By convention, females are placed to the left in human pedigrees, the opposite to the practice in animal pedigrees.

ALLELES

Alleles are members of a gene pair that occupy a particular site on homologous chromosomes. Most human genes are multiallelic, e.g., more than 100 alleles for the beta-polypeptide hemoglobin chain have been identified. Each diploid individual can receive only two alleles, one from each parent, no matter how great the number of alleles in the population. Examples include the alleles at the ABO blood group locus (A1, A2, A3, B1, B2, and O) and the alleles at the alpha-1-iduronidase locus. The Scheie and Hurler syndromes are caused by mutant alleles at the latter locus, but the Scheie allele produces a more normal enzyme protein. A number of allelic mutations have been found in the rhodopsin gene in patients with autosomal dominant retinitis pigmentosa; for example, the mutation Pro347Ser is a cytosine-to-thymidine transition in codon 347, changing the codon from specifying proline to

16.9 | Symbols used in human pedigree analysis.

one specifying leucine. Females can be either *homozygous* (two copies of the same allele) or *heterozygous* (two different alleles) for genes on the X chromosome. As males have only one X, they are said to be *hemizygous* for genes on this chromosome.

PATTERNS OF GENE TRANSMISSION

Classic Mendelian patterns of gene transmission (autosomal dominant and recessive, X-linked dominant and recessive) are somewhat arbitrarily defined on the basis of the ability to detect the results of the genetic variation in the heterozygote. In general, recessive traits result in enzyme deficiencies caused by mutations of the gene specifying the particular enzyme. Heterozygotes who have one normal gene therefore have roughly half the normal enzyme activity and usually are not clinically different from normal *(wild-type)* individuals, but specific laboratory tests can detect the deficiency at the enzyme level. Appropriate testing can detect heterozygotes in homocystinuria, galactosemia, galactokinase deficiency, gyrate atrophy (hyperornithinemia), Tay–Sachs disease, and others.

Dominant traits are usually caused by mutations affecting structural proteins such as cell receptor proteins (familial hypercholesterolemia); these may cause membrane defects (myotonic dystrophy), or subunit defects (unstable hemoglobins).

In some conditions, such as the ABO and MN blood groups, both alleles are expressed and detectable and neither allele modifies the function of the other; this is termed *codominance*.

AUTOSOMAL DOMINANT TRAITS

These traits produce a clearly definable abnormality in the heterozygote; homozygosity often is lethal before birth. The trait appears in every generation (*vertical transmission pattern* on pedigree drawings) and is transmitted by an affected person to 50% of the offspring if the trait is manifested in all who receive the mutant gene (expressed as *penetrance*, from 0% to 100%). Sex incidence is equal (Fig. 16.10). Ophthalmic examples include typical pigmentary retinopathy, aniridia, congenital cataract, Marfan syndrome, corneal dystrophies, and heterochromia iridis.[4]

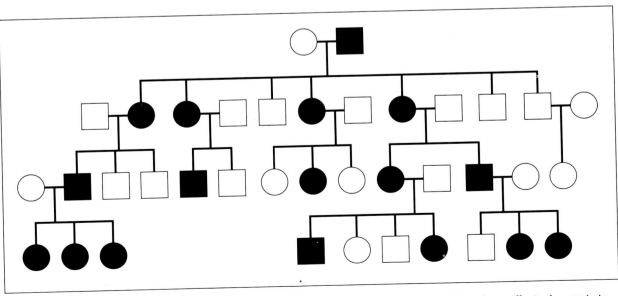

16.10 | Autosomal dominant transmission. Note vertical transmission pattern, equally-effected genders, and roughly 50% trait transmission from affected parents to their children.

AUTOSOMAL RECESSIVE TRAITS

Full clinical expression of the trait occurs only in the presence of a double dose of the mutant gene (homozygosity). Because the trait appears in siblings but usually not in parents or children, the pedigree shows a *horizontal transmission pattern* (Fig. 16.11). Parents of affected children are often consanguineous, and an equal sex incidence occurs. An average of one quarter of siblings are affected.

Ophthalmic examples include typical pigmentary retinopathy, oculocutaneous albinism, macular corneal dystrophy, microphthalmia, and Tay–Sachs disease.[4]

X-LINKED RECESSIVE TRAITS

Predominantly men are affected, and all their daughters, although unaffected, are carriers of the trait. Women can be affected if they are homozygous (often a lethal result), if they have only one X chromosome (Turner syndrome), or if random inactivation by the Lyon effect has suppressed a majority of the normal X chromosomes. The carrier does not usually manifest disease but may have a mild form, as in ocular albinism (sectors of depigmented retinal pigment epithelium) and gyrate atrophy (sectors of atrophic retina). Children of an affected father are never affected, unless the mother is a carrier. Affected men in a family are brothers or are related to each other through carrier women, i.e., maternal uncles. Pedigree analysis shows a *chess knight's move* pattern (Fig. 16.12). Ophthalmic examples include typical pigmentary retinopathy, Fabry disease, anomalous trichromacy, and retinoschisis.[4]

16.11 | Autosomal recessive transmission. Note horizontal transmission pattern, equally-affected genders, and roughly 25% trait transmission from carrier parents to their children.

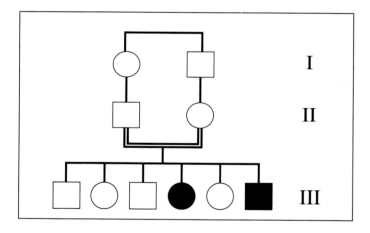

In this pattern, heterozygous men and women are affected equally. All daughters of affected men, but no sons, are affected. Distinction between autosomal dominant and X-linked dominant transmission patterns can be made only by looking at children of affected males. Affected women transmit to both sons and daughters with equal frequency, but affected men transmit only to daughters, not to sons (who receive the Y chromosome). Therefore, the incidence of the trait is twice as frequent in daughters as in

X-LINKED DOMINANT TRAITS

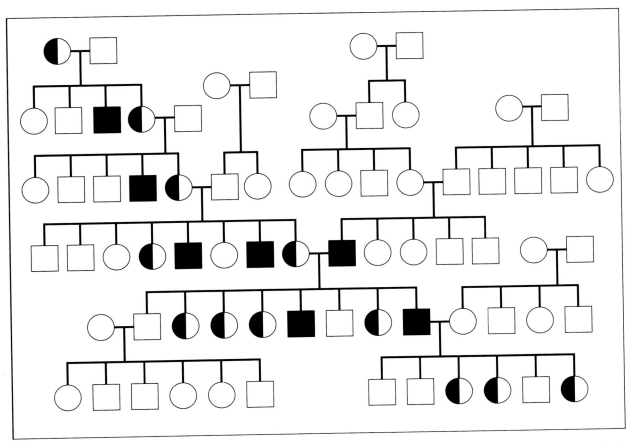

16.12 | X-linked recessive transmission. Note diagonal ("knight's move") transmission pattern, only males affected, and lack of father-son transmission. All daughters of affected fathers are carriers. The half-filled circle is the symbol for carrier female.

sons, unlike autosomal recessive traits which are equally as frequent (Fig. 16.13). Often these traits are lethal in hemizygous men. Ophthalmic examples include Aicardi syndrome and incontinentia pigmenti.[4]

CYTOPLASMIC INHERITANCE

All mitochondria are contributed by the maternal ovum; the sperm contributes only genetic material to the fertilized ovum. Mitochondria supply the cell with energy from aerobic respiration and contain one circular DNA of 17,000 base pairs called *chromosome M,* which codes for 20 proteins, a few ribosomes, and RNA. The mitochondrion is postulated to be a descendant of ancient bacteria-like organisms that entered a commensal-like relationship with eukaryotic cells, providing energy in exchange for a venue. The mitochondrial DNA is similar to that of bacteria, being circular, not bound by a nuclear envelope, and serviced by ribosomes smaller than human ribosomes.[5]

A feature of cytoplasmic transmission is that affected men never transmit a trait; their sisters may transmit to both sexes equally and may be variably affected themselves (Fig. 16.14). Ophthalmic examples include the Leber optic neuropathy and Kearns–Sayre syndrome.[6]

MULTIFACTORIAL TRAITS

These common conditions are caused by a mixture of genetic contribution and environment and should not be confused with polygenic traits, which are due to a contribution of more than one gene. A single organ is usually involved, and gene expression is often triggered by an environmental agent. Sex may be relevant, and the risk of occurrence is higher in relatives of patients, and higher still when more than one family member is involved or when the manifestation is severe. Consanguinity of parents may contribute to increased offspring risk; similar occurrence and severity in twins show that

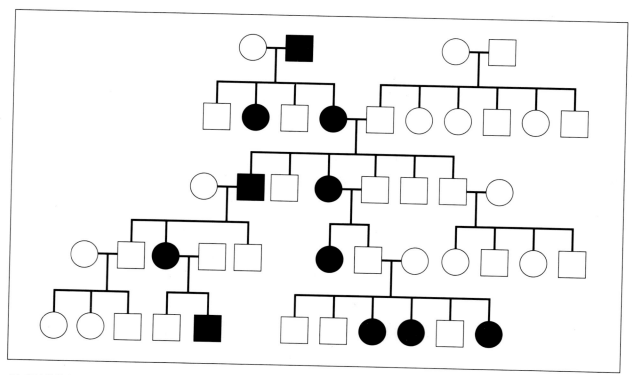

16.13 | X-linked dominant transmission. Note that both genders are affected, the presence of affected females, and no father-to-son transmission.

the trait has a genetic component. The risk to relatives decreases sharply with progressively distant relationship. Ophthalmic examples include strabismus, congenital glaucoma simplex, and primary open-angle glaucoma.[7]

Occurring in 1 of 500 live births, translocations involve breakage of two or more chromosomes and exchange of parts. Reciprocal translocations between chromosomes may involve loss of material *(unbalanced)* or conservation of chromosomal fragments *(balanced)*. Both types may be inherited or may occur de novo. A special type of translocation, entitled *Robertsonian* or *centric fusion translocation,* involves the acrocentric pairs 13, 14, or 15 and 21 or 22. A Robertsonian translocation yields a small and a large chromosome; the small fragment is often lost during cell division (Fig. 16.15).

STRUCTURAL CHROMOSOMAL MODIFICATIONS
TRANSLOCATIONS

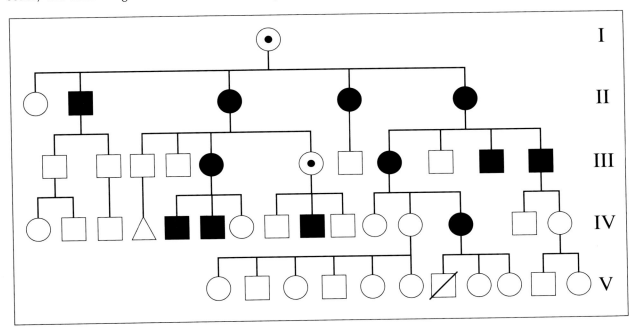

16.14 | Cytoplasmic inheritance. As ova contains almost all transmitted mitochondrial DNA, affected males cannot transmit trait, but their affected or carrier sister can.

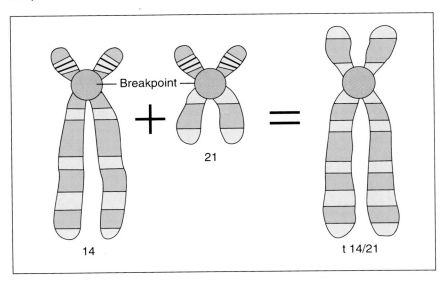

16.15 | Robertsonian translocation. The small chromosomal fragments with telomeres (extremities) are lost.

Chromosomal breakage is not random but occurs at "hot spots" along certain chromosomes.

DELETIONS

When fragments of a broken chromosome are lost, back-mutations to the normal wild-type cannot occur. As a rule, fragments lacking a centromere are lost because they are unable to align on the spindle plate during mitosis. Diagnosis of deletions is possible by the use of banding techniques during meiosis I metaphase. Deletions can be located at the end of the chromosome *(terminal deletion)* or along the chromosome length *(interstitial deletion)*.

Pertinent ophthalmic examples include the following. The Prader–Willi syndrome of mental retardation, short stature, obesity, binge eating, and wide mood swings is found in 1:25,000 live births (del 15q11–13). The cri-du-chat (cat cry) syndrome of severe mental retardation, unusual cry, and abnormal facies (especially fused eyebrows) is seen in 1:50,000 live births and is twice as frequent in males as in females (5p-). The 13q- syndrome involves mental and growth retardation, anal atresia, scalp defects, microcephaly, congenital heart disease, hypertelorism, microphthalmia, epicanthal fold, ptosis, antimongoloid lid slant, strabismus, congenital cataracts, uveal colobomas, optic nerve hypoplasia, retinal dysplasia and retinoblastoma. The 11p- syndrome is characterized by aniridia and Wilms tumor, genitourinary anomalies, mental retardation in some, and optic nerve hypoplasia.

INVERSIONS

These require two breaks in one chromosome, with the intervening fragments rotating 180 degrees and reinserting in the original location. Pericentric inversions include the centromere, whereas paracentric inversions do not. Gene regulation may be lost because the genetic material is out of order on the chromosome.

ISOCHROMOSOMES

Usually lethal, these anomalies occur when the centromere divides transversely instead of longitudinally, leading to metacentric daughter chromosomes, one with two long arms and the other with two short arms. Isochromosome X is seen in a Turner-like syndrome.

RING CHROMOSOMES

Also usually lethal, these are occasionally seen in retarded newborns. A break occurs near the long and short arms of a single chromosome, and the sticky ends attach. Faulty chromosomal division occurs at mitosis, with frequent loss of material. Chromosomes 5, 10, 13, 18, and 22 are most frequently involved.[8(p165-169)]

OTHER GENE PROPERTIES

Segregation is a property of two allelic genes occupying the same locus on two homologous chromosomes. During meiosis the two genes separate and therefore cannot occur together in a single offspring. Genes on different (nonhomologous) chromosomes may or may not separate during meiosis, in a random process termed *independent assortment.* Genes at different locations on the same chromosome may assort at meiosis due to crossing-over.

The closer together two loci are on the same chromosome, the less likelihood that they be separated by crossing-over during meiosis. Linkage between loci can be determined by identification of morphologically variant chromosomes, gene dosage methods, and separation of gene products and chromosomes in clones of somatic cell hybrids.

A genetic polymorphism exists when two or more alleles occur at a locus with appreciable frequency and no deleterious effect. Roughly one third of all structural genes are polymorphisms.[8(p92-93)]

Causes of chromosomal aberrations have been mentioned briefly above. Increased maternal age has been associated with trisomies caused by nondisjunction, which consists either of failure of sister chromatids to disengage in mitosis or meiosis II, or of homologous chromosomes to disengage in meiosis I. Increased paternal age has been associated with increased incidence of autosomal dominant traits such as achondroplasia, Waardenberg syndrome, and craniosynostosis. Autoimmune phenomena, such as the presence of antithyroid antibody, have been found more frequently in young mothers who have children with Down syndrome or Turner syndrome. Chromosome instability leading to an increased incidence of chromosome breakage has been identified in cultured cells of patients with such breakage. Environmental agents (clastogens) that increase mutations include chemicals, radiation, and ultraviolet light.

Many causes remain unknown. We do not understand why fetal trisomy 16 is present in one third of spontaneous abortions not related to advanced maternal age, or why the incidence of trisomy 4 decreases with increasing maternal age.[8(p40-46)]

By term, 99.4% of all conceptions with abnormal chromosome number or structure have been spontaneously aborted. Virtually all autosomal *aneuploidies* (abnormal chromosome number) have intrauterine growth retardation and mental retardation. Half of all persons with IQ of less than 50 have autosomal aneuploidy, and one quarter of those with IQ from 50 to 70. Of those with an IQ of less than 70, 12% have a "fragile-X" chromosome.

This most common of viable autosomal aneuploidies occurs in 1:1,000 live births and is markedly associated with advanced maternal age. One woman in 40 at age 44 will give birth to such a child, whereas 80% of conceptions are spontaneously aborted. Most (95%) are due to 47 chromosomes, trisomy 21 (Fig. 16.16), of which 78% represent maternal nondisjunction events and 22% paternal nondisjunction. Of the remainder, 2.5% are 46/47 mosaics who tend to have higher intellectual function, 1.2% are caused by nonherita-

CAUSES OF CHROMOSOMAL ABERRATIONS

SPECIFIC CHROMOSOME ANOMALIES

TRISOMY 21 (DOWN SYNDROME)

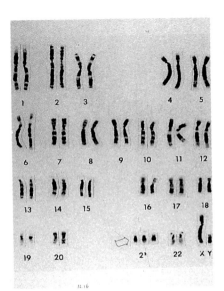

16.16 | Trisomy 21 karyotype. (Courtesy of Dr. Jorge Yunis, Hahnemann University, Philadelphia.)

ble chromosomal translocations and have 46 chromosomes, and 1.2% are caused by unbalanced translocations associated with risk of transmission. Low-set ears, flat face, hypotonia, palmar crease, epicanthal folds, and frequent cardiac problems are noted (Fig. 16.17). Most affected persons live into the third decade and have IQs ranging from 25 to (rarely) 100. Ophthalmic findings include lid slant, chronic blepharitis, ectropion, esotropia, iris stromal hypoplasia, Brushfield iris spots (Fig. 16.18), keratoconus, cataracts (Fig. 16.19), myopia, and aberrant retinal vessels.[8](176-180)

16.17 | Facies of adult with trisomy 21. (Courtesy of Dr. Myron Yanoff.)

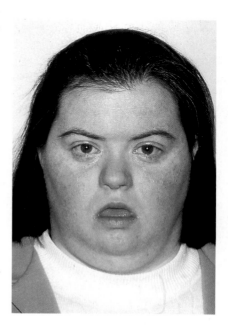

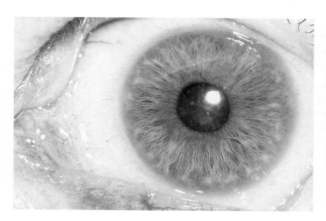

16.18 | Brushfield iris spots in patient with trisomy 21. (Courtesy of Dr. Myron Yanoff.)

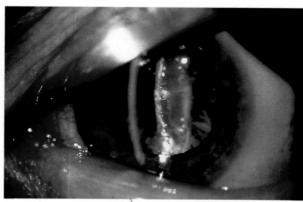

16.19 | Typical cerulean cataract in patient with trisomy 21. (Courtesy of Dr. Myron Yanoff.)

This second most common viable autosomal trisomy occurs in 1:8,000 live births. Nondisjunction causes 80%, 10% are caused by translocation, and 10% by mosaicism. Most affected infants die before the age of 4 months, rarely living to 15 years; three times as many girls as boys are affected. Systemic findings include mental retardation, growth failure, protruding occiput, micrognathia, misshapen ears, flexion deformities (Fig. 16.20), rocker-bottom feet, omphalocele, and myelomeningocele. Ophthalmic abnormalities include epicanthal folds, blepharophimosis, thick lower lid, ptosis, hypertelorism, congenital glaucoma, corneal opacities, microphthalmia, and uveal colobomas.[8(p181-183)]

TRISOMY 18 (EDWARDS SYNDROME)

Seen in 1:10,000 live births, this devastating disorder is caused by nondisjunction in 70% of cases, translocation with partial trisomy in 20%, and mosaic genotype in 10%. Systemic anomalies include severe midline central nervous system malformations, bilateral cleft lip and palate, heart and renal problems, polydactyly, clenched fists, and rocker-bottom feet. Ophthalmologic abnormalities include hypotelorism, synophthalmos or cyclopia (Fig. 16.21), corneal

TRISOMY 13 (PATAU SYNDROME)

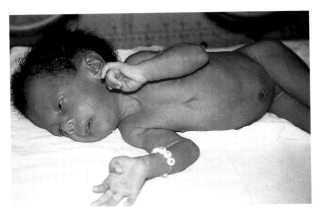

16.20 | Infant with trisomy 18. Note flexion contractures. (Courtesy of Dr. Myron Yanoff.)

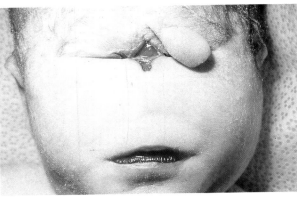

16.21 | Infant with cyclopia with trisomy 13. (Courtesy of Dr. Myron Yanoff.)

clouding, cataracts, persistent hyperplastic primary vitreous, optic atrophy, uveal colobomas, retinal dysplasia, and, uniquely, cartilage in a ciliary body coloboma (Fig. 16.22).[8(p180-181)]

TRISOMY 22 (CAT EYE SYNDROME)

This rare disorder consists of bilateral uveal colobomas, antimongoloid lid slant, and variable intelligence and fertility.

XO (TURNER SYNDROME)

This common disorder is seen in 1:2,500 live births, but 95% of affected fetuses are spontaneously aborted before term (Fig. 16.23). Of all aborted fetuses, 20% are XO, and it is suspected that true monosomy for the X chromosome is always lethal in utero; it may therefore be that all viable XO patients are XO/XX mosaics. No Barr body is present in buccal cells. These phenotypic girls are of short stature. Most are of normal intelligence (although difficulties of spatial perception are usually present), are sterile, and have a webbed neck (Fig. 16.24) and a high incidence of aortic stenosis. Ophthalmologic difficulties include pigmented eyelids, epicanthal folds, corectopia, vertically oval corneas, ptosis, nystagmus, blue sclera, strabismus, anterior axial embryonal cataracts, and the same incidence of X-linked recessive traits as in boys.[8(p193-201)]

MULTIPLE X SYNDROME

Patients with a 47, XXX chromosomal configuration have two Barr bodies, irregular menses, premature menopause, and normal offspring; this syndrome occurs in 1:1,000 live births. With an increasing number of X chromosomes (47, XXXX or greater) there is an increased tendency towards mental retardation and sterility.

XXY (KLINEFELTER SYNDROME)

These phenotypic boys have a Barr body, gynecomastia with a eunuchoid habitus, frequent mild mental retardation, and variable genital development. Sterility is usual. This syndrome is present in 1:400 males and many variations and mosaics occur, such as 48, XXXY.

XYY SYNDROME

Present in 1:300 boys, this syndrome is associated with increased androgen secretion and acne, and may possibly be accompanied by increased aggressive behavior. This phenomenon may result from nondisjunction in meiosis II.[8(p205-208)]

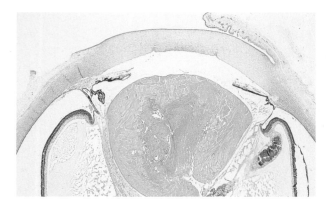

16.22 | Retinal dysplasia present at the lower right edge of a cataractous lens with trisomy 13. (Courtesy of Dr. Myron Yanoff.)

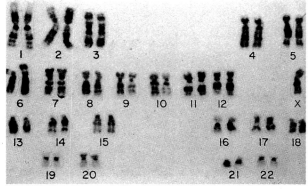

16.23 | Karyotype of XO Turner syndrome.

HUMAN CHROMOSOME MAPPING TECHNIQUES

RECOMBINANT ANALYSIS

Recombinant analysis is helpful in plant and animal genetics but is not as useful in human genetics because of small family size and inability to control matings. A 1% recombination at meiosis is defined a 1 map unit or centiMorgan and consists of roughly 1 million DNA base pairs. Thus, 50 map units is a 50% recombination rate and can represent genes on separate chromosomes or genes so far apart on the same chromosome that crossing-over occurs in each cell during meiosis I. Specialized statistical techniques can amplify the power of this recombinant analysis to aid in chromosome mapping.

CHROMOSOME STRUCTURE

Some patients have chromosomes that exhibit unusual morphology, allowing mapping of genes to that chromosome if the genes are transmitted together with the morphologically unusual chromosome. A classic example is the localization of the Duffy blood group to chromosome 1 by recognition of the "unwinder" locus on that chromosome.

SOMATIC CELL HYBRIDIZATION

By use of the Sendai virus and polyethylene glycol, human and mouse chromosomes can be fused (Fig. 16.25). As human chromosomes are progressively lost, gene products are measured and assigned to the appropriate chromosome.

RESTRICTION SITE MAPPING

Endoproteases are used to cut chromosomes into predictable pieces. Hybridization of known messenger RNA fragments identifies the part of the chromosome that made the messenger RNA. These fragments are isolated on agarose gel. Unfortunately, only 5% or so of the genome codes for a gene product, the remainder of the DNA being silent.

It is typical to find one nucleotide difference in every 250 nucleotides among healthy individuals, representing polymorphism.

RESTRICTION FRAGMENT LENGTH POLYMORPHISM

Specific enzymes are available that can cut DNA into characteristic strand lengths. If there is a mutation at a cutting site, the enzyme skips to the next site and differing lengths of DNA fragments result. One can separate the DNA fragments with selected messenger RNA attached to "silent" lengths of chromosome, identifying the location of genes by linkage to restriction fragment length polymorphisms.[9]

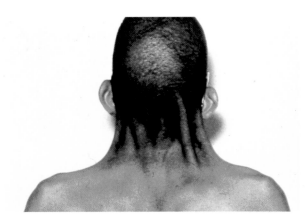

16.24 | Webbed neck of patient with XO Turner syndrome. (Courtesy of Dr. Myron Yanoff.)

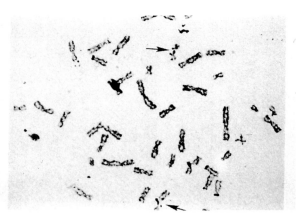

16.25 | Fusion of human and mouse chromosome with Sendai virus.

NEW TECHNIQUES IN MOLECULAR GENETICS
TRANSGENESIS

Transgenesis is the use of gene manipulation to modify animal cells permanently. DNA has been injected into the nucleus of mammalian germ cells using an SV40 virus DNA vector. If a functional gene is inserted at random, it will not be linked to a mutant and will likely segregate from it at meiosis. Thus, gene replacement can only be effective if a strategy for targeting the correct insertion site is available and successfully employed.

Despite these limitations, a growth hormone gene has been introduced into dwarf mice and produced growth hormone in the recipient rat's liver. These rats grew to three times their littermates' size, although undesirable side effects did appear. Replacement of poorly functioning enzymes in human diseases such as the mucopolysaccharidoses has been attempted with laboratory—but limited clinical—improvement.

BLOT TECHNIQUES

These permit the detection in an agarose gel of fragments which are complementary to a given DNA or RNA sequence. The Southern blot technique for detection of DNA restriction fragments has been extended to RNA and protein fragments (Northern and Western blotting techniques, respectively). DNA fragments in gel are denatured to single-stranded form by alkali and the gel is laid on top of buffer-saturated filter paper. The top gel surface is covered with nitrocellulose filter membrane and overlaid with multilayers of dry filter paper.

Buffer passes through the gel, drawn by capillary action, elutes the denatured DNA from the gel to the nitrocellulose, and is fixed by baking. The filter is placed in radioactive RNA, single-stranded DNA, or potentially complementary oligodeoxynucleotide. The membrane is washed, and the regions of hybridization are detected radiographically.

17 | CATARACTS IN CHILDREN

Gary R. Diamond

If one defines a cataract as any opacity of the lens sufficient to cause visual impairment, 0.3% of all children are thus afflicted.[1] The visual impact of the lens opacity is related to its location, time of onset, unilaterality versus bilaterality, and density. Successful visual rehabilitation of an eye that has a visually significant lens opacity depends on early diagnosis and surgical treatment and on rigorous optical correction and management of amblyopia.

CAUSE

Approximately half of childhood cataracts are of unknown cause and are unassociated with other abnormalities. They can be of many morphologic forms (see Volume 3, Chapter 8 of *Textbook of Ophthalmology*). Congenital infections, the paradigm being congenital rubella syndrome,[2] can cause significant cataracts. The congenital rubella cataract is bilateral, with a pearly white nucleus and less dense cortical opacity; the peripheral lamellae may be clear. These opacities are believed to represent direct viral lens invasion in the first trimester of gestation before the lens capsule is formed; disrupted maturation of lenticular epithelial cells has been demonstrated (Fig. 17.1).

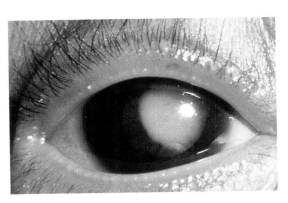

17.1 | Rubella cataract.

Congenital varicella, *herpes simplex* virus, toxoplasmosis, and cytomegalic inclusion virus have also been associated, although not consistently, with the appearance of cataracts at birth or at an early age.

In one study, transient bilateral lens vacuoles located just anterior to the posterior lens capsule were noted in 2.7% of low-birth-weight infants at roughly 16 days of age (Fig. 17.2). These were completely resolved over a 1- to 16-week period.[3]

Cataracts can occur secondary to a myriad of diseases in early childhood, some of which are listed in Figure 17.3. These cataracts are believed to be due to metabolic or mechanical disturbances. Of interest are cataracts associated with chronic headbanging, felt to be due to an alteration in lens capsule permeability.[4]

Posterior subcapsular cataracts caused by oral or topical steroid use are well documented; one series associated cataracts with oral use of more than 0.23 mg/kg prednisone per day.[5] These cataracts do not regress with discontinuation of the steroid (Fig. 17.4). Chlorpromazine-induced lamellar cataracts may reverse upon discontinuation of the medication.[6] Ergot, dinitrophenol, naphthalene, and triparanol are also cataractogenic.[7]

Chromosomal disorders are often associated with cataracts in childhood. Trisomy 21 (Down syndrome) may cause four patterns of lens opacity

17.2 | Transient lens vacuoles in the premature infant.

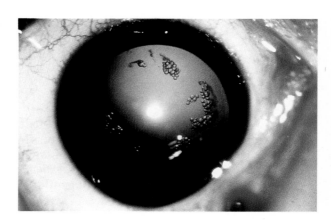

Figure 17.3. Syndromes Associated with Childhood Cataracts

DISEASE	BIOCHEMICAL DEFECT	INHERITANCE	OTHER OPHTHALMIC MANIFESTATIONS
Renal			
Lowe	Unknown	X-linked recessive	Glaucoma
Alport	Unknown	Autosomal dominant	Anterior lenticonus and polar cataract, myopia, spherophakia
Central nervous system			
Marinesco–Sjögren	Unknown	Autosomal dominant or recessive	
Connective tissue			
Conradi	Unknown	Unknown	Heterochromia iridis, optic atrophy
Marfan	Fibrillin	Autosomal dominant	Subluxed lenses, flat corneas, retinal detachment
Mandibulofacial			
Hallerman–Streiff	Unknown	Unknown	Microphthalmia, blue sclerae
Pierre Robin	Unknown	Unknown	Microphthalmia, retinal detachment, glaucoma
Treacher Collins	Unknown	Unknown	Lid pseudocolobomas
Skin			
Incontinentia pigmenti	Unknown	X-linked dominant	Corneal opacities, PHPV, optic atrophy, retinal detachment
Congential ectodermal dysplasia	Unknown	X-linked dominant or recessive	Sparse eyelashes and eyebrows
Rothmund–Thomson	Unknown	Autosomal recessive	Corneal opacities, microphthalmia, myopia, colobomas
Werner	Unknown	Autosomal recessive	Corneal opacities, blue sclerae, pigmented retinal dystrophy
Chromosomal			
Trisomy 13			Microphthalmia, colobomas, cartilage in ciliary body, retinal dysplasia
Trisomy 18			Colobomas, phimotic lid fissures
Trisomy 21			Brushfield spots, chronic conjunctivitis, strabismus, keratoconus
XO (Turner)			Strabismus
Metabolic			
Galactosemia	Gal 1-phosphate uridyl transferase	Autosomal recessive	
Galactokinase deficiency	Galactokinase	Autosomal recessive	
Pseudohypoparathyroidism	G-protein	Autosomal dominant or recessive	
Hypoparathyroidism	Unknown	Unknown	
Wilson disease	Unknown	Autosomal recessive	Kayser–Fleischer corneal ring
Fabry disease	α-galactosyl hydrolase	X-linked recessive	Venous aneurysmal dilatations of conjunctival and retinal vessels, vortex corneal dystrophy
Refsum disease	Phytanic acid α-hydroxylase	Autosomal recessive	Atypical pigmentary retinopathy, miosis, nyatagmus
Homocystinuria	Cystathionine synthetase	Autosomal recessive	Ectopia lentis, retinal detachment

(Figs. 17.5 and 17.6). The incidence observed with slit-lamp biomicroscopy increases from 60% in young children to almost 100% in adolescents.[8] Trisomies 13, 18, and Turner syndrome (XO) are also known to have a frequent association with early childhood cataracts.

A characteristic cataract with onset in late childhood or early adolescence has been described in juvenile diabetes, consisting of bilateral, multiple anterior or posterior subcapsular white "snowflake" dots located over a network of vacuoles. These cataracts rarely interfere with vision[9] (Fig. 17.7). Two inborn errors of galactose metabolism, galactosemia and galactokinase deficiency, result in elevated serum galactose; this substance can freely diffuse into lenses but is promptly reduced by aldose reductase to dulcitol, which cannot diffuse out of the lens. Osmotic hydration occurs, which leads to lens fiber destruction and cataract. Patients with galactosemia undergo cessation and sometimes reversal of cataract formation when galactose is eliminated from their diet. Cataracts are the only known manifestation of galactokinase deficiency. Heterozygotes may be more susceptible to cataracts in later adulthood, but homozygotes for this recessive trait have bilateral lamellar cataract formation in utero or early infancy.[10]

Patients with hypoparathyroidism, if untreated for a few years, may develop small, discrete bilateral lamellar opacities often associated with multicolored crystalline formations; these are rarely visually significant. Patients with pseudohypoparathyroidism may exhibit similar opacities. The Lowe oculocerebrorenal syndrome, believed to be transmitted as an X-linked recessive trait, is associated with bilateral total, nuclear, or posterior polar lens opacities present at birth or developing in early infancy.[11]

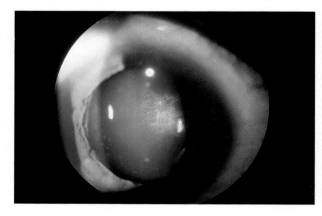

17.4 | Posterior subcapsular cataracts in child taking oral prednisone.

Figure 17.5. Trisomy 21 Cataract Patterns

Arcuate equatorial lens opacities
Embryonic sutural opacities
Congenital posterior polar opacities
Acquired cataracts

All neonates should undergo red reflex evaluation before they are taken home. Those with syndromes known to be associated with congenital cataract, or whose parents, siblings, or close relatives have early-onset cataracts, should undergo a dilated examination by an ophthalmologist as soon after birth as is feasible. A retinoscope is very useful for detection of subtle lens opacities, and direct ophthalmoscopy will permit estimation of density. In some children with dense opacities, the indirect ophthalmoscope is the only instrument that permits a view of the fundus. When the lens opacity is total, recourse to ultrasonography is essential to ascertain the status of the posterior structures of the globe.

After taking a complete history, consisting of age of onset, family history, systemic status of the infant, and presence of photophobia, nystagmus, or leukocoria as noted by others, the ophthalmologist should evaluate the infant's general appearance for any obvious signs of known syndromes. Visual acuity should be determined as precisely as possible, whether by fixational ability, preferential looking techniques, presence of optokinetic nystagmus, or by visual evoked response techniques. The corneas should be measured, pupil size noted, any anterior segment anomalies described, and pupillary responses tested; any direct or indirect afferent pupillary defect suggests the presence of pathology in addition to the cataract. The infant should be held to the slit lamp both before and after pupillary dilation to gauge the extent and location of the lens opacity. The extent of iris dilation should be noted. A central lens opacity of 3 mm or greater is considered visually significant and capable of causing amblyopia.[12] Microcornea and visible ciliary processes suggest persistent hyperplastic primary vitreous, in which case the vitreous and retina should be examined if possible.

DIAGNOSIS

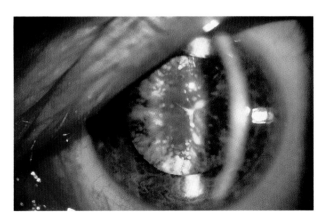

17.6 | Cerulean cataract in patient with trisomy 21.

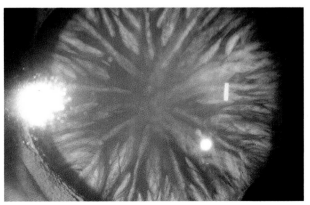

17.7 | Juvenile diabetes mellitus lens opacities.

Laboratory tests are usually indicated only for bilateral cataracts. These tests include karyotype analysis, urine for glucose, amino acids, and galactose, serum for calcium, glucose and, if indicated, for galactokinase. Serum assays for infectious agents are available, and viral lens cultures have been helpful in patients with rubella syndrome.

NONSURGICAL MANAGEMENT

Many small lens opacities do not require surgical lens removal. Amblyopia, when present, can be treated by occlusion of the other eye if it is uninvolved, as organic lesions may be associated with a superimposed amblyopia which is potentially reversible. An occasional child with a small central lens opacity may benefit from pupillary dilation with 2.5% phenylephrine three times a day. Optical iridectomy does not provide sufficient visual improvement and has been abandoned.

SURGICAL TREATMENT

Surgery should be performed on a visually significant unilateral congenital cataract as soon as the infant is sufficiently stable to tolerate general anesthesia, certainly within the first 3 weeks of life. For visually significant bilateral congenital cataracts, surgery should be performed before 8 weeks of life for best visual results.[13] Most ophthalmologists are more comfortable approaching the lens from the limbus, but some prefer a posterior approach through the region of the pars plana. The most common technique in use today involves removal of the lens from the anterior capsule posteriorly, after a large capsulectomy. An irrigation–aspiration device, usually mechanized, is capable of removing the soft nucleus and cortex of most congenital cataracts. A calcified or fibrotic lens fragment can be removed with a vitrectomy device or can be captured and manually removed with an intraocular forceps (Figs. 17.8–17.10).

Removal of the posterior capsule at the time of initial surgery remains controversial. Because these capsules always opacify in the neonate and because their amblyopia-producing capacities are difficult to evaluate, many surgeons perform a posterior capsulectomy and anterior vitrectomy at initial surgery. Others are concerned with the risks of cystoid macular edema, delayed retinal detachment, and vitreous in the anterior chamber. In older

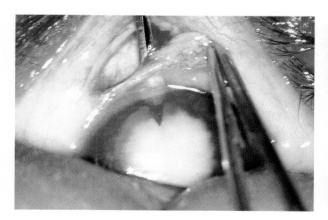

17.8 | A limbal-based conjunctival flap and limbal scleral incision have been constructed and the anterior chamber has been entered with a 2.2-mm blade. This blade then incises the anterior lens capsule.

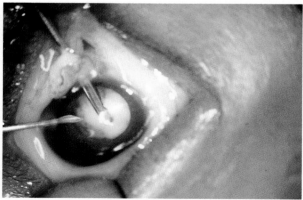

17.9 | An infusion port has been placed through clear cornea at nine o'clock. A suction-cutting instrument is placed in the lens and the lensectomy is started.

children, most surgeons would initially leave the posterior lens capsule intact, later performing an office-based YAG laser photodisruption, or secondary discission if the capsule becomes opacified.

VISUAL REHABILITATION

At present, four methods of visual rehabilitation are commonly utilized for aphakic children: glasses, contact lenses, epikeratophakia, and intraocular lenses.

Because of image size differences, glasses are most commonly used to provide optical correction in bilaterally aphakic children. Single-vision aphakic glasses fit as closely as possible to the cornea and overplussed for a reasonable near working distance are fitted to children below the age of 5 years. A typical approach is to add roughly 4.00 diopters of hyperopic correction to the distance correction for children under 1 year of age, 3.50 diopters for children from 1 to 3 years of age, and 3.00 diopters for children over 3 years of age. At age 5 years or so, a bifocal can be provided or, because binocularity is rarely obtained, one eye can be corrected for distance fixation and the other for near. Occasionally, a monocularly aphakic child can be visually rehabilitated with aphakic glasses.

Contact lenses remain the mainstay of visual rehabilitation for most children, and may consist of hard, soft, rigid gas-permeable, or silicone material. Hard lens fittings require particular attention to corneal curvature or the lens will not center over the pupil, and lens tolerance must be gradually increased. However, the lenses are small and are therefore relatively easy to place, remove, and manipulate. They can be manufactured to any specification and are sturdier. Corneal abrasions and punctate keratitis from overwear and hypoxia are potential concerns and require careful follow-up examinations. Soft lenses have a variable water content but tend to be quite oxygen-permeable. They do not require lengthy periods to acquire tolerance, but are relatively large, difficult to manipulate, and have a high incidence of loss or tearing. Soft lenses are available in defined parameters that vary according to the manufacturer. Rigid gas-permeable lenses are firmer than soft lenses but more flexible than hard lenses. They have high oxygen permeability, readily provide tolerance to wear, are sturdier than soft lenses, and can be custom-fashioned. Silicone lenses share many of the features of rigid gas-permeable lenses but are hydrophobic and, despite specialized treatment, can become firmly adherent to the cornea. Oxygen permeability is extremely high.

17.10 | At the completion of cortex removal, the surgeon may elect to remove or retain the posterior lens capsule.

Because of the ability to alter the strength and fitting parameters of a contact lens as the eye grows, and the noninvasive nature of the lens, contact lenses have earned a place as the most common method of childhood aphakic correction. Fusion can occur in patients who have binocularity, who acquire cataracts after birth, and who are fitted with contact lenses. Children under 5 years of age are overplussed as described above; when school age is reached, many are given contact lenses fit with a distance correction and reading glasses to be used for near work. Another approach in nonbinocular children is to provide one lens for distance work and the other for near.

Intraocular lenses are rarely placed in aphakic neonatal eyes because of the very proliferative nature of residual lens cortex in the neonate and the rapid growth of the eye and resultant changing refractive error during the first 2 years of life. However, intraocular lenses have been successfully placed in children of 3 years or older who acquire visually disabling cataracts from trauma or other cause. Many are secondary implantations after contact lens failure, or in circumstances of simultaneous corneal injury and presumed inability to wear a contact lens successfullly. Some contraindications include microphthalmos, glaucoma, uveitis, retinal detachment, and optic nerve defects or atrophy. Iris-fixated and anterior chamber lenses have been used in the past, but most surgeons prefer posterior chamber lenses placed in the residual capsular bag. Most children require a YAG laser photodisruption of the lens capsule shortly after lens placement. The selection of lens power is somewhat arbitrary, and most children require a distance glass correction as well as correction for near work. In a series reported by Hiles, 10% of patients developed corneal clouding and 13% a residual distance refractive error greater than 3.00 diopters.[14] However, 61% of children who had traumatic cataracts achieved 20/20 to 20/40 acuity, and 16% of those with congenital cataracts achieved this degree of acuity.

Epikeratophakia involves freezing of donor cornea and carving of this frozen tissue to form a lens which is sutured directly to the anterior host stroma. Central epithelium and a peripheral annular ring of the Bowman membrane must be removed from the recipient cornea. After implantation the donor tissue is invaded by host keratocytes and the graft becomes epithelialized. The dioptric strength and curvature of the donor tissue lens must be individualized and computed on the basis of axial length measurements, keratometry, and the desired postoperative refractive error. Because the central Bowman membrane remains, the donor lens can be replaced, if necessary, by one with different parameters. In a recent large series, 335 procedures performed in 314 eyes of children under 8 years of age were 89% successful after the first operation, 95% successful with repeated procedures, and 73% of the eyes were within 3.00 diopters of emmetropia. Visual acuity showed improvement in most cases.[15] Originally recommended for unilaterally aphakic children who were not contact lens compliant, the indications have been extended to include those who have corneal lacerations. Neonates have not been included because of potential delay in visual rehabilitation with graft healing and graft–host interface opacity and the usually excellent compliance with contact lenses in the very young. In addition, it may be difficult to obtain an appropriate tissue lens for the small eye and steep cornea of a typical neonate. In cases of noncompliance with contact lens wear, epikeratophakia permits optical correction without recourse to an intraocular procedure. Perhaps the only absolute contraindication is the child with chronic tear insufficiency or other corneal surface pathology.

The visual prognosis in children with congenital cataracts is improving because of recognition of the benefit of early surgery and visual rehabilitation, availability of better intraocular instrumentation, and improved means of optical correction. Before 1980 the visual outcome in patients with monocular congenital cataracts was so poor that many experienced ophthalmologists felt strongly they should not be removed. In 1981, Beller et al presented eight patients who underwent surgery before 42 days of age, all of whom, by visual evoked response testing, demonstrated better than 20/80 acuity and five of whom had 20/30 acuity or better.[16] Since that report, others have shown that approximately half of infants who undergo surgery for unilateral congenital cataracts before 6 weeks of age can develop 20/80 or better acuity when provided with rapid optical correction, occlusion of the noninvolved eye, and rigorous follow-up care.[17]

Occlusion therapy in patients with unilateral aphakia should be provided for all but one waking hour during the immediate postoperative period; the very young newborn may be awake only 10 hours a day. This can be decreased to roughly 6 hours a day in the older child once maximal visual potential has been realized. Most children require significant occlusion until about 9 years of age, at which time the patching can often be discontinued with acuity maintenance.

Bilateral congenital cataracts have always been associated with better visual prognosis because the sensory deficit is usually balanced, and therefore one eye usually is not granted fixation preference. Recent studies of children who underwent surgery before 8 weeks of age show normal visual development on a preferential looking test; Gelbart et al obtained acuity of 20/60 or better in 60% of 48 eyes that contained bilateral congenital cataracts.[13] Despite excellent acuities obtainable with early surgery, several studies have shown that few patients achieve binocular function.[16,18] Patching is necessary only when one eye develops a fixation preference.

RESULTS OF CATARACT SURGERY IN CHILDREN

SPECIAL FORMS OF CATARACT

Posterior lentiglobus (often termed lenticonus) is a unilateral congenital weakness in the posterior capsule of the lens that seldom causes opacity early in life. As the lens ages, the capsule becomes opaque and disc-shaped plaques may form. A persistent hyaloid artery is frequently observed, and the lens nucleus may be displaced backward towards the lentiglobus. Other anomalies of the eye such as uveal coloboma, microphthalmos, and anterior lentiglobus have occasionally been described. No hereditary tendency has been shown. Most cases present between the ages of 4 and 7 years with decreased visual acuity or strabismus in the involved eye; slit-lamp examination or retinoscopy will aid in the diagnosis. The visual prognosis is better than that for typical unilateral congenital cataract because there is a delayed onset of decreased vision and binocularity is present. Usually, the posterior capsule ruptures at time of lensectomy.

Zonular lamellar cataracts usually have a clear fetal nucleus surrounded by zones of peripheral nuclear or cortical opacity. In general, the peripheral cortex is clear and the condition is bilateral (Fig. 17.11). Because most children develop better acuity (especially at near fixation) than predicted by the lens appearance, caution should be exercised before removing these lenses. These children should be followed closely and intervention considered only when near acuity is less than 20/70. Even without lensectomy many of these children develop sufficient acuity to attend normal school classes.

17.11 | Zonular lamellar cataract. Note surrounding clear cortex.

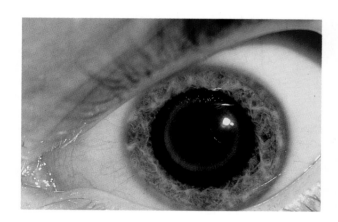

RETINOBLASTOMA

James J. Augsburger
and Myron Yanoff

EPIDEMIOLOGY AND INHERITANCE

Retinoblastoma is an uncommon malignant ocular neoplasm of childhood[1,2] that, if untreated, is almost uniformly fatal within 1–2 years of diagnosis. In spite of its rarity (frequency is about 1 in 18,000 live births), it is the most common primary intraocular malignancy of childhood. It arises from the retina and has the potential to prove fatal by direct extension from the eye into the brain or by widespread hematogenous metastasis to other organs of the body.[3] It affects only one eye in approximately 70%–80% of affected children, but it involves both eyes in about 20%–30% of cases. Retinoblastoma is a disorder of young children. The average age at the time of diagnosis is approximately 1.5 years in bilaterally affected children and 2 years in children who have monocular disease (about 89% of all cases of retinoblastoma are diagnosed before the age of 3 years).[2] However, it is occasionally detected within the first few weeks of life, and exceptional cases are diagnosed initially in children over 6 years of age.[4]

Retinoblastoma affects boys and girls with equal frequency and has no known racial predilection. Retinoblastoma usually is a sporadic condition (i.e., no prior affected family members). Most children who have the sporadic form of retinoblastoma are affected monocularly.[2] In contrast, a small portion of patients have a prior family history of this disease. In this situation, one of the parents usually is a survivor of retinoblastoma. The affected child in hereditary cases usually, but not always, has multiple tumors in both eyes.[2] Transmission of the disease in such families seems to follow genetic rules of autosomal dominant inheritance.[3]

Recent investigations into the genetics of retinoblastoma using molecular biology techniques of gene amplification and DNA sequence analysis[5] have shown that retinoblastoma arises as a result of two mutational events. If both mutations occur in the same somatic (postzygotic) cell, a single, unilateral, noninheritable retinoblastoma results. In the *hereditary form* the first mutation occurs in a germinal (prezygotic) cell (which, therefore, would mean that the mutation would be present in all resulting somatic cells), and the second mutation would occur in a somatic (postzygotic) cell, resulting in multiple retinal tumors (multifocal in one eye or bilateral tumors), and in primary tumors elsewhere in the body, *e.g.*, pineal tumors and sarcomas. The probability in the inherited form that the patient will develop the tumor (*i.e.*, will be genotypically and phenotypically abnormal) is 95 in 100. Occasionally, a generation may be skipped and the retinoblastoma may be transmitted to a genotypically abnormal but phenotypically normal family member.

The chromosomal region 13_q14 regulates the development of normality. If both chromosomal 13_q14 regions are normal, no retinoblastoma will develop. If one of the two 13 chromosomes has a 13_q14 deletion (heterozygous), a retinoblastoma still will not result. If both 13_q14 regions are deleted (homozygous), retinoblastoma results. Retinoblastoma, therefore, is inherited as an autosomal recessive at the cellular level, but clinically retinoblastoma follows genetic rules of an autosomal dominant inheritance pattern with approximately 90% penetrance.

About 5% of all retinoblastomas are inherited. The remaining 95% of all retinoblastomas develop by mutation (sporadic cases) with 25% of this total representing a genetic mutation in a germinal cell that can transmit the retinoblastoma to offspring and 75% a somatic mutation that cannot. The retinoblastoma in sporadic, somatic mutation cases is unifocal in one eye; in the sporadic genetic mutation cases it is multifocal in one eye or bilateral, or both.

All children who have retinoblastoma and their parents and siblings should probably be evaluated by modern molecular biology techniques to assess their risk of transmitting the disease to their offspring.[6] Genetic testing now is being developed as a prenatal test for parents-to-be who are survivors of genetic retinoblastoma. Children who have genetic retinoblastoma must be advised of their potential to transmit the disease when they become of reproductive age.

SIGNS AND SYMPTOMS

The most common sign of retinoblastoma is a white-appearing pupil (leukokoria) (Figs. 18.1, 18.2). This appearance, which is often referred to as a "glazed look" by the child's parents or guardians, is caused by reflection of

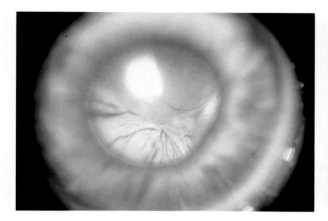

18.1 | Leukokoria in retinoblastoma with exophytic growth pattern.

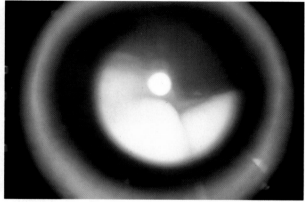

18.2 | Leukokoria in retinoblastoma with endophytic growth pattern. Note smooth, avascular appearance of intraocular tumor

light from the white intraocular tumor. Depending upon the intraocular extent of the tumor and its laterality, one or both eyes may exhibit this appearance. Less frequently encountered signs include strabismus (esotropia or exotropia), a red eye with buphthalmos and corneal clouding due to elevated intraocular pressure, discoloration of the iris in the involved eye (usually on the basis of neovascularization of the iris), loss of the fundus reflection in the affected eye on the basis of intraocular bleeding from the tumor, clumping or layering of white tumor cells on the iris or in the aqueous humor,[7] and spontaneous hyphema.

EXAMINATION

Although slit lamp biomicroscopy of young children sometimes is quite difficult, every effort should be made to perform this examination in the office at the time of initial patient assessment. If one is successful in this technique, one can assess the anterior chamber and iris in detail for evidence of tumor cells or iris neovascularization, and one can evaluate the clarity of the lens and the retrolental vitreous. In almost all children who have retinoblastoma, even those who have advanced intraocular tumors filling most of the globe, the lens is completely clear. Slit lamp examination also can disclose finely dispersed cells or tumor cell clumps (seeds) in the vitreous. In eyes with gross leukokoria, one also can determine whether any retina and retinal vessels can be seen (suggestive of an exophytic growth pattern) (Fig. 18.1) or whether only a fluffy white mass is visible (endophytic pattern) (Fig. 18.2). In some eyes, elements of both growth patterns can be detected.

With indirect ophthalmoscopy, one can further evaluate the extent of the intraocular tumor and related retinal abnormalities, including the extent of retinal detachment and the presence and extent of intravitreal or subretinal blood. In eyes with less advanced disease, well-defined individual tumor foci can be identified, often in association with prominent dilated and tortuous retinal blood vessels. Indirect ophthalmoscopy in the office requires the instillation of topical dilating and anesthestic drops, use of a lid speculum, and scleral depression (both to turn the eye as well as to indent the peripheral fundus for visualization). With suitable restraint of the child's arms and legs, such an examination can be performed comprehensively on both eyes in the office in a matter of minutes. Small tumors along the ora serrata and finely dispersed vitreous cells usually can be detected during such an examination.

Discrete intraretinal tumors appear as white, round to oval, dome-shaped retinal tumors (Fig. 18.3). Even relatively small tumors tend to attract

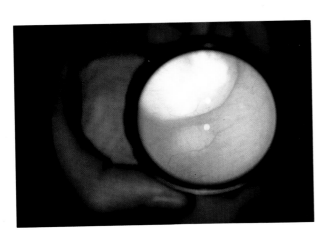

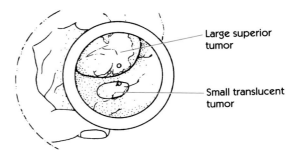

18.3 | Indirect ophthalmoscopic appearance of multifocal retinoblastoma. Larger superior lesion appears more opaque white, while smaller adjacent lesion appears relatively translucent.

Large superior tumor

Small translucent tumor

retinal blood vessels, which ramify prominently on the surface of the lesion. Very small lesions sometimes appear as translucent thickenings of the retina without substantial depth (Fig. 18.4A). Examination of the fundus with a green filter (red-free light) often helps accentuate such subtle lesions.

DIAGNOSTIC TESTS

Most relatively large tumors (those more than 10–15 mm in diameter) typically have evident white clumps of intralesional calcification. If one performs B-scan ultrasonography on an eye containing such a tumor,[8] the intralesional calcification will cause pronounced orbital shadowing (Fig. 18.5). The tumor itself will appear nodular and highly reflective. When one reduces the gain of the instrument, the reflections from the calcific particles within the tumor will persist.

Computed tomography (CT) scanning is helpful in confirming the diagnosis, especially in eyes filled with tumor in which uncertainty exists as to whether leukokoria is due to retinoblastoma or a simulating disorder such as Coats' disease.[9,10] Because retinoblastoma tumors characteristically are calcified, they can show up quite vividly and with good definition on the CT images (Fig. 18.6). Even relatively small tumors that show no prominent cal-

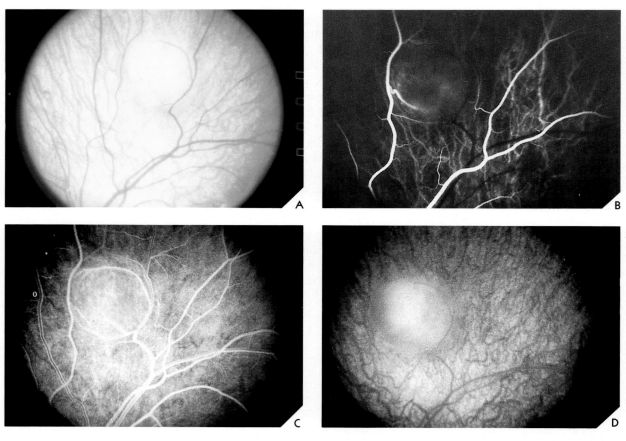

18.4 | Fluorescein angiography of small retinoblastoma. *A:* Translucent focal retinoblastoma with slightly prominent feeder and drainer retinal blood vessels. *B:* Arterial phase frame showing early filling of intralesional blood vessels from the retinal arterial system. *C:* Laminar venous phase frame showing fluorescent network of intralesional blood vessels. *D:* Late phase frame showing staining of retinal tumors.

cification ophthalmoscopically often appear very bright on CT because of their calcification. A small proportion of children who have retinoblastoma, however, fail to have intralesional calcification. Children who have the diffuse infiltrating form of retinoblastoma[11] characteristically develop tumors multicentrically within the retina and exhibit extensive seeding of the vitreous without associated calcification.

If fluorescein angiography is performed on a discrete intraretinal retinoblastoma (Fig. 18.4B–D), the angiogram shows rapid filling of the feeder artery, prompt filling of the intralesional vasculature, and rapid draining via the efferent vein. The intralesional capillaries tend to leak fluorescein, so that the tumor characteristically stains brightly in the late frames.[12,13] However, retinoblastoma lesions typically do not show substantial leakage into the overlying vitreous.

Many conditions can mirror retinoblastoma (Fig. 18.7), however, the principal differential diagnosis ("pseudogliomas") includes Coats' disease, persistent hyperplastic primary vitreous, and ocular toxocariasis. **Coats' disease**

DIFFERENTIAL DIAGNOSIS

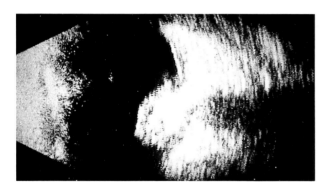

18.5 | B-scan ultrasonography of retinoblastoma. Retinal tumor appears extremely bright (intensely sonoreflective). Note shadowing of orbital pattern because of intralesional calcification.

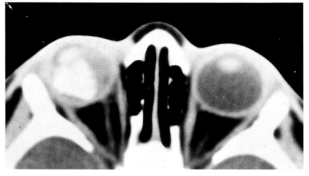

18.6 | CT scan of retinoblastoma showing dense intraocular tumor filling two thirds of right eye.

Figure 18.7. Differential Diagnosis of Retinoblastoma

Leukokoria
Coats' disease
Persistent hyperplastic primary vitreous
Ocular toxocariasis
Retinal dysplasia (13 trisomy)
Retinopathy of prematurity
Norrie's disease
Incontinentia pigmenti (Bloch-Sulzberger)
Massive retinal fibrosis

Metastatic retinitis
Congenital nonattachment of retina
Secondary retinal detachment
Juvenile retinoschisis
Medulloepithelioma
Congenital cataract
Coloboma of choroid

Discrete lesions
Tuberous sclerosis
Neurofibromatosis
Von Hippel
Myelinated nerve fibers
Retinochoroiditis
Coats' disease
Posterior toxocariasis
Proliferative RPE lesions

(Fig. 18.8) is an idiopathic retinal disorder without systemic associations characterized by retinal telangiectasia and secondary intraretinal and subretinal exudation. In advanced cases, the telangiectasia involves several quadrants of the retina and results in a total bullous exudative retinal detachment associated with thick, yellow subretinal fluid. Such cases very closely resemble advanced exophytic retinoblastoma. Ultrasonography and CT usually are helpful in distinguishing the noncalcified subretinal fluid of Coats' disease from the retinal detachment associated with calcified exophytic tumors in retinoblastoma.[8,9]

Persistent hyperplastic primary vitreous (PHPV) (Fig. 18.9) is an uncommon, usually unilateral congenital anomaly of the eye characterized by persistence of hyaloid vascular elements that subsequently undergo hyperplasia and contraction. The affected eye typically has a smaller corneal diameter than the unaffected eye. Its anterior chamber often is shallower than normal, and the lens posteriorly frequently becomes clouded, due to fibrovascular ingrowth of the vascular hyaloid tissue posteriorly, while the remainder of the lens remains clear, even in the face of a broken posterior capsule. Contraction of the retrolenticular hyaloid tissue also characteristically causes elongation of the ciliary processes, which appear prominently in some cases when one dilates the pupil. Ultrasonography, CT scanning, and magnetic resonance imaging (MRI) can help distinguish questionable cases of PHPV from retinoblastoma,[9,10] but in most cases ophthalmic physical examination is sufficient to make the diagnosis.

Ocular toxocariasis (Fig. 18.10) tends to be a disorder of slightly older children. Several forms of this nematode-related disease have been described. The varieties that most commonly cause problems in the differential diagnosis of retinoblastoma include:

1. The peripheral granulomatous pattern with secondary retinal traction and tractional retinal detachment.

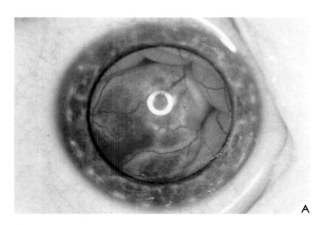

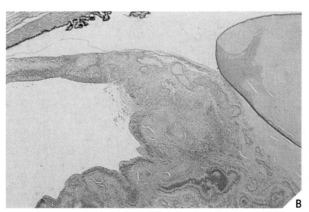

18.8 | *A:* The telangiectatic vessels on the surface of the retina have resulted in marked exudation and an exudative, bullous, retinal detachment. *B:* A histologic section of another case shows large, telangiectatic vessels in the peripheral retina. The vessels have leaked fluid, especially into the outer layers of the retina, causing a spreading and necrosis of the outer retina. (From Yanoff M, Fine BS: *Ocular Pathology*, ed 2. New York: Gower Medical Publishing, 1992, 18.10.)

2. The endophthalmitic form characterized by diffuse seeding of inflammatory cell clumps into the vitreous with occasional spillover into the aqueous.

Ultrasound and CT scanning will fail to show any calcified mass in such cases. Unfortunately, it is frequently difficult if not impossible to distinguish endophthalmitic toxocariasis from diffuse infiltrating retinoblastoma.[11] If one is in substantial doubt about the diagnosis, one should con-

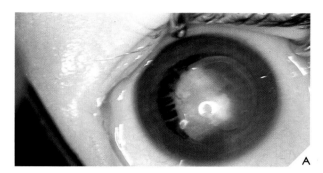

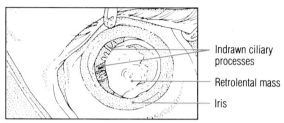

Indrawn ciliary processes

Retrolental mass

Iris

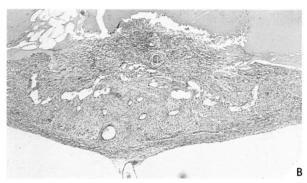

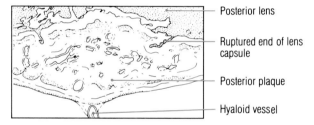

Posterior lens

Ruptured end of lens capsule

Posterior plaque

Hyaloid vessel

18.9 | Persistent hyperplastic primary vitreous (PHPV). *A:* Clinically, characteristically the ciliary processes are drawn inward and a posterior lens opacity is noted. *B:* A histologic section shows abundant mesenchymal fibrovascular tissue just behind and within the posterior lens. Note the ends of the ruptured lens capsule. A per- sistent hyaloid vessel also is present. (*A,* from Yanoff M, Fine BS: *Ocular Pathology,* ed 2. New York: Gower Medical Publishing, 1992, 18.6. *B,* courtesy of Dr. BW Streeten and reported in Caudill JW, Streeten BW, Tso MOM: *Ophthalmology 1985; 92:1153.*)

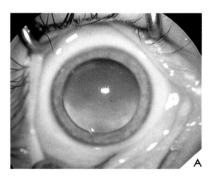

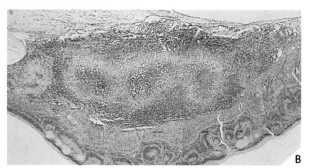

18.10 | Toxocariasis. *A:* An 8-year-old boy presented with leukokoria. The eye was white; other than loss of vision, no additional symptoms were present. *B:* A histologic section of another eye shows a peripheral retinal mass that contains an eosinophilic abscess. Often the worm itself is not found, but the eosinophils are evidence for its presence prior to dissolution. (From Yanoff M, Fine BS: *Ocular Pathology,* ed 2. New York: Gower Medical Publishing, 1992, 18.9.)

sider aqueous aspiration (in eyes that contain clinically detectable aqueous cells) or translimbal, transiridic vitreous aspiration for cytologic confirmation of the diagnosis.

Other less common causes of pseudoglioma include retinopathy of prematurity, Norrie's disease, incontinentia pigmenti (Bloch–Sulzberger syndrome), retinal dysplasia (13 trisomy), massive retinal fibrosis, metastatic retinitis, congenital nonattachment of the retina, secondary retinal detachment, juvenile retinoschisis, and medulloepithelioma.

MANAGEMENT AND PROGNOSIS

Factors influencing one's management recommendations for children with retinoblastoma include the size of the tumor or tumors, the location of the tumors, the laterality of the disease, the vision or vision potential in the affected eye, and the vision and visual potential in the unaffected eye (assuming the disease is unilateral). One should also take into account any associated ocular problems such as retinal detachment, vitreous hemorrhage, neovascularization of the iris, and secondary glaucoma. Finally, one must consider the age and general health of the child as well as personal preferences of the child's parents or legal guardians.

CLINICAL FACTORS AND PROGNOSIS

Untreated children who have retinoblastoma almost always die of intracranial extension or widely disseminated disease within approximately 2 years from the date of tumor detection. Recognized clinical prognostic factors for mortality[14] include younger age at detection and diagnosis (presumably because more advanced cases are detected earlier), unilaterality of the disease (apparently because unilateral cases tend to be detected later), extent of the intraocular tumor, and, most importantly, evidence of retrobulbar or extraocular tumor extension on CT or other imaging studies. In developed countries, the current prognosis for both unilaterally and bilaterally affected children who have retinoblastoma is approximately 90%.[2] Most of the retinoblastoma-related deaths that are going to occur do so within 2–4 years after the initiation of treatment, and few retinoblastoma-related deaths occur thereafter.

In view of the recognized natural history of retinoblastoma, observation without therapeutic intervention usually is not advocated. However, a number of circumstances exist where such an approach almost certainly is warranted. The most important circumstance is that of spontaneously arrested retinoblastoma. Spontaneously arrested lesions appear similar to regressed retinoblastoma lesions following irradiation but are detected in eyes without prior radiation therapy or other treatment (Fig. 18.11). The clinical term currently advocated for such lesions is retinoma (or retinocytoma).[15,16] Although retinomas convey the same implications for heredity of retinoblastoma as do viable lesions, such tumors usually remain dormant clinically and appear to have limited malignant potential.[16] Consequently, they usually can be observed on a regular interval basis without intervention unless they show evidence of renewed clinical activity.

The second circumstance in which continued observation is probably appropriate is that of true spontaneous regression of retinoblastoma.[15] Spontaneous regression is characterized by phthisis bulbi of the involved eye. If the entire tumor becomes necrotic, the prognosis for survival remains excellent. Unfortunately, viable tumor commonly persists in the optic nerve or orbit in such cases, and this viable retinoblastoma can eventually kill the affected patient.

Enucleation is the mainstay of treatment for retinoblastoma at this time.[17] This treatment is particularly applicable to children who have unilateral disease. It also is applicable for both eyes of some children who have bilateral, far-advanced disease not amenable to any eye-preserving therapy. Finally, it is commonly applicable to one eye (the more severely affected eye) in cases of asymmetric retinoblastoma. If enucleation is selected, the ophthalmic surgeon must attempt to obtain a long section of optic nerve at surgery. The principal route of exit of tumor cells from the eye is along the optic nerve.

At the cellular level, retinoblastomas are quite primitive and undifferentiated. Structures, such as Flexner-Wintersteiner and Homer Wright rosettes, as well as fleurettes, may be found (Figs. 18.12, 18.13). A patient whose tumor has abundant Flexner-Wintersteiner rosettes has a significantly better prognosis than a patient whose tumor has no rosettes. A tumor composed entirely of fleurettes also indicates an excellent prognosis. The mortality rate is around 25% if the tumor invades the choroid slightly; this rises to 65% when the invasion is massive. When the tumor does not invade the optic nerve, the mortality rate is approximately 8%. If invasion extends to the lamina cribrosa, but not beyond, the mortality rate rises to around 15%.

ENUCLEATION

CYTOLOGY AND PROGNOSIS

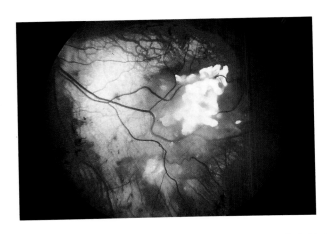

18.11 | Retinoma (spontaneously arrested retinoblastoma) consisting of calcific central nodule surrounded by extensive chorioretinal atrophy.

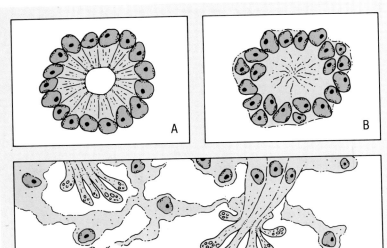

18.12 | Types of rosettes. *A:* The Flexner-Wintersteiner rosette consists of a central lumen lined by cuboidal tumor cells that contain nuclei positioned basally (away from the lumen). Delicate limiting membranes are seen at the apices of the cells that surround the lumen. *B:* Homer Wright rosettes are found more frequently in medulloblastomas and neuroblastomas than in retinoblastomas. In these rosettes, the cells line up around an acellular area that contains cobweb-like material. *C:* Fleurettes are flower-like groupings of tumor cells within the retinoblastoma. The cells of fleurettes show clear evidence of differentiation into photoreceptor elements. (From Yanoff M, Fine BS: *Ocular Pathology,* ed 2. New York: Gower Medical Publishing, 1992, 18.4.)

When the invasion is posterior to the lamina cribrosa, but not in the cut end of the nerve, the mortality rate is about 44%. If the invasion is to the point of surgical transection or to the posterior point of exit of the central retinal vessels from the optic nerve, the mortality rate is about 65%.

Prior pathologic studies have shown that enucleation usually is curative in retinoblastoma if an optic nerve section longer than 5 mm is obtained.[18] If possible, the ophthalmic surgeon should attempt to get an optic nerve section between 10 and 15 mm in length in every case. Contrary to some popular recommendations, insertion of an orbital implant probably

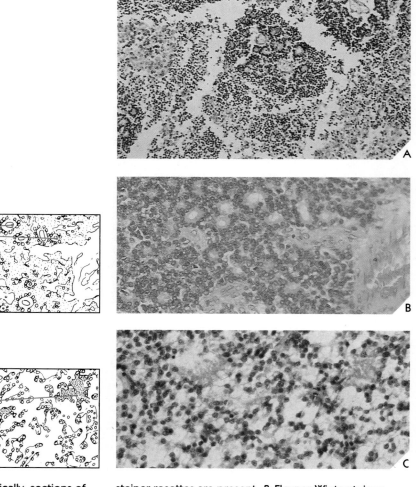

Flexner–Wintersteiner rosettes

Fleurettes

18.13 | Retinoblastoma. *A:* Characteristically, sections of retinoblastoma stained with hematoxylin and eosin and viewed under low magnification show some dark blue areas surrounded by light pink areas. The dark areas represent the viable cells and calcium deposition, and the light areas represent tumor necrosis. In this figure, the viable (dark blue) tumor cells are clustered around central blood vessels, and themselves surrounded by a mantle of necrotic (pink) cells. Numerous Flexner-Winter-steiner rosettes are present. *B:* Flexner-Wintersteiner rosettes show clear lumina lined by a delicate limiting membrane and cuboidal retinoblastoma cells with basally oriented nuclei. *C:* In this histologic section of a retinoblastoma, almost all of the cells show photoreceptor differentiation, indicated by the pale, eosinophilic acellular regions. The differentiated areas are forming rosettes. (From Yanoff M, Fine BS: *Ocular Pathology,* ed 2. New York: Gower Medical Publishing, 1992, 18.3,18.4.)

is appropriate, because orbital recurrence usually can be monitored in such situations quite effectively by CT scanning or MRI. The cosmetic results of enucleation generally are quite satisfactory as long as the child does not also require orbital radiation therapy.[19]

EXTERNAL BEAM RADIATION

The most commonly employed eye-preserving method of therapy for retinoblastoma is external beam radiation therapy.[20,21] This treatment usually is performed using a linear accelerator in a hospital radiation therapy department. Various radiotherapeutic set-ups for treatment of the whole eye have been devised, and the pros and cons of the different techniques are beyond the scope of this chapter. Standard target doses of radiation to the eye and orbit are in the range of 45–50 cGy given in divided fractions of approximately 150–200 cGy over 4–5 weeks.

External beam radiation therapy is highly effective in producing regression of vascularized retinal tumors (Fig. 18.14). Even very large cohesive retinoblastomas commonly show pronounced, prompt shrinkage with intensification of the intralesional calcification within a very short interval (several weeks) following the treatment. Two general patterns of postirradiation tumor regression have been identified. In the first pattern (Type I), the tumor regresses to an almost exclusively calcific, avascular residual mound (Fig. 18.14B). In the second pattern (Type II), the tumor regresses without prominent calcification but with a gray–tan "fish flesh" appearance. The dilated retinal vessels usually become markedly attenuated with both regression patterns. In some children, a combination of both regression patterns occurs, which is generally referred to as Type III regression.

External beam radiation therapy is applicable to eyes that contain one or more tumors involving the optic disc or macula, most eyes that have multiple tumors, both eyes in most children with bilateral disease, eyes that show diffuse vitreous seeding, and eyes failing prior local treatments such as photocoagulation or cryotherapy.

Vitreous seeds commonly do not respond well to radiation therapy, presumably because of their relatively hypoxic status.[21] As one also might expect, the larger the intraocular tumor, the less predictable the successful local response to treatment. The prognosis for preservation of the eye with at

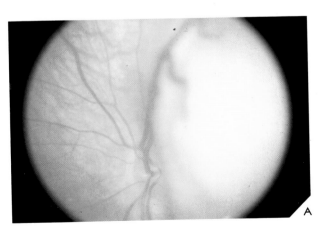
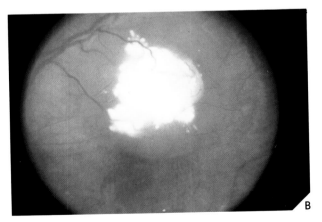

18.14 | External beam radiation therapy of retinoblastoma. A: Prominent macular and juxtapapillary retinoblastoma with dilated feeder and drainer retinal blood vessels. B: Same eye 11 months following external beam radiation therapy. Residual tumor is limited to superior macular region and consists of both calcific (Type I) and (Type II) fleshy portions (together called Type III regression pattern).

least some useful vision can be assessed with some degree of success using classifications such as the Reese–Ellsworth system[22] and the Essen prognosis classification.[23] The reader needs to be aware that neither of these classifications is appropriately applied to prognosis for survival. Other classifications, such as the tumor–node–metastasis (TNM) system[24] and the St. Jude's Hospital classification,[25] are more applicable to that sort of assessment.

If the whole eye is treated with external beam radiation therapy, a radiation-related cataract is likely to result.[26] Such a cataract typically begins as posterior subcapsular clouding, and in some children it may remain limited and stable in extent after development. In other children, it becomes progressively more pronounced, gradually obscuring details of the fundus and worsening vision. In such situations, cataract extraction usually is required.[27] Fortunately, the cataract often does not form for at least 6 months after the irradiation and often is delayed for as much as 1–1.5 years following the treatment. At the current target dose levels of radiation mentioned above, other significant intraocular radiation complications such as pronounced radiation retinopathy and neovascular glaucoma are extremely uncommon. A tendency for orbital bone growth arrest exists on the affected side, but such deformities are not nearly as pronounced now as they were in the past when higher doses of radiation therapy were employed and electron beam therapy was more commonly used.

EPISCLERAL PLAQUE RADIATION

In some children who have relatively large but localized retinoblastoma, even in the presence of limited localized vitreous seeding, episcleral plaque radiation therapy can be employed successfully.[28] Shielded plaques of iodine 125 or ruthenium 106 both are being used currently for such treatments. These types of plaques, by virtue of their shielding, prevent any substantial orbital dose from being delivered while effectively treating the local ocular disturbance. With plaque radiation therapy, a target dose of 40 Gy to the tumor apex generally is employed. Because of the physical dose distribution considerations of plaque radiotherapy, of course, the base of the tumor always receives a substantially higher dose than the apex. Such treatment is highly effective in bringing about prompt regression of treated tumors (Fig. 18.15). This form of therapy seems particularly applicable to eyes that con-

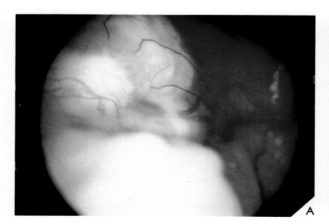
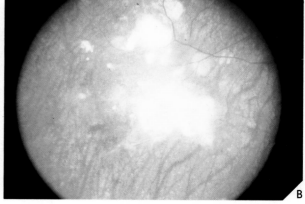

18.15 | Plaque radiation therapy of retinoblastoma. *A:* Multinodular retinoblastoma with prominent retinal vasculature prior to plaque treatment. *B:* Same lesion 6 months following episcleral plaque therapy. Residue of tumor consists almost exclusively of calcific tissue.

tain a solitary medium-to-large tumor that does not involve the optic disc or macula and that is associated with only a very limited amount of adjacent vitreous seeding. This form of therapy also can be used in eyes failing prior local therapy by photocoagulation or cryotherapy as well as some eyes locally failing prior external beam radiation therapy.

RETINAL PHOTOCOAGULATION

Retinal photocoagulation has been used for quite a number of years to treat eyes that contain one or a few small tumors, clear optical media, and no vitreous seeds.[29] Photocoagulation generally is not advocated for tumors involving the optic disc or macula. Tumors most amenable to this form of therapy are quite small, usually less than 7 mm in basal diameter and 2–3 mm in thickness. Xenon arc photocoagulation was the modality of photocoagulation generally employed until recently in retinoblastoma management. With the advent of the indirect ophthalmoscope laser delivery system that can be used in the operating room, such tumors now can be treated very effectively by laser therapy. The generally recommended approach to treatment is to create a confluent burn several burn widths around the base of the tumor, attempting to block off its feeding and draining retinal blood supply (Fig. 18.16A,B). Unless the entire tumor is small enough that it can be totally encompassed in a single laser burn, no treatment is directed to the tumor itself for fear of rupturing the internal limiting membrane and allowing shedding of tumor cells into the overlying vitreous. Treatment effectiveness usually is checked within 2 weeks and photocoagulation is repeated if necessary until the entire tumor is gone. Using scleral depression techniques, even tumors at the ora serrata now can be treated effectively and with relative ease by photocoagulation.

TRANSSCLERAL CRYOTHERAPY

Transscleral cryotherapy under indirect ophthalmoscopic visualization can be used to treat one to a few equatorial or preequatorial retinoblastoma tumors of small to medium size.[30] This therapy should not be used in eyes that have vitreous seeding. A double or triple freeze–thaw technique usually is employed, allowing an ice ball to encompass the entire tumor and overlying vitreous before being allowed to thaw at each site. As with photocoagulation,

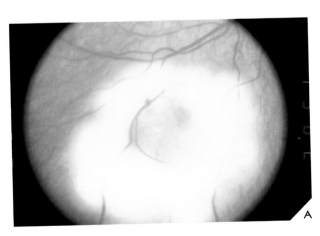

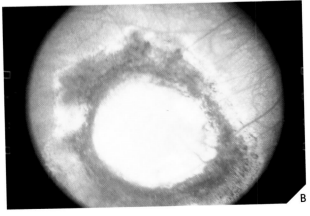

18.16 | Photocoagulation of retinoblastoma. *A:* Immediate postphotocoagulation fundus photograph showing intense white burn completely around retinal tumor with obliteration of feeder and drainer retinal blood vessels.

B: Same lesion 6 months following photocoagulation therapy. Treated lesion atrophic with hyperpigmented margins caused by retinal pigment epithelial hyperplasia.

this form of treatment generally should be repeated every 2–4 weeks until the entire tumor is gone.

As many as 20% of eyes in some series treated initially by one form of eye-preserving therapy eventually require some subsequent therapy by the same or another modality. In spite of the need for secondary treatments of a sequential type, the great majority of eyes that have small- to medium-sized tumors and no vitreous seeding can be salvaged with useful vision.

FOLLOW-UP

Following treatment of retinoblastoma, the child should be reexamined within about 2–4 weeks to assess treatment efficacy, and supplemental treatment should be performed if the prior therapy appears inadequate. Once treatment appears to have totally eradicated all intraocular tumors, children should be monitored at least every 3 months for at least 2 posttreatment years. Thereafter, children probably should be followed at about 6-month intervals until they are at least 6 years of age. Following that, children should continue to be followed at yearly intervals.

Some children have substantial orbital extension of tumor at the time of their initial diagnosis and treatment, and others develop subsequent orbital recurrence following enucleation. Although such cases were almost invariably fatal in the past, current evidence suggests that at least some of these children can now be salvaged by an aggressive regimen of tumor debulking, supplemental orbital irradiation, and systemic multidrug chemotherapy.[31,32] Unfortunately, the prognosis for children who have intracranial extension or widespread metastasis remains dismal at this point in time.

OTHER MALIGNANCIES

As mentioned earlier, approximately 90% of children who have retinoblastoma in this country currently survive their retinoblastoma. Unfortunately, these children now are known to have an increased risk of death from secondary nonretinoblastoma malignancies over the course of their lifetimes.[33,34] The exact probability of such an event currently is somewhat controversial, but the best available evidence suggests that at least 20% of retinoblastoma survivors will develop such malignancies (commonly osteogenic or soft tissue sarcomas) within 25 years after their retinoblastoma treatment. In addition, children who have bilateral or familial retinoblastoma seem to be at substantially increased risk for developing an ectopic intracranial retinoblastoma involving the pineal, suprasellar, or parasellar tissues (trilateral retinoblastoma).[35] Such lesions can cause obstructive hydrocephalus as well as seeding into the cerebrospinal fluid and implantation metastasis along the spinal cord. Unfortunately, cases of ectopic intracranial retinoblastoma almost always (if not always) are fatal in spite of aggressive treatment.

BENIGN TUMORS IN THE DIFFERENTIAL DIAGNOSIS OF RETINOBLASTOMA

James J. Augsburger
and Myron Yanoff

RETINAL ASTROCYTIC HAMARTOMA

The retinal astrocytoma (astrocytic hamartoma) is a benign tumor believed to arise from glial cells (astrocytes) of the inner retina. Lesions of this type occur in isolated (usually unifocal) and syndromic (usually multifocal and bilateral) varieties. The syndromic variety, which occurs in tuberous sclerosis (Bourneville's disease), is one of the phakomatoses (Fig. 19.1) and by far the more commonly recognized type.

Several clinical types of retinal astrocytoma have been described.[1] The classic retinal lesion is a white, dense, superficial retinal lesion that is 1-disc diameter or more in size and has a surface appearance resembling that of rock candy (Fig. 19.2A). A classic retinal astrocytic hamartoma evaluated by fluorescein angiography shows relatively slow filling of the intralesional vasculature, absence of dilated afferent and efferent retinal vascular channels, and late staining of the tumors (Fig. 19.2B–D). The second type of lesion is an opaque, white, inner retinal thickening that has a more smooth and soft surface appearance (Fig. 19.3). The third variety is a faint, translucent, intraretinal lesion which is smaller in size than the other two varieties.

Figure 19.1. Phakomatoses

Angiomatosis retinae (von Hippel's disease)	Tuberous sclerosis (Bourneville's disease)
Meningocutaneous angiomatosis (Sturge-Weber syndrome)	Ataxia telangiectasia (Louis-Bar syndrome)
Neurofibromatosis (von Recklinghausen's disease)	Arteriovenous communication of retina and brain (Wyburn-Mason syndrome)

Often the different types of lesions occur simultaneously in the same eye. The lesions tend to develop early in childhood and show some tendency for limited progression during the childhood years. However, these tumors do not have malignant potential and do not metastasize. If they occur in or adjacent to the foveola, they can cause visual loss on the basis of neurosensory retinal destruction. In most cases, however, they are associated with normal visual acuity.

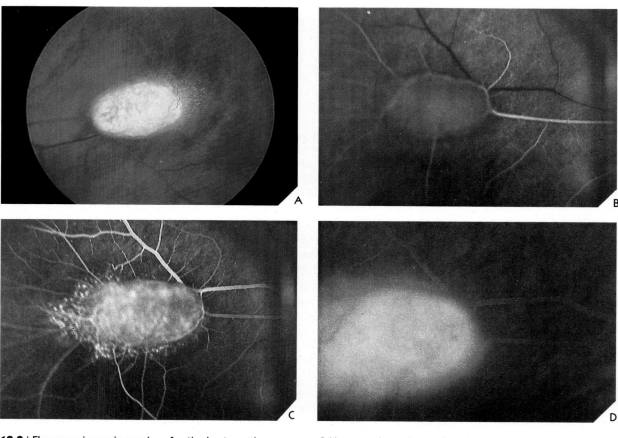

19.2 | Fluorescein angiography of retinal astrocytic hamartoma. *A:* Focal white "mulberry type" retinal astrocytic hamartoma. *B:* Arterial phase frame showing feeder retinal arteries and faint pseudofluorescence of tumor.

C: Venous phase frame showing prominent intralesional retinal vascular supply. *D:* Late phase frame showing staining of lesion without leakage into overlying vitreous.

19.3 | Multifocal retinal astrocytomas of different densities in patient with tuberous sclerosis.

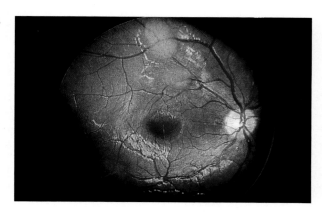

Multifocal, bilateral retinal astrocytomas occur most commonly in the context of tuberous sclerosis.[1] This disorder is a multisystem disease having a wide spectrum of clinical characteristics. Classic clinical features of the disorder include seizures, characteristic malar facial skin changes known as adenoma sebaceum (really angiofibromas), pale cutaneous lesions (ash leaf spots) that are most commonly found on the trunk, subungual fibromas of the digits, paraventricular astrocytomas of the central nervous system (CNS), cardiac rhabdomyomas, and other assorted lesions. Some individuals who have tuberous sclerosis are mentally retarded, but normal intelligence is not unusual in this syndrome. The optic nerve often shows a typical "mulberry lesion" (Fig. 19.4).

An atypical type of retinal astrocytoma is an isolated, nonsyndromic lesion[2] that occurs unilaterally in an otherwise unaffected individual (Fig. 19.5). Lesions of this type can attain a relatively large size and occasionally

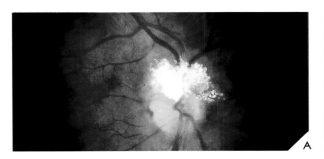

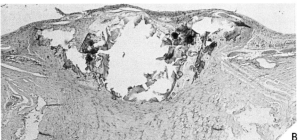

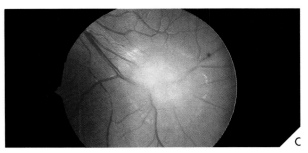

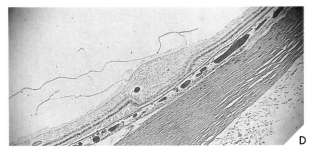

19.4 | Tuberous sclerosis. *A:* Fundus shows typical mulberry lesion involving the superior part of the optic nerve. *B:* Histologic section of another case shows a giant drusen of the optic nerve. *C:* The lesion, as seen in the fundus of a young child before it grows into the mulberry configuration, is quite smooth and resembles a

retinoblastoma. *D:* Histologic section of an early lesion shows no calcification but simply a proliferation of glial tissue. (*A–D*, from Yanoff M, Fine BS: *Ocular Pathology,* ed 2. New York: Gower Medical Publishing, 1992, 2.13. *C,* courtesy of Dr. DB Schaffer.)

19.5 | Isolated "exophytic" astrocytic hamartoma of retina with associated bullous nonrhegmatogenous retinal detachment.

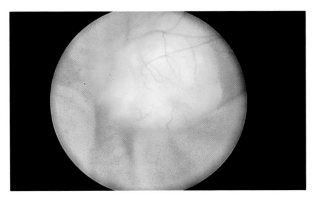

cause profound visual loss, usually on the basis of their location or accumulation of exudative subretinal fluid. Unless the possibility of an astrocytoma is considered clinically, eyes with this sort of tumor usually require enucleation because amelanotic choroidal melanoma or another malignant neoplasm cannot be excluded. Some lesions that appear to be retinal astrocytomas on initial histopathologic evaluation, however, are actually cases of massive gliosis of the retina.[3]

RETINAL CAPILLARY HEMANGIOMA

The retinal capillary hemangioma is a benign vascular tumor arising from the vasculature of the retina or optic disc. It generally is considered to be hamartomatous in nature.[4] As with the astrocytic hamartoma of the retina, the capillary hemangioma occurs in both syndromic and isolated clinical settings. In the syndromic form, retinal capillary hemangiomas occur as a manifestation of the von Hippel–Lindau syndrome.[5] In this disorder, the capillary hemangiomas generally are multifocal and bilateral (Fig. 19.6). As with retinoblastoma, the various tumors in this condition tend to be markedly dissimilar in size, even within a single affected eye. In the isolated, nonsyndromic form of the disease, a single retinal capillary hemangioma usually is detected in only one eye of an otherwise healthy individual. The syndromic

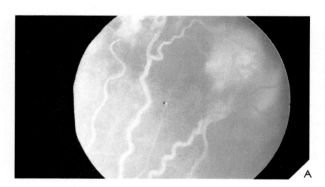

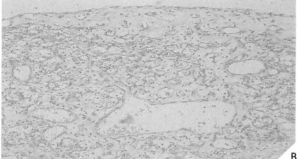

19.6 | von Hippel's disease. *A:* Superiorly, two round retinal lesions associated with von Hippel's disease (angiomatosis retinae) are apparent along with feeder vessels. *B:* Histologic section shows two distinct types of cells: endothelial cells lining the numerous capillaries,

and, present between the capillaries, stromal cells derived from vascular endothelium that appear "foamy." (*A,B,* from Yanoff M, Fine BS: *Ocular Pathology,* ed 2. New York: Gower Medical Publishing, 1992, 2.6. *B,* courtesy of Dr. DH Nicholson.)

19.7 | Small globular retinal capillary hemangioma with prominent dilated, tortuous afferent and efferent retinal blood vessels.

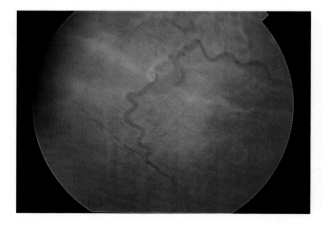

form of the disease tends to be inherited as an autosomal dominant condition, while the isolated form is usually sporadic (nonfamilial).

The typical capillary hemangioma of the retina or optic disc appears as a reddish, spherical lesion fed and drained by dilated, tortuous retinal vessels (Fig. 19.7). Prominent afferent and efferent vessels of this type commonly are noted even in eyes that contain tumors smaller than 0.5-disc diameter in size. Generally, the larger the tumor the more extensive the dilation and tortuosity of the corresponding retinal vessels. In many cases, the feeding arteries and draining veins also become irregularly segmented with fusiform dilations along their course. Such alterations often seem more pronounced on the arterial limb than on the venous side of the vascular loop. Intraretinal and subretinal exudation overlying and surrounding a retinal capillary hemangioma is common, particularly when the tumor is more than approximately 2–3 mm in diameter. In many eyes, the accumulation of intraretinal and subretinal exudates can be accentuated in the macular region, even if the hemangiomas responsible for the exudation are substantially distant from the macula. In eyes that contain extremely large capillary hemangiomas, a partial or even total retinal detachment and extensive subretinal accumulation of thick exudative fluid containing cholesterol and macrophages can develop (Fig. 19.8), a situation that frequently leads to iris neovascularization and secondary angle-closure glaucoma and a blind, painful or phthisical eye. In other eyes, vitreoretinal membrane formation can be a prominent feature of the fundus picture. The vitreous membranes commonly appear to be adherent to the hemangiomas, sometimes causing a centripetal tractional force on the equatorial retina.

Capillary hemangiomas arising on the optic disc[6] generally appear less well-defined and less globular than those arising in the extrapapillary retina (Fig. 19.9). The retinal blood vessels feeding and draining capillary hemangiomas of the disc generally are not prominent, and the development of exudative intraretinal and subretinal fluid around the lesion and disc can further obscure the lesion margins.

Fluorescein angiography of a typical retinal capillary hemangioma shows rapid filling of the afferent artery, brisk filling of the entire retinal vas-

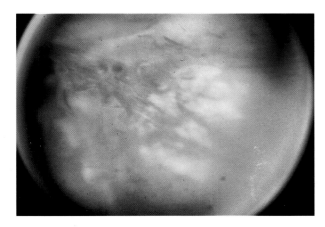

19.8 | Large retinal capillary hemangioma with prominent associated retinal blood vessels and extensive retinal detachment.

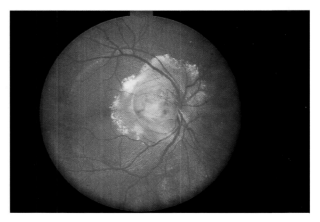

19.9 | Retinal capillary hemangioma of disc with associated circumpapillary exudates and macular subretinal fluid.

cular tumor, intense hyperfluorescence of the entire vascular lesion shortly thereafter, and subsequent rapid filling of the efferent vein (Fig. 19.10). The vascular tumor leaks fluorescein exuberantly into the overlying vitreous, and the late phase frames often are extremely hazy because of the diffuse vitreous fluorescence. Fluorescein also leaks into the subretinal fluid of an associated exudative retinal detachment.

Although some retinal capillary hemangiomas have been observed that remain stable for months or years, or even regress spontaneously without causing exudative phenomena,[7] many if not most capillary hemangiomas of the disc do enlarge to at least a limited degree during follow-up.

Capillary hemangiomas of the retina or optic disc usually are the earliest detected manifestation of von Hippel–Lindau syndrome.[5] The typical age at detection in this form of the condition is during the second to third decade of life. Important extraocular features of the von Hippel–Lindau syndrome include capillary hemangiomas ("hemangioblastomas") of the brain and spinal cord, renal cell carcinoma and pheochromocytoma of the kidney, and cystic lesions of other abdominal visceral organs.[5] The associated renal tumors and intracranial vascular tumors commonly prove fatal to affected individuals if not detected early. Consequently, all persons in whom a capil-

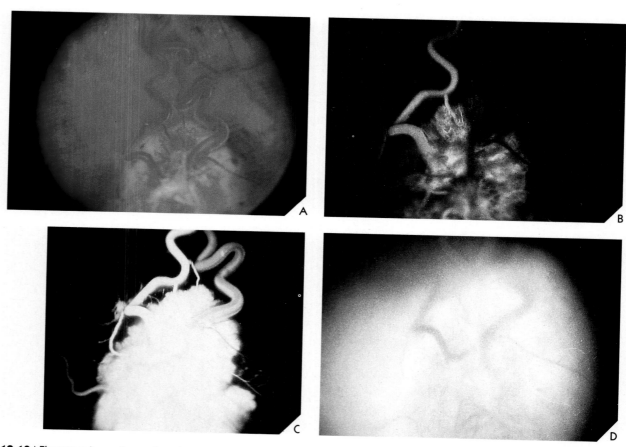

19.10 | Fluorescein angiography of retinal capillary hemangioma. *A:* Prominent retinal capillary hemangioma in inferior periphery with dilated, tortuous afferent and efferent retinal vessels. *B:* Arterial phase frame showing rapid filling of lesion from retinal arterial limb. *C:* Venous phase frame showing laminar filling of draining vein and intense diffuse fluorescence of entire hemangioma. *D:* Late phase frame showing prominent leakage of fluorescein from entire vascular lesion into overlying vitreous.

lary hemangioma of the optic disc or retina is identified should be considered potentially affected by the other manifestations of this syndrome. As mentioned previously, individuals who have multifocal or bilateral retinal capillary hemangiomas, a family history of capillary hemangiomas of the retina and disc, or a family history of individuals who have vascular CNS tumors or unusual kidney tumors should be particularly suspected of having von Hippel–Lindau syndrome. Such individuals probably should be evaluated by abdominal and CNS imaging studies [magnetic resonance imaging (MRI) or computed tomography (CT)]. If possible, family members also should be examined ophthalmically to see if any other individuals can be identified who have retinal capillary hemangioma.

Because capillary hemangiomas of the retina and optic disc have no intrinsic malignant potential, management decisions for such lesions should be based on the desire to preserve or restore vision in affected eyes. The most commonly employed method of management at this time is photocoagulation of the vascular tumor[8] (Fig. 19.11). This treatment is particularly effective against tumors that are up to 3–4 mm in diameter, but it is commonly less effective in larger tumors. Most individuals currently believe that the tumor should not be treated intensely in a single session but should rather be treated lightly with relatively large spot sizes and long exposure times on multiple occasions over several months. In addition, the retina surrounding the capillary hemangioma commonly is treated by scatter photocoagulation prior to treatment of the vascular tumor in an effort to prevent progression of exudative retinal detachment. The feeder artery leading to the vascular hemangioma also can be occluded by a series of burns along its course leading to the hemangioma.[9] In successfully treated cases, the hemangioma becomes atrophic and involuted, and the feeding and draining retinal vessels lose their dilation and tortuosity. The exudates commonly reabsorb gradually. Depending on the extent of macular scarring and thickness of the exudates, the vision may or may not recover.

In the case of some peripheral retinal capillary hemangiomas and some larger tumors, transconjunctival or transscleral cryotherapy can be employed

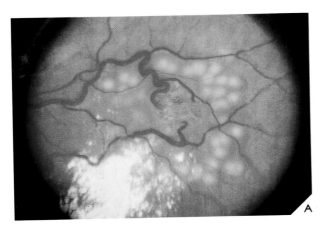
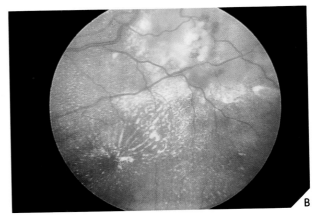

19.11 | Photocoagulation of retinal capillary hemangioma. *A:* Immediate posttreatment fundus photographs of localized retinal capillary hemangioma with associated macular exudates. First session of treatment was directed to marginal retina around lesion and not to lesion proper. *B:* After several additional sessions of laser treatment. Note almost total regression of hemangioma, return of afferent and efferent vessels to near normal caliber, and reduction in intraretinal exudates.

as an alternative to photocoagulation[10] (Fig. 19.12). With this form of treatment, one generally localizes the tip of the cryoprobe at the site of the retinal capillary hemangioma by using it as a scleral depressor during indirect ophthalmoscopy. One then performs double or even triple freeze–thaw therapy to the tumor, allowing the ice ball to come completely through the lesion into the overlying vitreous. This form of treatment also may have to be repeated at intervals of 4–6 weeks or more until the lesion is totally obliterated and the retinal feeder and drainer vessels return to normal caliber.

In some eyes that contain extremely large retinal capillary hemangiomas, a few experienced ophthalmic surgeons have employed aggressive techniques such as penetrating diathermy[11] or episcleral ruthenium 106 plaque radiation therapy to destroy the lesion. With improvements in vitreo-retinal surgical techniques, a number of eyes that contain large or numerous retinal capillary hemangiomas and exudative or tractional retinal detachment are now managed by an internal technique that typically includes pars plana vitrectomy coupled with endophotocoagulation or endodiathermy to the tumors.[12] Finally, some eyes that become blind and painful or phthisical eventually come to enucleation.

Patients who have a small retinal capillary hemangioma that is causing no exudative phenomena and those previously treated with satisfactory involution of their tumor or tumors must continue to be monitored periodically for local tumor activation or new tumor formation. Management of capillary hemangiomas of the optic disc is extremely problematic. If the tumor involves the temporal portion of the disc, its treatment by photocoagulation or another coagulative method commonly results in substantial further visual impairment, even though it is likely to be successful in causing tumor involution or stabilization. In contrast, the occasional capillary hemangioma that involves the nasal portion of the disc and causes exudative circumpapillary retinal detachment and visual loss often can be markedly improved by photocoagulation.

RETINAL CAVERNOUS HEMANGIOMA

The cavernous hemangioma of the retina and optic disc is a benign vascular lesion that is believed to be hamartomatous in nature.[3,4,13] Although occasionally associated with cutaneous vascular lesions and minimal nonprogressive intracranial vascular lesions,[14,15] this condition usually appears to be nonsyndromic in nature. It is most frequently identified in a unifocal

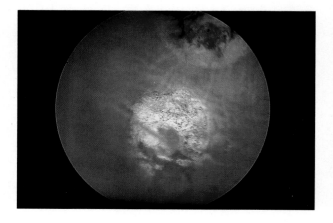

19.12 | Cryotherapy of retinal capillary hemangioma. Same lesion as shown in Fig. 19.7 three months following double freeze–thaw transscleral cryotherapy. The lesion is atrophic and feeder and drainer vessels have become attenuated. Adjacent atrophic focus is site of previously treated hemangioma.

nonfamilial situation, but occasional bilateral, familial cases have been reported.[15,16]

The typical cavernous hemangioma of the retina appears as a cluster of vascular saccules within the retina in association with an anomalous-appearing retinal venous channel (Fig. 19.13A). The clustering of intraretinal vascular saccules typically involves an area 1–4 disc diameters in size, while the individual vascular saccules making up the lesion generally range from microaneurysmal size to greater than a retinal vein width at the disc. Larger lesions commonly have associated whitish glial proliferation on their surfaces, which initially can be mistaken for exudative material. However, true subretinal and intraretinal exudates in association with such lesions are extremely uncommon and never massive in extent.

While the associated anomalous retinal vein in such lesions commonly is quite pronounced, this vessel usually is not dilated or tortuous. Similarly, any dilated or tortuous feeder arterioles usually are not present. Lesions of this type occurring on the optic disc[17] are quite similar in character, having the appearance of multiple vascular saccules containing dark venous blood.

Fluorescein angiography of a cavernous hemangioma of the retina or disc (Fig. 19.13B–D) typically shows slow filling of the lesion, which is

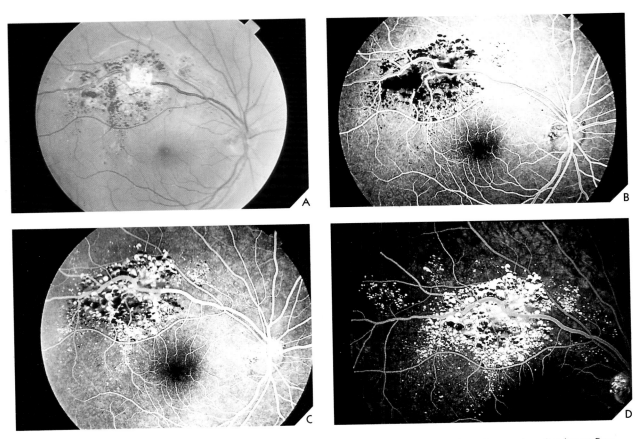

19.13 | Cavernous retinal hemangioma. *A:* Localized retinal hemangioma appears as cluster of small, red, intraretinal saccules with associated superficial whitish gliosis. Note prominent retinal vein passing through center of lesion. *B:* Laminar venous phase frame showing hypofluorescence of most vascular saccules comprising lesion. *C:* Late venous phase frame showing hyperfluorescence of some but not all vascular saccules. *D:* Late phase frame showing hypofluorescence of most vascular saccules comprising lesion. Note plasma–erythrocyte separation in some of the larger vascular saccules.

delayed substantially longer than the filling of the surrounding normal capillary bed. The vascular saccules comprising the lesion accumulate fluorescein gradually as the study progresses and remain brightly fluorescent long after most of the intravascular fluorescein has faded. If the component vascular saccules are quite large, one occasionally notes the phenomenon of "plasma–erythrocyte separation," which appears as bright fluorescein in the upper portion of the individual saccules and dark settled red blood cells in the lower portion.

Most eyes that contain a cavernous hemangioma of the retina or optic disc have no visual problem and require no treatment. The principal compli-

19.14 | Neurofromatosis. *A:* Iris shows multiple small spider-like melanocytic nevi, characteristic of neurofromatosis. *B:* The iris nevi, also called Lisch nodules, are caused by collections of nevus cells. *C:* The choroid is markedly thickened by the hamartomatous process. Numerous structures such as neural rosettes, tactile nerve endings, and nevi may be found within the thickened choroid. Note the thickened nerves (plexiform neurofibromas) in the sclera. In classic von Recklinghausen disease (type 1 neurofibromatosis or peripheral type) café au lait spots, peripheral neurofibromas, and Lisch nodules predominate. In type 2, or the central type, bilateral acoustic neuromas are characteristic. (From Yanoff M, Fine BS: *Ocular Pathology,* ed 2. New York: Gower Medical Publishing, 1992, 2.8.)

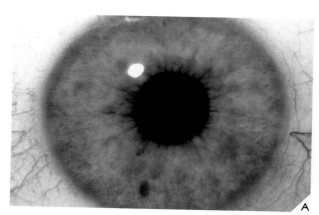

A

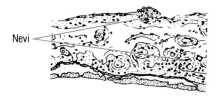

Nevi

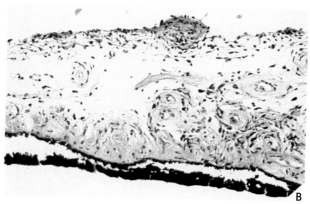

B

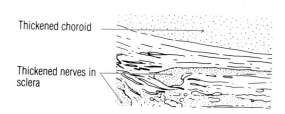

Thickened choroid

Thickened nerves in sclera

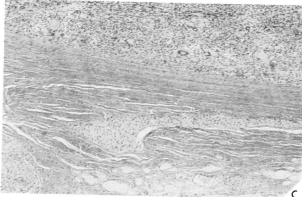

C

cation of cavernous hemangiomas of the retina or optic disc is vitreous hemorrhage, which tends to be most common and most severe in eyes with the largest lesions. If vitreous hemorrhage is recurrent and massive, transscleral cryotherapy or pars plana vitrectomy with endocoagulation may be required. In view of the lack of significant CNS or visceral lesions in most individuals with this form of retinal hemangioma, the appropriateness of routine CNS and abdominal imaging studies (CT or MRI) is uncertain.[18]

Phakomatoses, such as neurofibromatosis (Fig. 19.14), meningocutaneous angiomatosis (Sturge-Weber syndrome) (Fig. 19.15), ataxia telangiectasia (Louis-Bar syndrome), and arteriovenous communication of retina and brain (Wyburn Mason syndrome), rarely can be confused with retinoblastoma. Generally, however, the correct diagnosis is established from the systemic manifestations.

OTHER BENIGN TUMORS

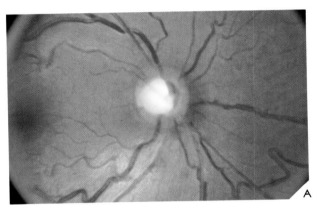

A

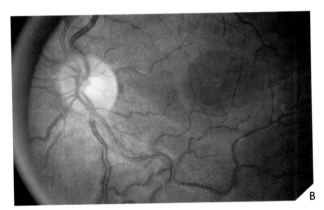

B

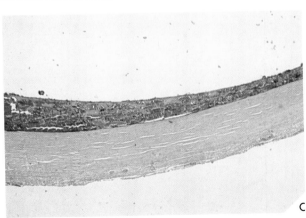

C

19.15 | Sturge-Weber syndrome. *A:* The fundus shows both the characteristic bright red appearance of the involved eye, caused by the choroidal hemangioma, and an enlarged optic nerve cup, secondary to increased intraocular pressure in that eye. *B:* The normal fundus of the patient's left eye is shown for comparison. *C:* In another case, the choroid is diffusely involved by a cavernous hemangioma. When a choroidal hemangioma occurs in the Sturge-Weber patient, it is diffuse, large, and difficult to distinguish from any normal choroid that might be present. When it occurs in a patient without the syndrome, it is focal, small, and easy to distinguish from the surrounding normal choroid. (*A–C,* from Yanoff M, Fine BS: *Ocular Pathology,* ed 2. New York: Gower Medical Publishing, 1992, 2.6. *C,* courtesy of Dr. R. Cordero-Moreno.)

MALIGNANT TUMORS IN THE DIFFERENTIAL DIAGNOSIS OF RETINOBLASTOMA

James J. Augsburger and Myron Yanoff

MEDULLOEPITHELIOMA

The medulloepithelioma is a tumor derived from neuroectoderm and usually arises intraocularly from the nonpigmented epithelium of the ciliary body.[1] In rare occasions, the lesions arise from the iris, sensory retina, or optic disc. They range from benign proliferations to frankly malignant neoplasms that have unequivocal invasive but very limited metastatic potential. Most medulloepitheliomas of the ciliary epithelium probably are congenital in nature. In many cases, they include heterotopic elements such as cartilage or bone which results in their pathologic categorization as teratomas (teratoid medulloepithelioma).[1]

Medulloepitheliomas of the ciliary body typically appear in children as tan to white lesions of the extreme peripheral fundus, occasionally with involvement of the peripheral iris (Fig. 20.1). Lesions of this type commonly have a prominent cystic character. Occasionally, the absence of zonules and resultant abnormalities of lens curvature (lens colobomas) have been observed in patients.

20.1 | Medulloep-ithelioma of iris and ciliary body with associated lens coloboma. Tumor is fleshy-pink in color and contains prominent intralesional blood vessels.

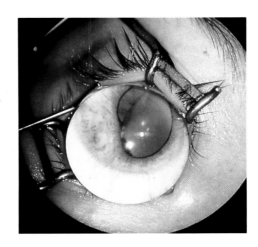

A common complication of medulloepitheliomas of the ciliary body is development of neovascular glaucoma.[1,2] In some cases, a glaucoma of this type develops even when the tumor is limited in extent. Because the eye is extremely firm, it may not be possible to depress the sclera sufficiently on a standard examination under anesthesia to visualize the tumor. Also, the far peripheral location of the lesion may preclude conventional contact B-scan from detecting such a tumor. In the face of unexplained neovascular glaucoma and a satisfactory view of the posterior fundus, one should consider the possibility of medulloepithelioma and evaluate the eye further by alternative methods of ocular imaging (computed tomography or magnetic resonance imaging) (Fig. 20.2) or perform a paracentesis at examination under anesthesia followed by reexamination of the peripheral fundus with scleral depression.

Medulloepithelioma, even in its benign varieties, tends to be a relentlessly progressive tumor. Furthermore, if it extends through the sclera, which is quite rare, it can prove fatal on the basis of either local invasive growth or metastasis.[1,2] Although local resection of the tumor by iridocyclectomy and even episcleral plaque radiotherapy have been employed in a number of cases,[1,2] such treatments have rarely been entirely successful in eradicating the tumor. Most cases eventually come to enucleation, and cases that have massive orbital extension may even require exenteration. As long as the tumor is still contained within the eye at the time of enucleation, survival is generally assured.

Histologically, medulloepithelioma consists of poorly differentiated neuroectodermal tissue that in some areas resembles embryonic retina (Fig. 20.3). The cells often are arranged in a double layer, and the innermost layer secretes hyaluronic acid ("vitreous"). Cartilage is present in 20% of cases. Also rhabdomyoblasts may be present. When heteroplastic elements, such as cartilage or rhabdomyoblasts, are present, the tumor is referred to as a teratoid medulloepithelioma.

LEUKEMIC INFILTRATIONS

Some individuals who have leukemia have infiltrative leukemic fundus lesions at the time of initial diagnosis;[3] others develop such lesions during the course of their hematologic malignancy.[4,5] Much more common than true neoplastic infiltrations of the retina, optic disc, choroid, or vitreous,

20.2 | CT scan of medulloepithelioma of ciliary body. Nasal ciliary body lesion in left eye appears prominently elevated with indentation of the lens in its equatorial region.

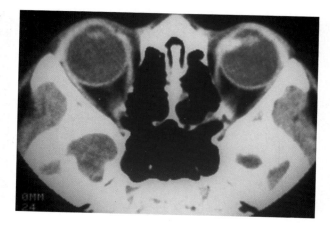

however, are hemorrhagic fundus lesions; these are usually linear and blot-like retinal hemorrhages (Figs. 20.4, 20.5), occasionally with white centers, and are attributable to the commonly associated anemia and thrombocytopenia.[3–5]

Nonhemorrhagic fundus lesions in leukemia appear to be relatively uncommon. Recognized intraocular leukemic lesions include cellular infil-

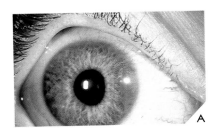

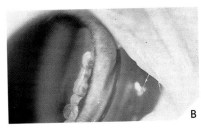

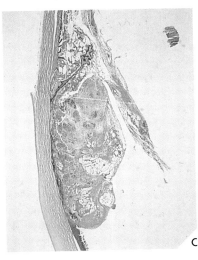

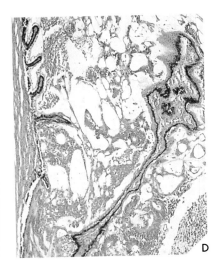

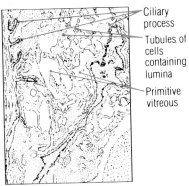

20.3 | Benign medulloepithelioma. *A:* The tumor seen in the anterior chamber angle nasally had originated in the ciliary body, best seen in *B* (after pupillary dilatation). *C:* A histologic section of another case shows structures that resemble primitive medullary epithelium, ciliary epithelium, and retina. The tumor arises from nonpigmented ciliary epithelium. *D:* Increased magnification shows the tubules of cells. Structures analogous to external limiting membrane of the retina appear on one surface of the tubules (in some areas forming lumina), while the less well defined opposite surface is in contact with a primitive vitreous. When these tumors contain heteroplastic elements, e.g., cartilage or brain tissue, they are called teratoid medulloepitheliomas. (*A–D,* from Yanoff M, Fine BS: *Ocular Pathology,* ed 2. New York: Gower Medical Publishing, 1992, 17.6. *A,B,* courtesy of Dr. JA Shields. *C,D,* courtesy of Dr. JS McGavic.)

Ciliary process
Tubules of cells containing lumina
Primitive vitreous

20.4 | Leukemic retinopathy with typical retinal hemorrhages.

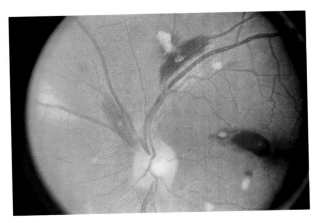

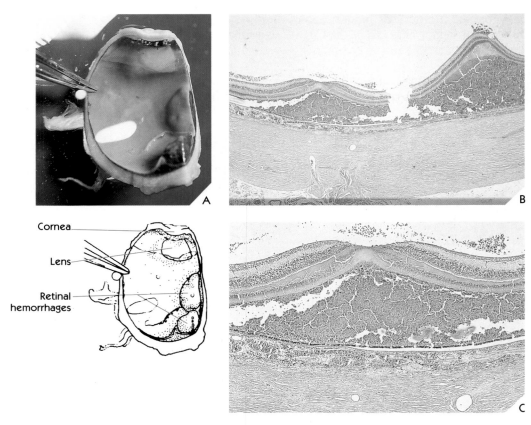

Cornea

Lens

Retinal
hemorrhages

20.5 | *A:* Cut gross eye from a patient who died of acute leukemia shows intra- and sub-retinal hemorrhages and leukemic infiltrates.

B: Histology of same eye demonstrates involvement of fovea (shown in higher magnification in *C*) and adjacent retina.

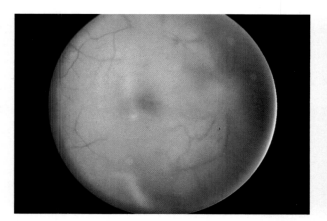

20.6 | Vitreous haze due to cellular infiltration of vitreous by leukemic cells in relapsed acute lymphocytic leukemia.

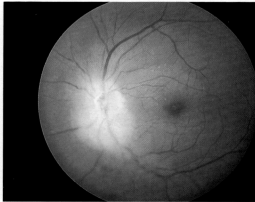

20.7 | Disc involvement in chronic myelogenous l Some vitreous cells were also present overlying t optic disc.

tration of the vitreous[6] (Fig. 20.6), intraretinal infiltrations (which can occur as "sheathing" along retinal vessel walls or as fluffy solid confluent infiltrates),[3-5] optic disc infiltrations (Fig. 20.7),[7] retinal pigment epithelial detachments,[8] and nonrhegmatogenous retinal detachments.[9] Leukemia also occasionally can present as a localized or diffuse choroidal infiltration, a neoplastic hypopyon, or an iris infiltration.[10] In patients who have chronic myelogenous leukemia, peripheral retinal capillary obstruction and microaneurysm formation have also been observed. In a few patients who have leukemia, neovascularization of the optic disc or retina has been reported.[11,12]

Leukemic infiltrative fundus lesions usually are not a presenting feature of the underlying hematologic malignancy. Fewer than 5% of patients who have leukemia have any identifiable infiltrative leukemic fundus lesions at the time of initial leukemic diagnosis.[3] The detection of leukemic fundus lesions, however, can and commonly does appear to correlate with relapse from remission and appears to be an extremely poor prognostic sign for long-term survival.

Because patients who have leukemia commonly are immunosuppressed (either on the basis of their malignancy or more often by virtue of the effects of chemotherapy), it is sometimes difficult, if not impossible, to tell clinically whether a fundus lesion is truly a leukemic infiltration or an infectious lesion caused by an opportunistic organism.[5,6] In such cases, fine needle aspiration biopsy may be of great value in establishing the correct diagnosis.

Ophthalmic treatment of infiltrative leukemic disease generally consists of external beam radiation therapy to the involved eye or eyes.[5,6] Retinal lesions typically respond promptly and completely to this treatment. Massive optic disc infiltration that causes visual loss also commonly responds to such treatment, but vision often does not improve. In addition, systemic chemotherapy appropriate to the particular type of leukemia almost always is required in these cases.

REFERENCES

1. Bach C, Seefelder M: *Atlas zur Entwicklungsgeschehen der Menschen Auges.* Leipzig: Wilhelm Engelmann, 1914.
2. Rabl L: *Über der Bau und Entwicklung der Linse.* Leipzig: Wilhelm Engelmann, 1930.
3. Noden D: Periocular mesenchyme: Neural crest and mesodermal interactions, in Jakobiec F (ed): *Ocular Anatomy, Embryology and Teratology.* Philadelphia: Harper & Row, 1982, 97–120.
4. Yamasuki N: Embryologic development of lens substance. *Yokohama Med Bull 1957;8:251–257.*
5. Kupfer C, Kaiser–Kupfer MI: A new hypothesis on anterior chamber developmental anomalies with glaucoma. *Trans Ophthalmol Soc UK 1978;98:213–217.*
6. Barber A: *Embryology of the Human Eye.* St. Louis: CV Mosby, 1955.
7. Mann I: Development of the human retina. *Am J Ophthalmol 1928;II:515–523.*
8. Versari I: Hyaloid vessel growth and remodeling. *Ric Morfol 1923;3:1–16.*
9. Michaelson I: The mode of development of the vascular system of the retina and some observations on its significance for certain retinal diseases. *Trans Ophthalmol Soc UK 1948;68:137–193.*
10. Balazs E: Fine structure of developing vitreous. *Int Ophthalmol Clin 1975;15:53–71.*
11. Gartner J: Elektron microskopische Untersuchungen zur Struktur der Zonule beim Rittenembryo. *Berl Zusammenkunft Dtsch Ophthalmol Ges 1968;69:551–561.*
12. Breathnach A, Wyllie L: Ultrastructure of retinal pigment epithelium of the human fetus. *J Ultrastruct Res 1966;16:584–593.*
13. Lercke W: Elektronmikroskopische Beobachtungen an der Bruckschen Membran des menschlichen Auges. *Berl Zusammenkunft Dtsch Ophthalmol Ges 1963;65:384–392.*
14. Kanazawa S: Electron microscopic study of the human fetal optic nerve. *Nippon Ganka Gakkai Zasshi 1969;73:1330–1342.*
15. Wulle K-G: The development of the productive and drainage system of the aqueous humor in the human eye. *Adv Ophthalmol 1972;26:269–275.*
16. Anderson H, Ehlers N, Matthiessen M, Claesson M: Histochemistry and development of the human eyelids II. *Acta Ophthalmol 1967;45:288–291.*

CHAPTER 1
OCULAR EMBRYOLOGY

1. Robinson RJ: Assessment of gestational age by neurologic examination. *Arch Dis Child 1966;41:437-443.*
2. Goldhammer Y: Paradoxical pupillary light reaction, in Smith JL (ed): *Neuro-ophthalmology Update.* New York: Masson, 1977, 39-42.
3. Yee RD, Balon RW, Hanrubia Y: Study of congenital nystagmus. *Br J Ophthalmol, 1980;64:926-930.*
4. Albin RV, Salpatek P: Saccadic localization of peripheral targets by the very young human infant. *Percep Psychophys 1975;17:293-297.*
5. Gorman JJ, Cogan DG, Gellis SS: An apparatus for grading the visual acuity of infants on the basis of opticokinetic nystagmus. *Pediatrics 1957;9:1088-1091.*
6. Berlyne DE: The influence of the albedo and complexity of stimulus on visual fixation in the human infant. *Br J Psychol 1958;49:315-318.*
7. Marg E, Freeman DN, Peltzman P, Goldstein PJ: Visual acuity development in human infants: evoked potential measurements. *Invest Ophthalmol Vis Sci 1976;15:150-154.*
8. Beller R, Hoyt CS, Marg E, Odom JV: Good visual fixation after neonatal surgery for congenital monocular cataracts. *Am J Ophthalmol 1981;91:559-564.*
9. Lombrosco CT, Duffy FH, Ross RM: Selective suppression of cerebral evoked potentials to patterned light in amblyopia exanopsia. *Electroenceph Clin Neurophysiol 1969;27:238-243.*
10. Spelmann R, Gross RA, Ho SU, et al: Visual evoked potentials and postmortem findings in a case of cortical blindness. *Ann Neurol 1977;2:531-534.*

CHAPTER 2
EVALUATING VISION IN PREVERBAL AND PRELITERATE INFANTS AND CHILDREN

11. Fantz RL: Pattern vision in young infants. *Psychol Res 1958;8:43-50.*

12. Atkinson J, Bradick O, Moar K: Development of contrast sensitivity in the first three months of life in the human infant. *Vis Res 1977;17:1057-1060.*

13. Dobson V, Mayer DL, Lee CP: Visual acuity screening of preterm infants. *Invest Ophthalmol Vis Sci 1980;19:1498-1503.*

14. Teller D, McDonald M, Preston K, et al: Assessment of visual acuity in infants and children: the acuity card procedure. *Dev Med Child Neurol 1986;28:779-784.*

15. Hollenberg MJ, Spira AW: Human retinal development: ultrastructure of the retina. *Am J Anat 1973;137:357-369.*

16. Magoon EH, Robb RM: Development of myelin in human optic nerve and tract. A light and electron microscopic study. *Arch Ophthalmol 1981;99:655-664.*

17. Mellor DH, Fielder AR: Dissociated visual development: electrodiagnostic studies in infants who are 'slow to see.' *Dev Med Clin Neurol 1980;22:307-314.*

18. Lambert SR, Kriss A, Taylor D: Delayed visual development. *Ophthalmology 1989;96:524-529.*

CHAPTER 3
ANATOMY
AND PHYSIOLOGY

1. Gilbert PW: The origin and development of the human extrinsic ocular muscle. *Contrib Embryol Carnegie Inst 1957;36:59–78.*

2. Mann I: *The Development of the Human Eye,* ed 2. New York: Grune & Stratton, 1950.

3. Koornneef L: The development of the connective tissue in the human orbit. *Acta Morphol Neerl Scand 1976;14:263–290.*

4. Duke–Elder S, Wybar KC: *System of Ophthalmology.* Vol 11. *The Anatomy of the Visual System.* St. Louis: CV Mosby, 1961.

5. Howe L: *The Muscles of the Eye.* New York: Putnam, 1907.

6. Whitnall SE: *The Anatomy of the Human Orbit.* London: Oxford Medical Publications, 1921.

7. Wolff E: *Anatomy of the Eye and Orbit,* ed 5. Revised by RJ Last. Philadelphia: WB Saunders, 1961.

8. Hesser C: Der Bindegewebsapparat und die glatte Muskulatur der Orbita beim Menschen im normalen Zustande. *Anatom Hefte 1913;49:1–302.*

9. Fuchs E: Beitrage zur normalen Anatomie des Augapfels. *Graefes Arch Clin Exp Ophthalmol 1884;30:1–60.*

10. Volkmann AW: Zur mechanik der Augenmuskeln. *Berl Verheilk Konige Sachs Ges Wochenschr 1869;20:28–69.*

11. Schneller: Anatomisch-physiologische Untersuchungen über die Augennuskeln Neugeborener. *Graefes Arch Clin Exp Ophthalmol 1899;41:178–226.*

12. Tillaux P: *Traite d'Anatomie Topographique,* ed 6. Paris: Asselin et Houzeau, 1890, 166.

13. Fink WH: A study of the anatomical variations in the attachments of the oblique muscles of the eyeball. *Trans Am Acad Ophthalmol Otolaryngol 1947;7:500–513.*

14. Fink WH: *Surgery of the Oblique Muscles of the Eye.* St. Louis: CV Mosby, 1951.

15. Muhlendyck H: Wachstum und Lange der ausseren Augenmuskeln. *Berl Dtsch Ophthalmol Ges 1978;75:449–452.*

16. Tenon JR: *Mémoires et d'Observations sur l'Anatomie, la Pathologie et la Chirurgie, et Principalement sur l'Organe de l'Oeil.* Paris: Nyon, 1806, 193–203.

17. Koornneef L: Details of the orbital connective tissue system in the adult. *Acta Morphol Neerl Scand 1977;15:1–34.*

18. Valu L: Uber die normale Struktur und Alternenderungen der Bindegewebsfasern der aussern Augenmuskeln. *Graefes Arch Clin Exp Ophthalmol 1976;169:272–284.*

19. Wohlfart G: Untersuchungen uber die Gruppierring von Muskelfasern verschiedener Grosse und Struktur innerhalb der primaren Muskelfaserbundel in der Skeletmuskulatur, sowie Beobachtungen uber die Inner-

vation diesen Bundel. *Z Mikrosk Anat Forsch 1935;37:621–642.*

20. Thulin I: Histologie des muscles oculaires chez l'homme et les singes. *Compt Rend Soc Biol 1914;76:490–493.*

21. Dietert SE: The demonstration of different types of muscle fibers in human extraocular muscle by electron microscopy and cholinesterase staining. *Invest Ophthalmol 1965;4:51–63.*

22. Brandt DE, Leeson CR: Structural differences of fast and slow fibers in human extraocular muscle. *Am J Ophthalmol 1966;62:478–487.*

23. Hess A: The structure of slow and fast extrafusal muscle fibers in the extraocular muscles and their nerve endings in guinea pigs. *J Cell Comp Physiol 1961;58:63–80.*

24. Hess A, Pilar G: Slow fibers in the extraocular muscles of the cat. *J Physiol (Lond) 1963;169:780–798.*

25. Mayr R: Structure and distribution of fiber types in the external eye muscles of the rat. *Tissue Cell 1971;3:433–462.*

26. Pachter BR, Davidowitz J, Breinin GM: Light and electron microscopic serial analysis of mouse extraocular muscle: morphology, innervation and topographical organization of component fiber populations. *Tissue Cell 1976;8:547–560.*

27. Martinez AJ, Hay S, McNeer KW: Extraocular muscles, light microscopy and ultrastructural features. *Acta Neuropathol (Berl) 1976;34:237–253.*

28. Cheng K: Cholinesterase activity in human extraocular muscles. *Jpn J Ophthalmol 1963;7:174–183.*

29. Hess A: Further morphological observations of "en plaque" and "en grappe" nerve endings on mammalian extrafusal muscle fibers with the cholinesterase technique. *Rev Can Biol 1962;21:241–248.*

30. Mukuno K: Fine structure of the human extraocular muscles. Part 3. Neuromuscular junctions in the normal human extraocular muscles. *Acta Soc Ophthalmol Jpn 1968;72:104–121.*

31. Ringel SP, Wilson WB, Barden MT, Kaiser KK: Histochemistry of human extraocular muscle. *Arch Ophthalmol 1978;96:1067–1072.*

31. Cooper S, Daniel PM: Muscle spindles in human extrinsic eye muscles. *Brain 1949;72:1–24.*

32. Merrillees NCR, Sunderland S, Haylow W: Neuromuscular spindles in the extraocular muscles in man. *Anat Rec 1950;108:23–30.*

33. Ruskel GL, Wilson J: Spiral nerve endings and dapple motor end plates in monkey extra-ocular muscles. *J Anat (Lond) 1983;136:85–95.*

34. Ciaccio GV: Sur les plaques nerveuses finales dans des vértibres. *Arch Ital Biol 1891;14:31–57.*

35. Sas J, Appeltauer C: Atypical muscle spindles in the extrinsic eye muscles of man. *Acta Anat 1963;55:311–322.*

36. Wolter J: Morphology of the sensory nerve apparatus in striated muscle of the human eye. *Arch Ophthalmol 1955;53:201–207.*

37. Cooper S, Eccles JC: The isometric responses of mammalian muscles. *J Physiol (Lond) 1930;69:377–385.*

38. Duke–Elder WS, Duke–Elder PM: The contraction of the extrinsic muscles of the eye by choline and nicotine. *Proc R Soc (Ser B) 1930;107:332–343.*

39. Goldberg SJ, Lennerstrand G, Hall CD: Motor unit responses in the lateral rectus muscle of the cat: intracellular current injection of abducens nucleus neurons. *Acta Physiol Scand 1976;96:58–63.*

40. Lennerstrand G: Motor units in eye muscles, in Lennerstrand G, Bach-y-Rita P (eds): *Basic Mechanisms of Ocular Motility and Their Clinical Implications.* Oxford: Pergamon Press, 1975, 119–143.

41. Fuchs AF, Luschei ES: Development of isometric tension in simian extraocular muscle. *J Physiol (Lond) 1971;219:155–166.*

42. Barmack NH, Bell CC, Rence BG: Tension and rate of tension development during isometric responses of extraocular muscle. *J Neurophysiol 1971;34:1072–1079.*

43. Robinson DA, O'Meara DM, Scott AB, Collins CC: Mechanical components of human eye movements. *J Appl Physiol 1969;26:548–553.*

44. Collins CC, Scott AB, O'Meara D: Muscle tension during unrestrained human eye movements. *J Physiol (Lond) 1975;245:351–369.*

45. Collins CC: The human oculomotor control system, in Lennerstrand G, Bach-y-Rita P (eds): *Basic Mechanisms of Ocular Motility and Their Clinical Implications*. Oxford: Pergamon Press, 1975, 145–180.

46. Collins CC: Orbital mechanics, in Bach-y-Rita P, Collins CC, Hyde JE (eds): *The Control of Eye Movements*. New York: Academic Press, 1971, 283–325.

47. Robinson DA: The mechanics of human saccadic eye movement. *J Physiol (Lond) 1964;174:245–264.*

48. Park R, Park G: The center of ocular rotation in the horizontal plane. *Am J Physiol 1933;104:545–552.*

49. Fry GA, Hill WW: The center of rotation of the eye. *Am J Optom 1962;39:581–595.*

50. Donders FC: Beitrag zur Lehre von den Bewegungen des menschlichen Auges. *Holl Beitr Anatom Physiol Wissenschr 1846;1:105–145, 379–383.*

51. Westheimer G, McKee SP: Failure of Donder's law during smooth pursuit eye movements. *Vis Res 1973;13:2145–2153.*

52. Listing JB, cited in Reute CGT: *Lehrbuch der Ophthalmologie fur Aerzte und Studirende*, Vol 1, ed 2. Braunschweig: F Vieveg & Sohn, 1855, 37 (Listing did not publish his law).

53. Landolt E: Table of torsion measurements with convergence in the horizontal plane and in planes above and below. Cited in Aubert H: physiologische optik, in Graefe A, Saemisch T (eds): *Handbuch der Gesammten Augenheilkunde*, Vol 2. Leipzig: Engelmann, 1876, 662.

54. Quereau JVD: Rolling of the eye around its visual axis during normal movements. *Arch Ophthalmol 1955;53:807–810.*

55. Nakayama K: Coordination of extraocular muscles, in Lennerstrand G, Bach-y-Rita P (eds): *Basic Mechanisms of Ocular Motility and Their Clinical Implications*. Oxford: Pergamon Press, 1975, 193–207.

56. Goodwin AW, Fender DH: Recognition of component differences in two-dimensional oculomotor tracking tasks. *Vis Res 1973;13:1905–1913.*

57. Robinson DA: Oculomotor unit behavior in the monkey. *J Neurophysiol 1970;33:393–404.*

58. Schiller PH: The discharge charactenstics of single units in the oculomotor and abducens nuclei of the unanesthetized monkey. *Exp Brain Res 1970;10:347–362.*

59. Henneman E, Somjen G, Carpenter DO: Functional significance of cell size in spinal motoneurons. *J Neurophysiol 1965;28:560–580.*

60. Henneman E, Somjen G, Carpenter DO: Excitability and inhibitability of motoneurons of different sizes. *J Neurophysiol 1965;28:599.*

61. Strachan IM, Brown BH: Electromyography of extraocular muscles in Duane's syndrome. *Br J Ophthalmol 1972;56:594–599.*

62. Sherrington CS: Experimental note on two movements of the eye. *J Physiol 1894;17:27–29.*

63. Hering E: *Die Lehre vom Binocularen Sehen*. Leipzig: Engelmann, 1868. English translation by Bridgeman B, Stark L: *The Theory of Binocular Vision*. New York: Plenum, 1977.

64. Bahill AT, Cuiffreda KJ, Kenyon R, Stark L: Dynamic and static violations of Herring's Law of equal innervation. *Am J Optom Physiol Opt 1976;53:786–796.*

65. Krewson WE: The action of the extraocular muscles. *Trans Am Ophthalmol Soc 1950;48:443–486.*

66. Boeder P: The co-operation of extraocular muscles. *Am J Ophthalmol 1961;51:469–481.*

67. Robinson DA: A quantitative analysis of extraocular muscle cooperation and squint. *Invest Ophthalmol 1975;14:801–825.*

68. Miller JM, Robinson DA: A model of the mechanics of binocular alignment. *Comput Biomed Res 1984;17:436–470.*

69. von Helmholtz H: *Handbuch der Physiologischen Optik*, ed 3. Hamburg: Voss, 1910. English translation by Southall JPC for the Optical Society of America, 1925.

70. Robinson DA: The functional behavior of the peripheral ocular motor apparatus: a review. Disorders of ocular motility, neurophysiological and clinical aspects, in Kommerell G (ed): *Symposium of the Deutsches*

Ophthalmologischen Gesellschaft, Disorders of Ocular Motility, April 1977, Freiburg. Munich: Bergman, 1978, 43–61.

1. Tscherning H: *Optique Physiologique.* Paris: Georges Carre et C. Naud, 1898.
2. Donders FC: *On the Anomalies of Accommodation and Refraction of the Eye.* London: The New Sydenham Society, 1864.
3. Brodie SE: Photographic calibration of the Hirschberg test. *Invest Ophthalmol Vis Sci 1987;28:736–742.*
4. Krimsky E: The binocular examination of the young child. *Am J Ophthalmol 1943;26:624–625.*
5. Guyton DL: Remote optical systems for ophthalmic examinations. *Trans Am Ophthalmol Soc 1986;84:869–919.*
6. Ludvigh E: Amount of eye movement objectively perceptible to the unaided eye. *Am J Ophthalmol 1949;32:649–650.*
7. Thompson JT, Guyton DL: Ophthalmic prisms: measurement errors and how to minimize them. *Ophthalmology 1983;90:204–210.*
8. Kestenbaum A: *Clinical Methods of Neuro-Ophthalmic Examination,* ed 2. New York: Grune & Stratton, 1961.
9. Ellerbrock VJ: Experimental investigations of vertical fusional movements. *Am J Optom 1949;26:327–333.*
10. Hofmann FB, Bielschowsky A: Die Verwertung der Kopneigung zur Diagnose der Augenmuskellahmungen. *Graefes Arch Ophthalmol 1900;51:174–185.*
11. Ellerbrock VJ: The aftereffect of aniseikonia on the ampiltude of vertical divergence. *Am J Optom 1952;29:403–408.*

CHAPTER 4
EVALUATION OF OCULAR ALIGNMENT AND EYE MOVEMENTS

1. Adler FH: *Physiology of the Eye.* St. Louis: CV Mosby, 1959.
2. Burian HM: The sensorial retinal relationships in comitant strabismus. *Arch Ophthalmol 1947;37:336–340.*
3. Jampolsky A: Characteristics of suppression in strabismus. *Arch Ophthalmol 1955;54:683–689.*
4. Parks MM: The monofixation syndrome, in Dabezies O: *Strabismus. Transactions New Orleans Academy of Ophthalmology.* St. Louis: CV Mosby, 1971.
5. Arthur BW, Smith JT, Scott WE: Long term stability of alignment in the monofixation syndrome. *J Pediatr Ophthalmol Strabismus 1989;26:224.*
6. Parks MM: Stereoacuity as an indicator of bifixation, in Knapp P: *Strabismus Symposium.* New York: Karger, 1968.
7. Ogle KN: Fixation disparity. *Am Orthop J 1954;4:35–40.*

CHAPTER 5
SENSORY ADAPTATIONS IN STRABISMUS

1. Wheatstone C: Contributions to the physiology of vision. Part I. On some remarkable, and hitherto unobserved, phenomena of binocular vision. *R Soc Lond Philos Trans 1838;128:371–394.*
2. Mitchell DE: Retinal disparity and diplopia. *Vis Res 1966;6:441–451.*
3. Mitchell DE: Properties of stimuli eliciting vergence eye movements and stereopsis. *Vis Res 1970;10:145–162.*
4. Schor CE, Tyler CW: Spatio-temporal properties of Panum's fusional area. *Vis Res 1981;21:683–692.*
5. Wheatstone C: Contributions to the physiology of vision. Part II. On some remarkable, and hitherto unobserved, phenomena of binocular vision (continued). *London, Edinburgh, Dublin Phil Mag J Sci 1852;3:504–523.*
6. Hillebrand F: *Lehre von den Gesichtsempfindungen.* Vienna: Springer, 1929.
7. Ogle KN: *Researches in Binocular Vision.* Philadelphia: WB Saunders, 1950.
8. Amigo G: A vertical horopter. *Optica Acta 1974;21:277–292.*
9. Nakayama K: Geometrical and physiological aspects of depth perception, in Benton S (ed): *Three Dimensional Imaging. (Proc Soc Photo-Optical Instrument Engineers 1977;120:2–9.)*

CHAPTER 6
EVALUATION OF SENSORY STATUS IN STRABISMUS

10. Julesz B: Binocular depth perception of computer-generated patterns. *Bell Syst Tech J* 1967;46:1203–1221.

11. Julesz B: *Foundations of Cyclopean Perception.* Chicago: University of Chicago Press, 1971.

12. Ogle KN, Weil MP: Stereoscopic vision and the duration of the stimulus. *Arch Ophthalmol* 1958;48:4–12.

13. Ogle KN: Disparity limits of stereopsis. *Arch Ophthalmol* 1952;48:50–60.

14. Ogle KN: On the limits of stereoscopic vision. *J Exp Psychol* 1952;44:253–259.

15. Blakemore C: The range and scope of binocular depth discrimination in man. *J Physiol (Lond)* 1970;211:599–622.

16. Rawlings SC, Shipley T: Stereoscopic acuity and horizontal angular distance from fixation. *J Opt Soc Am* 1969;59:991–993.

17. Mitchell DE, Blakemore C: Binocular depth perception and the corpus callosum. *Vis Res* 1970;10:49–54.

18. McKee SP, Levi DM, Bowne SF: The imprecision of stereopsis. *Vis Res* 1990;30:1763–1779.

19. Bishop PO: Stereopsis and the random element in the organization of the striate cortex. *Proc R Soc Lond [B]* 1979;204:415–434.

20. Joshua DE, Bishop PO: Binocular single vision and depth discrimination. Receptive field disparities for central and peripheral vision and binocular interaction on peripheral single units in cat striate cortex. *Exp Brain Res* 1970;10:389–416.

21. Barlow HB, Blakemore C, Pettigrew JD: The neural mechanism of binocular depth discrimination. *J Physiol Lond* 1967;193:327–342.

22. Fischer B, Poggio GF: Depth sensitivity of binocular cortical neurons of behaving monkeys. *Proc R Soc Lond [B]* 1979;204:409–414.

23. Poggio GF, Fischer B: Binocular interaction and depth sensitivity in striate and prestriate cortex of behaving rhesus monkey. *J Neurophysiol* 1977;40:1392–1405.

24. Freeman RD, Ohzawa I: On the neurophysiological organization of binocular vision.*Vis Res* 1990;30:1661–1676.

25. Richards W: Stereopsis and stereoblindness. *Exp Brain Res* 1970;10:380–388.

26. Richards W: Anomalous stereoscopic depth perception. *J Opt Soc Am* 1971;61:410–414.

27. Richards W, Regan D: A stereo field map with implications for disparity processing. *Invest Ophthalmol* 1973;12:904–909.

28. Jones R: Anomalies of disparity detection in the human visual system. *J Physiol (Lond)* 1977;264:621–640.

29. Nakayama K: DaVinci stereopsis: depth and subjective occluding contours from unpaired image points. *Vis Res* 1990;30:1811–1825.

30. Regan D, Beverley KI, Cynader M: Stereoscopic subsystems for position in depth and for motion in depth. *Proc R Soc Lond [B]* 1979;204:485–501.

31. Pirenne MH: Binocular and uniocular thresholds in vision. *Nature* 1943;152:698–699.

32. Horowitz MW: An analysis of the superiority of binocular over monocular visual acuity. *J Exp Psychol* 1949;39:581–596.

33. Blake R, Sloane M, Fox R: Further developments in binocular summation. *Percep Psychophys* 1981;30:266–276.

34. Travers T: Suppression of vision in squint and its association with retinal correspondence and amblyopia. *Br J Ophthalmol* 1938;22:557–604.

35. Bagolini B: Presentazione di una sbarra di filtri a densita scalare assorbenti i raggi luminosi. *Boll Ocul* 1957;36:638–651.

36. Aulhorn E: Phasedifferenz-Haploskopie. Eine neue Methode zur Trennung der optischen Eindrucke beider Augen. *Klin Monatsbl Augenheilk* 1966;148:540–544.

37. Cüppers C: Moderne Schielbehandlung. *Klin Monatsbl Augenheilk* 1956;129:579–604.

38. Lang J: A new stereotest. *J Pediatr Ophthalmol Strabismus* 1983;20:72–74.

REFERENCES

1. Jampolsky A: Ocular divergence mechanisms. *Trans Am Ophthalmol Soc 1970;68:730–822.*
2. Cass EE: Divergent strabismus. *Br J Ophthalmol 1937;21:538–559.*
3. Gregersen E: The polymorphous exo patient. Analysis of 231 consecutive cases. *Acta Ophthalmol 1969;47:579–590.*
4. Duane A: A new classification of the motor anomalies of the eyes based upon physiological principles, together with their symptoms, diagnosis and treatment. *Ann Ophthalmol Otolaryngol 1896;5:969–1008; 1897;6:84–122; 1897;6:247–260.*
5. Burian HM, Smith DR: Comparative measurement of exodeviations at twenty and one hundred feet. *Trans Am Ophthalmol Soc 1971;69:188–199.*
6. Burian HM, Franceschetti AT: Evaluation of diagnostic methods for the classification of exodeviations. *Trans Am Ophthalmol Soc 1970;68:56–71.*
7. Wirtschafter JD, von Noorden GK: The effect of increasing luminance on exodeviations. *Invest Ophthalmol Vis Sci 1964;3:549.*
8. Jampolsky A: Characteristics of suppression in strabismus. *Arch Ophthalmol 1955;54:683–696.*
9. Pratt–Johnson J, Wee HS: Suppression associated with exotropia. *Can J Ophthalmol 1969;4:136–144.*
10. Campos EC: Binocularity in comitant strabismus: binocular visual field studies. *Doc Ophthalmol 1982;53:249–281.*
11. Sidikaro Y, von Noorden GK: Observations in sensory heterotropia. *J Pediatr Ophthalmol Strabismus 1982;19:12–19.*
12. Sireteanu R: Binocular vision in strabismic humans with alternating fixation. *Vision Res 1982;22:889–896.*
13. Moore S, Cohen RL: Congenital exotropia. *Am Orthopt J 1985;35:68–70.*
14. von Noorden GK, Brown DJ, Parks M: Associated convergence and accommodative insufficiency. *Doc Ophthalmol 1973;34:393–403.*
15. Hardesty HH, Boynton JR, Keenan JP: Treatment of intermittent exotropia. *Arch Ophthalmol 1978;96:268–274.*
16. Haase W, deDecker W: Binokulare sensorische Defekte beim Strabismus divergens intermittens. *Klin Monatsbl Augenheilk 1981;179:81–84.*
17. Raab EL, Parks MM: Recession of the lateral recti: Early and late postoperative alignments. *Arch Ophthalmol 1969;82:203–208.*
18. Bedrossian EH: Surgical results following the recession-resection operation for intermittent exotropia. *Am J Ophthalmol 1962;53:351–359.*
19. Moore S: The prognostic value of lateral gaze measurements in intermittent exotropia. *Am Orthopt J 1969;19:69–71.*
20. Hermann JS: Surgical therapy for convergence insufficiency. *J Pediatr Ophthalmol 1981;18:28–31.*
21. Parinaud H: Clinique nerveuse: Paralysie des mouvements associes des yeux. *Arch Neurol (Paris) 1883;5:145–172.*
22. Duane A: Congenital deficiency of abduction associated with impairment of adduction, retraction movements, contraction of the palpebral fissure and oblique movements of the eye. *Arch Ophthalmol 1905;4:133–159.*
23. Huber A: Electrophysiology of the retraction syndrome. *Br J Ophthalmol 1974;58:293–300.*
24. Scott AB: Upshoot and downshoot, in Sousa–Dias C (ed): *Smith–Kettlewell Symposium on Basic Sciences in Strabismus.* Guaruja, Brazil, October 16–17, 1976.
25. Miller JM, Robinson DA: A model of the mechanics of binocular alignment. *Comput Biomed Res 1984;17:436–470.*
26. Hotchkiss MG, Miller NR, Clark AW, Green WM: Bilateral Duane's retraction syndrome. A clinical-pathological case report. *Arch Ophthalmol 1980;98:870–874.*
27. Hoyt WF, Nachtigäller H: Anomalies of the ocular motor nerves: Neuroanatomic correlates of paradoxical innervation in Duane's syndrome and related congenital ocular motor disorder. *Am J Ophthalmol 1965;60:443–448.*
28. Miller NR, Kiel SM, Green W, Clask AW: Unilateral Duane's retraction syndrome (type 1). *Arch Ophthalmol 1982;100:1468–1472.*

CHAPTER 7
EXOTROPIA

CHAPTER 8
ESOTROPIA

1. Archer SM, Sondhy N, Helveston EM: Strabismus in infancy. *Ohpthalmology 1989;96:133–138.*
2. Ing MR: Early surgical alignment for congenital esotropia. *Trans Am Ophthalmol Soc 1981;79:625–633.*
3. Waardenburg PJ: Squint and heredity. *Doc Ophthalmol 1954;7:422–494.*
4. Costenbader F: Infantile esotropia. *Trans Ophthalmol Soc UK 1970;59:397–429.*
5. Hiles DA, Watson A, Biglan AW: Characteristics of infantile esotropia following early bimedial rectus recession. *Arch Ophthalmol 1980; 98:697–703.*
6. Helveston EM: Dissociated vertical deviation, a clinical and laboratory study. *Trans Am Ophthalmol Soc 1981; 78:734–779.*
7. von Noorden GK: The nystagmus blockage syndrome. *Trans Am Ophthalmol Soc 1976; 74:220–236.*
8. Ing MR: Early surgical alignment for congenital esotropia. *Trans Am Ophthalmol Soc 1981; 79:625–663.*
9. Szymd SM, Nelson LB, Calhoun JC, Spratt C: Large bimedial rectus recessions in congenital esotropia. *Br J Ophthalmol 1985; 69:271–274.*
10. Magoon EH: Infantile esotropes treated under age one with botulinum chemodenervation routinely show motor fusion. *Invest Ophthalmol Vis Sci 1984; 25:74–78.*
11. Baker JD, Parks MM: Early-onset accommodative esotropia. *Am J Ophthalmol 1980; 90:11–18.*
12. Burian M: Cyclic esotropia, in Allen H (ed): *Strabismus Ophthalmic Symposium II.* St. Louis: CV Mosby, 1958.
13. Costenbader F, Manuel D: Cyclic esotropia. *Arch Ophthalmol 1964; 71:150–154.*
14. Richter C: *Biologic Clocks in Medicine and Psychiatry.* Springfield: CC Thomas, 1965.
15. Henderson JC: The congenital facial diplegia syndrome: Clinical features, pathology and aetiology. A review of 61 cases. *Brain 1939; 62:381–403.*
16. Parks MM: Ophthalmoplegic syndromes and trauma, in Duane TD, Jaeger E (eds): *Clinical Ophthalmology.* Philadelphia: JB Lippincott, 1985.
17. Gadoth N, Biedner B, Torde G: Möbius syndrome and Poland anomaly: case report and review of the literature. *J Pediatr Ophthalmol Strabismus 1978;16:374–376.*
18. Hotchkiss MG, Miller NR, Clark AW, et al: Bilateral Duane's retraction syndrome. A clinical-pathologic report. *Arch Ophthalmol 1980; 98:870–874.*
19. Huber A: Electrophysiology of the retraction syndrome. *Br J Ophthalmol 1974;58:293–300.*
20. Pressman SH, Scott WE: Surgical treatment of Duane's syndrome. *Ophthalmology 1986;93:29–38.*

CHAPTER 9
OBLIQUE MUSCLE
DYSFUNCTIONS

1. Gobin MH: Sagitallization of the oblique muscles as a possible cause for the "A," "V," and "X" phenomena. *Br J Ophthalmol 1968;52:13–21.*
2. Wilson ME, Parks MM: Primary inferior oblique overaction in congenital esotropia, accommodative esotropia, and intermittent exotropia. *Ophthalmology 1989;96:7–11.*
3. Capo H, Mallette RA, Guyton DL: Overacting of oblique muscles in exotropia: A mechanical explanation. *J Pediatr Ophthalmol Strabismus 1988;25:281–285.*
4. Elliot RL, Mankin SJ: Anterior transposition of the inferior oblique. *J Pediatr Ophthalmol Strabismus 1981;18:3–7.*
5. Del Monte MA, Parks MM: Denervation and extirpation of the inferior oblique. An improved weakening procedure for marked overaction. *Ophthalmology 1983;90:1178–1181.*
6. Diamond GR, Parks MM: The effect of superior oblique weakening procedures on primary position horizontal alignment. *J Pediatr Ophthalmol Strabismus 1981;18:1–3.*

1. Urrets–Zavalia A, Solares–Zamora J, Olmos H: Anthropological studies on the nature of cyclovertical squint. *Br J Ophthalmol 1961;45:578–596.*
2. Helveston E: *Atlas of Strabismus Surgery.* St. Louis: CV Mosby, 1977, 4.
3. Knapp P: Vertically incomitant horizontal strabismus: The so-called "A" and "V" syndromes. *Trans Am Ophthalmol Soc 1969;67:304–310.*
4. Romano P, Roholt P: Measured graduated recessions of the superior oblique muscles. *J Pediatr Ophthalmol Strabismus 1983;20:134–139.*

CHAPTER 10
ALPHABET PATTERN STRABISMUS

CHAPTER 11
CONGENITAL, COMITANT, AND PARETIC VERTICAL STRABISMUS

1. Duke–Elder S, Wybar K: *Systems of Ophthalmology,* Vol 6. *Ocular Motility and Strabismus.* St. Louis: CV Mosby, 1973, 736–740.
2. Khodadoust AA, vonNoorden GK: Bilateral vertical retraction syndrome: a family study. *Arch Ophthalmol 1967;78:606–612.*
3. Bielschowsky A: Disturbances of the vertical motor muscles of the eyes. *Arch Ophthalmol 1938;20:175–200.*
4. Keane JR: Ocular skew deviation. *Arch Neurol 1975;32:185–190.*
5. Ellis FD, Helveston EM: Superior oblique palsy. *Int Ophthalmol Clin 1976;16:127–135.*
6. vonNoorden GK, Murray E, Wong SY: Superior oblique paralysis. A review of 270 cases. *Arch Ophthalmol 1986;104:1771–1776.*
7. Rucker CW: The causes of paralysis of the third, fourth, and sixth cranial nerves. *Am J Ophthalmol 1966;61:1293–1298.*
8. Rush JA, Younge BR: Paralysis of cranial nerves III, IV, and VI: causes and prognosis in 1,000 cases. *Arch Ophthalmol 1981;99:76–79.*
9. Knapp P: Diagnosis and surgical treatment of hypertropia. *Am Orthopt J 1971;21:29–37.*
10. Moore S, Stockbridge L: Diagnostic observation on acquired unilateral and bilateral superior oblique paresis, in Mein J, Bierlaagh JJ, Brummelkamp–Dons TEA (eds): *Orthoptics.* Amsterdam: Excerpta Medica, 1972, 266–269.
11. Kraft SP, Scott WE: Masked bilateral superior oblique palsy. Clinical features and diagnosis. *J Pediatr Ophthalmol Strabismus 1986;23:264–272.*
12. Hermann JS: Masked bilateral superior oblique paresis. *J Pediatr Ophthalmol Strabismus 1981;18:43–48.*
13. Robinson DA: Bielschowsky head-tilt test-II. Quantitative mechanics of the Bielschowsky head-tilt test. *Vis Res 1985;25:1983–1988.*
14. Jampolsky A: Management of acquired (adult) muscle palsies, in *Symposium on Neuro-Ophthalmology. Transactions of the New Orleans Academy of Ophthalmology.* St. Louis: CV Mosby, 1976, 148–167.
15. Parks MM: Isolated cyclovertical muscle palsy. *Arch Ophthalmol 1958;60:1027–1035.*
16. Helveston EM: Two-step for diagnosing paresis of vertically acting extraocular muscle. *Am J Ophthalmol 1967;64:914–915.*
17. Knapp P, Moore S: Diagnosis and surgical operations in superior oblique surgery. *Int Ophthalmol Clin 1976;16:137–149.*
18. Harada M, Ito Y: Surgical correction of cyclotropia. *Jpn J Ophthalmol 1964;8:88–96.*
19. Miller N: Solitary oculomotor nerve palsy in childhood. *Am J Ophthalmol 1977;83:106–111.*
20. Victor DI: The diagnosis of congenital unilateral third nerve palsy. *Brain 1976;99:711–718.*
21. Loewenfeld IE, Thompson HS: Oculomotor paresis with cyclic spasms. A critical review of the literature and a new case. *Surv Ophthalmol 1975;20:81–124.*
22. Heinze J: Cranial nerve avulsion and other neural injuries in road accidents. *Med J Aust 1969;2:1246–1249.*
23. Metz HS, Mazow M: Botulinum treatment of acute sixth and third nerve palsy. *Graefes Arch Clin Exp Ophthalmol 1988;226:141–144.*
24. Odel JG, Winterkorn JM, Behrens MM: The sleep test for myasthenia gravis. A safe alternative to Tensilon. *J Clin Neuro-Ophthalmol 1991;11:288–292.*

CHAPTER 12
OTHER VERTICAL STRABISMUS

1. Bielschowsky A: Die einseitigen und gegensinnigen ("dissoziierten") Vertikalbewegungen der Augen. *Graefes Arch Ophthalmol 1930;25: 493–553.*

2. MacDonald AL, Pratt-Johnson JA: The suppression patterns and sensory adaptations to dissociated vertical divergent strabismus. *Can J Ophthalmol 1974;9:113–119.*

3. Sprague JB, Moore S, Eggers HM, Knapp P: Dissociated vertical deviation. Treatment with the Faden operation of Cuppers. *Arch Ophthalmol 1980;98:465–468.*

4. vonNoorden GK: Indication of the posterior fixation suture. *Ophthalmology 1978;85:512–520.*

5. Magoon E, Cruciger M, Jampolsky A: Dissociated vertical deviation: an asymmetric condition treated with large bilateral superior rectus recession. *J Pediatr Ophthalmol Strabismus 1982;19:152–156.*

6. Parks MM: The weakening surgical procedures for eliminating overaction of the inferior oblique muscle. *Am J Ophthalmol 1972;73:107–122.*

7. Jampel RS, Fells P: Monocular elevation paresis caused by a central nervous system lesion. *Arch Ophthalmol 1968;80:45–55.*

8. Knapp P: The surgical treatment of double elevator paralysis. *Trans Am Ophthalmol Soc 1969;67:304–323.*

9. Brown HW: True and simulated superior oblique tendon sheath syndromes. *Doc Ophthalmol 1973;34:123–136.*

10. Moore AT, Walker J, Taylor D: Familial Brown's syndrome. *J Pediatr Ophthalmol Strabismus 1988;25:202.*

11. Zipf RF, Trokel SL: Simulated superior oblique tendon sheath syndrome following orbital floor fracture. *Am J Ophthalmol 1973;75:700–705.*

12. Hermann JS: Acquired Brown's syndrome of inflammatory origin. *Arch Ophthalmol 1978;96:1228–1232.*

13. Killian PJ, McClain B, Lawless OJ: Brown's syndrome. An unusual manifestaton of rheumatoid arthritis. *Arthritis Rheum 1977;20:1080–1084.*

14. Wang FM, Wertenbaker C, Behrens MM, Jacobs JJ: Acquired Brown's syndrome in children with juvenile rheumatoid arthritis. *Ophthalmology 1984;91:23–26.*

15. Girard LJ: Pseudoparalysis of the inferior oblique muscle. *South Med J 1956;49:342–346.*

16. Crawford JS, Orton R, Labow–Daily L: Late results of superior oblique muscle tenotomy in true Brown's syndrome. *Am J Ophthalmol 1980;89:824–829.*

17. Eustis HS, O'Reilly C, Crawford JS: Management of superior oblique palsy after surgery for true Brown's syndrome. *J Pediatr Ophthalmol Strabismus 1987;24:10–16.*

18. Brown HW: Congenital structural muscle anomalies, in Allen JH (ed): *Strabismus Ophthalmic Symposium.* St. Louis: CV Mosby, 1950: 205–236.

19. Harley RD, Rodrigues MM, Crawford JS: Congenital fibrosis of the extraocular muscles. *Trans Am Ophthalmol Soc 1978;76:197–226.*

20. Hansen E: Congenital general fibrosis of the extraocular muscles. *Acta Ophthalmol 1968;46:469–476.*

21. Hötte HHA: *Orbital Fractures.* Springfield, IL: Charles C Thomas, 1970.

22. Emery JM, vonNoorden GK, Schlernitzauer DA: Orbital floor fractures: long–term follow–up of cases with and without surgical repair. *Am J Ophthalmol 1972;74:299–306.*

23. Dunnington JH, Berke RN: Exophthalmos due to chronic orbital myositis. *Arch Ophthalmol 1943;30:446–466.*

24. Manor RS, Kurz O, Lewitus Z: Intraocular pressure in endocrinologic patients with exophthalmos. *Ophthalmologica 1974;168:241–252.*

25. Simonsz HJ, Kommerell G: Increased muscle tension and reduced elasticity of affected muscles in recent-onset Graves' disease caused primarily by active muscle contraction. *Doc Ophthalmol 1989;72:215–224.*

26. Ward DM: The heavy eye phenomenon. *Trans Ophthalmol Soc UK 1967;717–726.*

27. Johnson LV: Adherence syndrome: pseudoparalysis of the lateral or superior rectus muscle. *Arch Ophthalmol 1950;44:870–878.*

1. Yuodelis C, Hendrickson A: A qualitative and quantitative analysis of the human fovea during development. *Vision Res 1986;26:847–855.*
2. Hutenlocher PR, DeCourten C, Garey LJ, Van Der Loos H: Synaptogenesis in human visual cortex—evidence for synapse elimination during normal development. *Neurosci Lett 1982;33:247–252.*
3. LeVay S, Wiesel TN, Hubel DH: The development of ocular dominance columns in normal and visually deprived monkeys. *J Comp Neurol 1980;19:1–51.*
4. Derrington A: Effects of visual deprivation on the development of spatial frequency selectivity in kitten visual cortex. *Proc Physiol Soc 1980;33:62P.*
5. DeValois RL, Albrecht DG, Thorell LG: Spatial frequency selectivity of cells in macaque visual cortex. *Vision Res 1982;22:545–559.*
6. Wiesel TN, Hubel DH: Single-cell responses in striate cortex of kittens deprived of vision in one eye. *J Neurophysiol 1963;26:1003–1017.*
7. Hubel DH, Wiesel TN: Receptive fields of cells in striate cortex of very young, visually inexperienced kittens. *J Neurophysiol 1963;26: 994–1002.*
8. Hubel DH, Wiesel TN, LeVay S: Plasticity of ocular dominance columns in monkey striate cortex. *Phil Trans R Soc Lond (Biol) 1977;278:377–409.*
9. Guillery RW: Binocular competition in the control of geniculate cell growth. *J Comp Neurol 1972;144:117–130.*
10. Eggers HM, Blakemore C: Physiological basis of anisometropic amblyopia. *Science 1978;201:264–267.*
11. Hubel DH, Wiesel TN: The period of susceptibility to the physiological effects of unilateral eye closure in kittens. *J Physiol (Lond) 1970; 206:419–436.*
12. Hubel DH, Wiesel TN: Binocular interaction in striate cortex of kittens reared with artificial squint. *J Neurophysiol 1965;28:1041–1059.*
13. Blakemore C: The conditions required for the maintenance of binocularity in the kitten's visual cortex. *J Physiol (Lond) 1976;261:423–444.*
14. Eggers HM, Gizzi MS, Movshon JA: Spatial properties of striate cortical neurons in esotropic macaques. *Invest Ophthalmol Vis Sci 1984;(suppl 25):278.*
15. Blakemore C: Genetic instructions and developmental plasticity in the kitten's visual cortex. *Phil Trans R Soc Lond [B] 1977;278:425–434.*
16. Mitchell DE, Freeman RD, Millodot M, Haegerstrom G: Meridional amblyopia: Evidence for modification of the visual system by early visual experience. *Vision Res 1973;13:535–558.*
17. Movshon JA, Eggers HM, Gizzi MS, et al: Effects of early unilateral blur on the macaque's visual system. III. Physiological observations. *J Neurosci 1987;7:1340–1351.*
18. von Noorden GK, Crawford MLJ, Middleditch PR: Effect of lid suture on retinal ganglion cells in Macaca mulatta. *Brain Res 1977; 122:437–444.*
19. Hendrickson AE, Movshon JA, Eggers HM, et al: Effects of early unilateral blur on the macaque's visual system. II. Anatomical observations. *J Neurosci 1987;7:1327–1339.*
20. Levitt JB, Movshon JA, Sherman SM, Spear PD: Effects of monocular deprivation on macaque LGN. *Invest Ophthalmol Vis Sci 1989;(suppl 30):296.*
21. von Noorden GK, Crawford MLJ, Levacy RA: The lateral geniculate nucleus in human anisometropic amblyopia. *Invest Ophthalmol Vis Sci 1983;24:788–790.*
22. Hendry SHC, Jones EG: Reduction in number of immunostained GABAergic neurons in deprived-eye dominance columns of monkey area 17. *Nature 1986;320:750–752.*
23. Demer JL, von Noorden GK, Volkow ND, Gould KL: Imaging of cerebral blood flow and metabolism in amblyopia by positron emission tomography. *Am J Ophthalmol 1988;105:337–347.*
24. Kushner BJ: Functional amblyopia associated with organic disease. *Am J Ophthalmol 1981;91:39–45.*

CHAPTER 13
AMBLYOPIA

25. Freeman RD, Bradley A: Monocularly deprived humans: nondeprived eye has supernormal vernier acuity. *J Neurophysiol 1980;43:1645–1653.*

26. Levi DM, Klein SA: Differences in vernier discrimination for gratings between strabismic and anisometropic amblyopes. *Invest Ophthalmol Vis Sci 1982;23:398–407.*

27. Gstalder RJ, Green DG: Laser interferometric acuity in amblyopia. *J Pediatr Ophthalmol 1971;8:251–256.*

28. Levi DM, Klein SA, Aitsebaomo AP: Vernier acuity, crowding and cortical magnification. *Vis Res 1985;25:963–977.*

29. Abraham SV: Accommodation in the amblyopic eye. *Am J Ophthalmol 1961;52:197–200.*

30. Ciuffreda KJ, Hokoda SC, Hung GK, Semmlow JL: Accommodative stimulus/response function in human amblyopia. *Doc Ophthalmol 1984;56:303–326.*

31. Bangerter A: *Amblyopiebehandlung,* ed 2. Basel: Karger, 1953.

32. von Noorden GK, Mackensen G: Phenomenology of eccentric fixation. *Am J Ophthalmol 1962;53:642–661.*

33. Cüppers C: Moderne Schielbehandlung. *Klin Monatsbl Augenheilk 1956;129:579–604.*

34. Aulhorn E: Die gegenseitige Beeinflussung abildungsgleicher Netzhaustellen bei normalen und gestortem Binocularsehen. *Doc Ophthalmol 1967;23:26–61.*

35. Francois J, Verriest G, Verluyten P: Comparison of the results of static and kinetic perimetry in the central region of the visual field of the amblyopic eye, in Arruga A (ed): *Strabismus.* (Symp. Giessen, August 1966.) Basel: Karger, 1968, 45–50.

36. von Noorden GK, Burian HM: Visual acuity in normal and amblyopic patients under reduced illumination. I. Behavior of visual acuity with and without neutral density filters. *Arch Ophthalmol 1959;61:533–535.*

37. Mackensen G: Das Fixationsverhalten amblyopischer Augen; Elektroculographicsche Untersuchungen. *Arch F Ophthal 1957;159:200–211.*

38. von Noorden GK, Burian HM: An electro-ophthalmographic study of the behavior of the fixation of amblyopic eyes in light- and dark-adapted states. A preliminary report. *Am J Ophthalmol 1958;46:68–72.*

39. Schor C: A directional impairment of eye movement control in strabismic amblyopia. *Invest Ophthalmol 1975;14:692–697.*

40. Bedell HE, Flom MC: Bilateral oculomotor abnormalities in strabismic amblyopes: evidence for a common central mechanism. *Doc Ophthalmol 1985;59:309–321.*

41. Awaya S, Miyake Y, Imaizumi Y, et al: Amblyopia in man suggestive of stimulus deprivation amblyopia. *Jpn J Ophthalmol 1973;17:69–82.*

42. Hess RF, France TD, Tulunay–Keesey U: Residual vision in humans who have been monocularly deprived of pattern stimulation in early life. *Exp Brain Res 1981;44:295–311.*

43. Harrad RA, Graham CM, Collin JR: Amblyopia and strabismus in congenital ptosis. *Eye 1988;2:625–627.*

44. Zipf R: Binocular fixation pattern. *Arch Ophthalmol 1976;94:401–405.*

45. von Noorden GK, Frank JW: Relationship between amblyopia and the angle of strabismus. *Am Orthop J 1976;26:31–33.*

46. Helveston EM: Relationship between degree of anisometropia and depth of amblyopia. *Am J Ophthalmol 1966;62:757–759.*

47. von Noorden GK, Avilla C, Sidikarno Y, LaRoche R: Latent nystagmus and strabismic amblyopia. *Am J Ophthalmol 1987;103:87–89.*

48. Hardesty HH: Occlusion amblyopia. Report of a case. *Arch Ophthalmol 1959;62:314-316.*

49. Vereecken EP, Brabant P: Prognosis for vision in amblyopia after loss of the good eye. *Arch Ophthalmol 1984;102:220–224.*

50. Haase W: Optische Penalization als therapeutisches Hilfsmittel beim frühkindlichen Strabismus. *Adv Ophthalmol 1978;35:26–44.*

51. Fletcher MC, Abbott W, Girard LJ, et al: Results of biostatistical study of the management of suppression amblyopia by intensive pleoptics versus conventional patching. *Am Orthopt J 1969;19:8–30.*

52. Campbell FW, Hess RF, Watson PG, Banks R: Preliminary results of a

physiologically based treatment of amblyopia. *Br J Ophthalmol 1978; 62:748–755.*

53. Eggers HM, Bunke A: An evaluation of the CAM vision stimulator. *Am Orthopt J 1982;31:13–18.*
54. Tytla ME, Labow–Daily LS: Evaluation of the CAM treatment for amblyopia: a controlled study. *Invest Ophthalmol Vis Sci 1981;20: 400–406.*
55. Mehdorn E, Mattheus S, Schuppe A, et al: Treatment for amblyopia with rotating gratings and subsequent occlusion: a controlled study. *Int Ophthalmol 1981;3:161–166.*
56. Sedan J:*Post-cure de l'Ambliope Medique.* Paris: Masson, 1958.
57. Fricker SJ, Kuperwaser MC, Stromberg AE, Goldman SG: Stripe therapy for amblyopia with a modified television game. *Arch Ophthalmol 1981;99:1596–1599.*
58. Vereecken EP, Brabant P: Prognosis for vision in amblyopia after the loss of the good eye. *Arch Ophthalmol 1984;102:220–224.*
59. Hamed LM, Glaser JS, Schatz NJ: Improvement of vision in the amblyopic eye following visual loss in the contralateral normal eye: a report of three cases. *Binoc Vis Quart 1991;6:97–100.*
60. Tommila V, Tarkkanen A:Incidence of loss of vision in the healthy eye in amblyopia. *Br J Ophthalmol 1981;65:575–577.*
61. Levi DM, Klein S: Hyperacuity and amblyopia. *Nature 1982; 298:268–270.*

CHAPTER 14
OTHER FORMS OF NONSURGICAL STRABISMUS MANAGEMENT

1. Sarniguet–Badoche J: Early medical treatment of strabismus, in Reinecke R (ed): *Strabismus II.* Orlando, FL: Grune & Stratton, 1984, 83–89.
2. Prism Adaptation Study Research Group: Efficacy of prism adaptation in the surgical management of acquired esotropia. *Arch Ophthalmol 1990;108:1248–1256.*
3. Berard P: Prisms: Their therapeutic use in strabismus, in *International Strabismus Symposium: An Evaluation of Present Status of Orthoptics, Pleoptics, and Related Diagnosis and Treatment Regimes.* New York: Karger, 1968, 339–344.
4. Scott A: Botulinum toxin injection of eye muscles to correct strabismus. *Trans Am Ophthalmol Soc 1981; 79:734–770.*
5. Biglan A, Burnstine R, Rogers G, Saunders R: Management of strabismus with botulinum A toxin. *Ophthalmology 1989;96:935–943.*
6. Lingua R: Sequelae of botulinum toxin injection. *Am J Ophthalmol 1985;100:305–307.*

CHAPTER 16
INTRODUCTION TO GENETICS

1. Thompson JS, Thompson MW: *Genetics in Medicine* (Chapter 2: The molecular structure and function of chromosomes and genes), ed 4. Philadelphia: WB Saunders, 1986, 29–43.
2. Thompson JS, Thompson MW: *Genetics in Medicine* (Chapter 3: The chromosomal basis of heredity), ed 4. Philadelphia: WB Saunders, 1986, 22–29.
3. Thompson JS, Thompson MW: *Genetics in Medicine* (Chapter 3: The chromosomal basis of heredity), ed 4. Philadelphia: WB Saunders, 1986, 7–22.
4. Schmeckel RD: The genetic basis of ophthalmic disease. *Surv Ophthalmol 1980;25:37–46.*
5. Grivell L: Mitochondrial DNA. *Sci Am 1983;248:78–89.*
6. Nikoskelaninen EK, Savontaus ML, Wanne OP: Leber's hereditary optic neuroretinopathy: a maternally inherited disease. *Arch Ophthalmol 1987;105:665–671.*
7. Thompson JS, Thompson MW: *Genetics in Medicine* (Chapter 6: Modes of heredity), ed 4. Philadelphia: WB Saunders, 1986, 111–119.
8. Emery AEH, Rimoin DL (eds): *Principles and Practice of Medical Genetics.* New York: Churchill Livingstone, 1983.
9. Bolstein D, White RL, Skoinick MM: Construction of a genetic linkage map in man using restriction fragment length polymorphisms. *Am J Human Genet 1980;32:314–321.*

CHAPTER 17
CATARACTS IN CHILDREN

1. McDonald AD: Congenital cataracts. *Dev Med Child Neurol* 1966;8:304–309.
2. Gregg NM: Congenital cataract following German measles in the mother. *Trans Ophthalmol Soc Aust* 1941;3:35–46.
3. Alden ER, Kalina RE, Hodson WA: Transient cataracts in low-birth-weight infants. *J Pediatr* 1973;82:314–318.
4. Spalter HE, Bemporad JR, Souls JA: Cataracts following chronic head-banging. *Arch Ophthalmol* 1970;83:182–186.
5. Bihari M, Grossman BJ: Posterior subcapsular cataracts: related to long-term corticosteroid treatment in children. *Am J Dis Child* 1968; 116:604–608.
6. Geiger LA, Lesser LI: Ocular side effects of chlorpromazine in a child. *JAMA* 1967;202:916–917.
7. Scheie HG, Albert DM: *Adler's Textbook of Ophthalmology.* Philadelphia: WB Saunders, 1969, 29.
8. Schub M: Corneal opacities in Down's syndrome with thyrotoxicosis. *Arch Ophthalmol* 1968;80:618–621.
9. Scheie HG, Alpert DM: *Adler's Texbook of Ophthalmology.* Philadelphia: WB Saunders, 1969, 439.
10. Gitzelmann R: Deficiency of erythrocyte galactokinase in a patient with galactose diabetes. *Lancet* 1965;2:670–671.
11. Holmes GE, Tucker V: Oculo-cerebro-renal syndrome. *Clin Pediatr* 1972;11:119–124.
12. Hiles DA: Infantile cataracts. *Pediatr Ann* 1983;12:556–573.
13. Gelbart S, Hoyt C, Jastrebski G, et al: Longterm visual results in bilateral congenital cataracts. *Am J Ophthalmol* 1982;93:615–621.
14. Hiles D: Intraocular lenses. *Surv Ophthalmol* 1990;34:371–379.
15. Morgan KS, McDonald MB, Hiles DA, et al: The nationwide study of epikeratophakia in children. *Am J Ophthalmol* 1987;103:366–374.
16. Beller R, Hoyt C, Marg E, et al: Good visual function after neonatal surgery for congenital monocular cataracts. *Am J Ophthalmol* 1981; 91:559–567.
17. Birch EE, Stager DR: Prevalence of good visual acuity following surgery for unilateral congenital cataract. *Arch Ophthalmol* 1988;106:40–47.
18. Pratt–Johnson JA, Tillson G: Unilateral congenital cataract: binocular status after treatment. *J Pediatr Ophthalmol Strabismus* 1989;26:72–75.

CHAPTER 18
RETINOBLASTOMA

1. Pendergrass TW, Davis S: Incidence of retinoblastoma in the United States. *Arch Ophthalmol* 1980; 98:1204–1210.
2. Sanders BM, Draper GJ, Kingston JE: Retinoblastoma in Great Britain 1969–80: Incidence, treatment and survival. *Br J Ophthalmol* 1988; 72:576–583.
3. MacKay CJ, Abramson DH, Ellsworth RM: Metastatic patterns of retinoblastoma. *Arch Ophthalmol* 1984; 102:391–396.
4. Takahashi T, Tamura S, Inoue M, et al: Retinoblastoma in a 26–year–old adult. *Ophthalmology* 1983; 90:179–183.
5. Letson RD, Ramsay NKC, Desnick RJ: Factors for improved genetic counseling for retinoblastoma based on a survey of 55 families. *Am J Ophthalmol* 1979; 87:449–459.
6. Yandell DW, Campbell TA, Dayton SH, et al: Oncogenic point mutations in the human retinoblastoma gene: Their application to genetic counseling. *N Engl J Med* 1989; 321:1689–1695.
7. Haik BG, Dunleavy SA, Cooke C, et al: Retinoblastoma with anterior chamber extension. *Ophthalmology* 1987; 94:367–370.
8. Verma N, Ghose S, Chandrasekhar G: Ultrasonic evaluation of retinoblastoma. *Jpn J Ophthalmol* 1984; 28:222–229.
9. Arrigg PG, Hedges TR, Char DH: Computed tomography in the diagnosis of retinoblastoma. *Br J Ophthalmol* 1983; 67:588–591.
10. Mafee MF, Goldberg MF, Cohen SB, et al: Magnetic resonance imaging versus computed tomography of leukocoric eyes and use of in vitro proton magnetic resonance spectroscopy of retinoblastoma. *Ophthalmology* 1989; 96:965–976.

11. Nicholson DH, Norton EWD: Diffuse infiltrating retinoblastoma. *Trans Am Ophthalmol Soc 1980; 78:265–285.*

12. Ohnishi Y, Yamana Y, Minei M, et al: Application of fluorescein angiography in retinoblastoma. *Am J Ophthalmol 1982; 93:578–588.*

13. Shields JA, Sanborn GE, Augsburger JJ, et al: Fluorescein angiography of retinoblastoma. *Trans Am Ophthalmol Soc 1982; 80:98–109.*

14. Rubenfeld M, Abramson DH, Ellsworth RM, et al: Unilateral vs bilateral retinoblastoma. Correlations between age at diagnosis and stage of ocular disease. *Ophthalmology 1986; 93:1016–1019.*

15. Gallie BL, Phillips RA, Ellsworth RM, et al: Significance of retinoma and phthisis bulbi for retinoblastoma. *Ophthalmology 1982; 89:1393–1399.*

16. Eagle RC, Shields JA, Donoso L, et al: Malignant transformation of spontaneously regressed retinoblastoma, retinoma/retinocytoma variant. *Ophthalmology 1989; 96:1389–1395.*

17. Abramson DH, Ellsworth RM: The surgical management of retinoblastoma. *Ophthalmic Surg 1980; 11:596–598.*

18. Kopelman JE, McLean IW, Rosenberg SH: Multivariate analysis of risk factors for metastasis in retinoblastoma treated by enucleation. *Ophthalmology 1987; 94:371–377.*

19. Markoe AM, Brady LW, Grant GD, et al: Radiation therapy of ocular disease, in Perez CA, Brady LW (eds): *Principles and Practice of Radiation Oncology.* Philadelphia: JB Lippincott, 1987, 453–472.

20. Abramson DH, Ellsworth RM, Tretter P, et al: Treatment of bilateral groups I through III retinoblastoma with bilateral radiation. *Arch Ophthalmol 1981; 99:1761–1762.*

21. Abramson DH, Ellsworth RM, Tretter P, et al: Simultaneous bilateral radiation for advanced bilateral retinoblastoma. *Arch Ophthalmol 1981; 99:1763–1766.*

22. Reese AB, Ellsworth RM: The evaluation and current concept of retinoblastoma therapy. *Trans Am Acad Ophthalmol Otolaryngol 1963; 67:164–172.*

23. Hopping W: The new Essen prognosis classification for conservative sight saving treatment of retinoblastoma, in Lommatzsch PK, Blodi FC (eds), *Intraocular Tumors.* Berlin: Akademie–Verlag, 1983, 497–505.

24. Campbell JR, Sobin L, Zimmerman LE: The TNM classification of malignant tumors of the eye and ocular adnexa. *Am J Ophthalmol 1985; 100: 83–84.*

25. Howarth C, Meyer D, Hustu HO, et al: Stage–related combined modality treatment of retinoblastoma. *Cancer 1980; 45:851–858.*

26. Egbert PR, Donaldson SS, Moazed K, et al: Visual results and ocular complications following radiotherapy for retinoblastoma. *Arch Ophthalmol 1978; 96:1826–1830.*

27. Brooks HL Jr, Meyer D, Shields JA, et al: Removal of radiation–induced cataracts in patients treated for retinoblastoma. *Arch Ophthalmol 1990; 108:1701–1708.* ,

28. Amendola BE, Markoe AM, Augsburger JJ, et al: Analysis of treatment results in 36 children with retinoblastoma treated by scleral plaque irradiation. *Int J Radiation Oncol Biol Phys 1989; 17:63–70.*

29. Shields JA, Shields CL, Parsons H, et al: The role of photocoagulation in the management of retinoblastoma. *Arch Ophthalmol 1990; 108: 205–208.*

30. Shields JA, Parsons H, Shields CL, et al: The role of cryotherapy in the management of retinoblastoma. *Am J Ophthalmol 1989; 108:260–264.*

31. Stevenson KE, Hungerford J, Garner A: Local extraocular extension of retinoblastoma following intraocular surgery. *Br J Ophthalmol 1989; 73:739–742.*

32. Goble RR, McKenzie J, Kingston JE, Plowman PN, et al: Orbital recurrence of retinoblastoma successfully treated by combined therapy. *Br J Ophthalmol 1990; 74:97–98.*

33. Draper GJ, Sanders BM, Kingston JE: Second primary neoplasms in patients with retinoblastoma. *Br J Cancer 1986; 53:661–671.*

34. Roarty JD, McLean IW, Zimmerman LE: Incidence of second neoplasms

in patients with bilateral retinoblastoma. *Ophthalmology 1988; 95:1583–1587.*

35. Kingston JE, Plowman PN, Hungerford JL: Ectopic intracranial retinoblastoma in childhood. *Br J Ophthalmol 1985; 69:742–748.*

CHAPTER 19
BENIGN TUMORS IN THE DIFFERENTIAL DIAGNOSIS OF RETINOBLASTOMA

1. Nyboer JH, Robertson DM, Gomez MR: Retinal lesions in tuberous sclerosis. *Arch Ophthalmol 1976; 94:1277–1280.*
2. Arnold AC, Hepler RS, Yee RW, et al: Solitary retinal astrocytoma. *Surv Ophthalmol 1985; 30:173–181.*
3. Yanoff M, Zimmerman LE, Davis R: Massive gliosis of the retina. A continuous spectrum of glial proliferation. *Int Ophthalmol Clin 1971; 11:211–229.*
4. Augsburger JJ, Shields JA, Goldberg RE: Classification and management of hereditary retinal angiomas. *Int Ophthalmol 1981; 4:93–106.*
5. Hardwig P, Robertson DM: von Hippel–Lindau disease: A familial, often lethal, multi-system phakomatosis. *Ophthalmology 1984; 91:263–270.*
6. Gass JD, Braunstein R: Sessile and exophytic capillary angiomas of the juxtapapillary retina and optic nerve head. *Arch Ophthalmol 1980; 98:1790–1797.*
7. Whitson JT, Welch RB, Green WR: von Hippel–Lindau disease: Case report of a patient with spontaneous regression of a retinal angioma. *Retina 1986; 6:25–3259.*
8. Lane CM, Turner G, Gregor ZJ, et al: Laser treatment of retinal angiomatosis. *Eye 1989; 3:33–38.*
9. Blodi CF, Russell SR, Pulido JS, et al: Direct and feeder vessel photocoagulation of retinal angiomas with dye yellow laser. *Ophthalmology 1990; 97:791–797.*
10. Watzke RC: Cryotherapy for retinal angiomatosis. *Arch Ophthalmol 1974; 92:399–401.*
11. Cardoso RD, Brockhurst RJ: Perforating diathermy coagulation for retinal angiomas. *Arch Ophthalmol 1976; 94:1702–1715.*
12. Schwartz PL, Fastenberg DM, Shakin JL: Management of macular puckers associated with retinal angiomas. *Ophthalmic Surg 1990; 21:550–556.*
13. Messmer E, Laqua H, Wessing A, et al: Nine cases of cavernous hemangioma of the retina. *Am J Ophthalmol 1983; 95:383–390.*
14. Colvard DM, Robertson DM, Trautmann JC: Cavernous hemangioma of the retina. *Arch Ophthalmol 1978; 96:2042–2044.*
15. Goldberg RE, Pheasant TR, Shields JA: Cavernous hemangioma of the retina. *Arch Ophthalmol 1979; 97:2321–2324.*
16. Pancurak J, Goldberg MF, Frenkel M, et al: Cavernous hemangioma of the retina. *Retina 1985; 5:215–220.*
17. Mansour AM, Jampol LM, Hrisomalos NF, et al: Cavernous hemangioma of the optic disc. *Arch Ophthalmol 1988; 106:22.*
18. Schwartz AC, Weaver, RG Jr, Bloomfield R, et al: Cavernous hemangioma of the retina, cutaneous angiomas, and intracranial vascular lesion by computed tomography and nuclear magnetic resonance imaging. *Am J Ophthalmol 1984; 98:483–487.*

CHAPTER 20
MALIGNANT TUMORS IN THE DIFFERENTIAL DIAGNOSIS OF RETINOBLASTOMA

1. Broughton WL, Zimmerman LE: A clinicopathologic study of 56 cases of intraocular medulloepitheliomas. *Am J Ophthalmol 1978; 85:407–418.*
2. Canning CR, McCartney ACE, Hungerford J: Medulloepithelioma (diktyoma). *Br J Ophthalmol 1988; 72:764–767.*
3. Schachat AP, Markowitz JA, Guyer DR, et al: Ophthalmic manifestations of leukemia. *Arch Ophthalmol 1989; 107:697–700.*
4. Rubenstein RA, Yanoff M, Albert DM: Thrombocytopenia, anemia, and retinal hemorrhage. *Am J Ophthalmol 1968; 65:435–439.*
5. Kincaid MC, Green WR: Ocular and orbital involvement in leukemia. *Surv Ophthalmol 1983; 27:211–232.*
6. Swartz M, Schumann GB: Acute leukemic infiltration of the vitreous diagnosed by pars plana aspiration. *Am J Ophthalmol 1980; 90:326–330.*

7. Nikaido H, Mishima H, Ono H, et al: Leukemic involvement of the optic nerve. *Am J Ophthalmol 1988; 105:294–298.*

8. Tang RA, Aguirre Vila–Coro A, Wall, S, et al: Acute leukemia presenting as a retinal pigment epithelium detachment. *Arch Ophthalmol 1988; 106:21–22.*

9. Stewart MW, Gitter KA, Cohen G: Acute leukemia presenting as a unilateral exudative retinal detachment. *Retina 1989; 9:110–114.*

10. Schachat AP, Jabs DA, Graham ML, et al: Leukemic iris infiltration. *J Pediatr Ophthalmol Strabismus 1988; 25:135–138.*

11. Delaney WV Jr, Kinsella G: Optic disc neovascularization in leukemia. *Am J Ophthalmol 1985; 99:212–213.*

12. Leveille AS, Morse PH: Platelet–induced retinal neovascularization in leukemia. *Am J Ophthalmol 1981; 91:640–643.*

INDEX

monofixation syndrome, 5.4–5.7, **5.4–5.7**
suppression and anomalous retinal
correspondence, 5.2–5.4, **5.2**
visual confusion and diplopia, 5.1, **5.1**
Sex determination, 16.6–16.7
Sherrington's law, 3.18
Simulated divergence excess, in exotropia,
7.2
Simulated sheath syndrome, 12.5
Skew deviation, 11.1
Sleep, and eye movements, 3.17
Slit lamp biomicroscopy, of
retinoblastoma, 18.3
Snellen acuity in amblyopia. *See*
Amblyopia.
Somatic cell hybridization, 16.21, **16.25**
Spatial frequency, in amblyopia,
13.3–13.6, 13.9–13.11
Spindles, extraocular muscles, 3.12, **3.16,
3.17**
Spiral of Tillaux, 3.4, **3.4**
Square-wave gratings, 2.3
Staining techniques for chromosomes,
16.3–16.5, **16.2–16.4**
Stereoacuity, 6.13
Stereopsis
clinical testing, 6.27–6.29, **6.30–6.32**
in exotropia, 7.3
physiology, 6.10–6.18, **6.15–6.23**
Stereothreshold, 6.15, **6.19**
Strabismus fixus, 8.15
Strabismus sursoadductorius, 12.2–12.3,
12.2
Streptococcal infections, and convergence
insufficiency, 7.5
Sturge-Weber syndrome, 19.11
Suckling difficulty, Mo[uml]bius
syndrome, 8.12
Suppression
and anomalous retinal correspondence,
5.2–5.4, **5.2, 5.3**
definition, 6.20
depth of, 6.24
in exotropia, 7.3, 7.4
Supramid, for ocular myasthenia gravis,
11.12
Supranuclear disorders. *See* Vertical
strabismus.
Surgical techniques, 15.1–15.18
for accommodative esotropia, 8.11–8.12
approach to inferior oblique muscle,
15.15–15.17, **15.75–15.92**
approach to superior oblique tendon,
15.17–15.18, **15.93–15.102**
and Brown syndrome, 12.5, 12.6
congenital cataracts, 17.6
for congenital esotropia, 8.5
for dissociated vertical divergence, 12.2
for Duane syndrome, 7.12
and esotropia, 8.12
for exotropia, 7.8–7.9
for fourth nerve paralysis, 11.8–11.9,
11.10
for Graves' ophthalmopathy, 12.8

for inferior oblique overaction, 9.4
posterior fixation suture, 15.13–15.15,
15.62–15.74
recession of rectus muscle, 15.3–15.7,
15.1–15.31
resection of rectus muscle, 15.7–15.12,
15.32–15.61
for superior oblique overaction, 9.6
V-pattern esotropia, 10.2–10.3
Suture, posterior fixation, 15.13–15.15,
15.62–15.74
Syndactyly, in Mo[uml]bius syndrome,
8.13

Tay-Sachs disease, 16.11, 16.12
Teenagers, accommodative esotropia, 8.12
Tenon's capsule
anatomy, 3.7–3.8, **3.9**
in strabismus surgery. *See* Surgical
techniques.
Third nerve palsy, 11.9–11.11, **11.11,
11.12**
and secondary exotropia, 7.10
13q- syndrome, 16.16
Thyroid disease, Graves' ophthalmopathy,
12.7–12.8
Titmus stereotest, 6.28
TNO stereotest, 6.29, **6.31**
Tongue, in Mo[uml]bius syndrome, 8.12
Torsion
extraocular muscles, 3.15–3.17
fourth nerve paralysis, 11.6
inferior oblique overaction, 9.3
Toxocariasis, ocular, 18.6–18.7, **18.10**
Toxoplasmosis, 17.2
Transgenesis, 16.22
Translocations of chromosomes,
16.15–16.16, **16.15**
Trauma, head
cyclic esotropia, 8.12
fourth nerve paralysis, 11.2
and secondary exotropia, 7.10, **7.5**
third nerve palsy, 11.9
Trichromacy, anomalous, 16.12
Triparanol, and cataracts in children, 17.2
Trisomy 13 (Patau syndrome),
16.19–16.20, 18.8, **16.21, 16.22**
cataracts, 17.4
Trisomy 18 (Edwards syndrome), 16.19,
16.20
cataracts, 17.4
Trisomy 21 (Down syndrome),
16.17–16.18
cataracts, 17.2–17.3, **17.5, 17.6**
Trisomy 22 (cat eye syndrome), 16.20,
16.23, 16.24
Trochlea
in Brown syndrome, 12.5, 12.6
fourth nerve paralysis, 11.2
Tropicamide, for accommodative
esotropia, 8.8
Tscherning's ophthalmophacometer, 4.2
Tuberous sclerosis 19.1–19.4
Tumbling E test, 2.5, **2.10**